T0329810

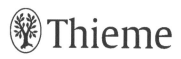

Early Onset Scoliosis

A Comprehensive Guide from the Oxford Meetings

Colin Nnadi, MBBS, FRCS (ORTH)
Consultant Spine Surgeon
Oxford University Hospitals NHS Trust
Oxford, United Kingdom

With contributions by

Ahmed Abdelaal, Behrooz A. Akbarnia, Ahmet Alanay, Andrew Baldock, Robert M. Campbell, Jr., Vivienne Campbell, Federico Canavese, Robert Crawford, Ozgur Dede, Evan M. Davies, Alain Dimeglio, Jean Dubousset, Hazem Elsebaie, Jeremy C.T. Fairbank, Adrian Gardner, Arvindera Ghag, Matthew J. Goldstein, Jaime A. Gómez, Michael Grevitt, N.S. Harshavardhana, Jayaratnam Jayamohan, Sandeep Jayawant, Nima Kabirian, David Marks, Richard E. McCarthy, S.M.H. Mehdian, Min Mehta, Jorge Mineiro, Ian W. Nelson, M.H. Hilali Noordeen, Howard Park, Nasir A. Quraishi, Harwant Singh, Laura Streeton, Anne H. Thomson, Athanasios I. Tsirikos, Peter D. Turnpenny, Michael G. Vitale, John K. Webb

240 illustrations

Thieme
Stuttgart • New York • Delhi • Rio de Janeiro

Library of Congress Cataloging-in-Publication Data

Early onset scoliosis : a comprehensive guide from the Oxford meetings / [edited by] Colin Nnadi.
   p. ; cm.
Includes bibliographical references.
ISBN 978-3-13-172661-2 (alk. paper) – ISBN 978-3-13-172671-1 (eISBN)
I. Nnadi, Colin, editor.
[DNLM: 1. Scoliosis–congenital. 2. Child. 3. Infant. 4. Scoliosis–surgery. 5. Spine–abnormalities. WE 735]
RD771.S3
616.7'3–dc23
2014044547

© 2016 Georg Thieme Verlag KG

Thieme Publishers Stuttgart
Rüdigerstrasse 14, 70469 Stuttgart, Germany
+49 [0]711 8931 421, customerservice@thieme.de

Thieme Publishers New York
333 Seventh Avenue, New York, NY 10001 USA
+1 800 782 3488, customerservice@thieme.com

Thieme Publishers Delhi
A-12, Second Floor, Sector-2, Noida-201301
Uttar Pradesh, India
+91 120 45 566 00, customerservice@thieme.in

Thieme Publishers Rio de Janeiro,
Thieme Publicações Ltda.
Edifício Rodolpho de Paoli, 25º andar
Av. Nilo Peçanha, 50 – Sala 2508
Rio de Janeiro 20020-906, Brasil
+55 21 3172 2297

Cover design: Thieme Publishing Group
Typesetting by DiTech

Printed in Germany by Aprinta Druck, Wemding

ISBN 978-3-13-172661-2

Also available as an e-book:
eISBN 978-3-13-172671-1

Important note: Medicine is an ever-changing science undergoing continual development. Research and clinical experience are continually expanding our knowledge, in particular our knowledge of proper treatment and drug therapy. Insofar as this book mentions any dosage or application, readers may rest assured that the authors, editors, and publishers have made every effort to ensure that such references are in accordance with **the state of knowledge at the time of production of the book.**

Nevertheless, this does not involve, imply, or express any guarantee or responsibility on the part of the publishers in respect to any dosage instructions and forms of applications stated in the book. **Every user is requested to examine carefully** the manufacturers' leaflets accompanying each drug and to check, if necessary in consultation with a physician or specialist, whether the dosage schedules mentioned therein or the contraindications stated by the manufacturers differ from the statements made in the present book. Such examination is particularly important with drugs that are either rarely used or have been newly released on the market. Every dosage schedule or every form of application used is entirely at the user's own risk and responsibility. The authors and publishers request every user to report to the publishers any discrepancies or inaccuracies noticed. If errors in this work are found after publication, errata will be posted at www.thieme.com on the product description page.

Some of the product names, patents, and registered designs referred to in this book are in fact registered trademarks or proprietary names even though specific reference to this fact is not always made in the text. Therefore, the appearance of a name without designation as proprietary is not to be construed as a representation by the publisher that it is in the public domain.

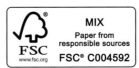

In memory of my father from whom I learnt so much.

–Colin Nnadi

Contents

Preface

On the 8th of September 2011, a group consisting of 22 spine surgeons, two pediatricians, a geneticist, and an anesthetist gathered in Christ Church, Oxford, for the inaugural early onset scoliosis meeting. Delegates from Europe, North America, and as far afield as Australia and Asia attended.

This was the first meeting of its kind in the United Kingdom. It was a unique occasion for several reasons. First, the breadth of knowledge and experience available amongst invited faculty was immeasurable in value. Second, the great and the good, from the practicing to the retired, came out in force to produce one of the most entertaining meetings I have ever had the privilege to attend. Third, and by no means last, was the holistic theme that ran through the meeting. There were lectures from surgeons, geneticists, occupational therapists, and nurses. For the first time, we heard a parent's view of dealing with the social consequences of early onset spinal deformity. Members of the audience and faculty alike were able to share practical challenges and broach solutions.

The beautiful ambience of Christ Church, which has been home to countless philosophers, scientists, scholars, and statesmen, provided a salient backdrop for exciting debate and discussion.

Early onset scoliosis is an evolving specialty with more exciting developments still to come. There is much we do not know but what we are now aware of is the importance of controlling spinal deformity to potentiate the development of other organs such as the lungs and heart. We have a better understanding of spinal growth and its impact on the growing child. We have not found conclusive ways to treat this problem but there are interesting new strategies being developed all the time. The one theme that constantly rears its head in relation to this condition is the need for teamwork. Due to the often multi-systemic nature of early onset scoliosis, multi-disciplinary input is a prerequisite for good management. This philosophy formed the basis of the holistic theme of the meeting.

It is hoped that by reading this book the individual will develop a better understanding of what early onset scoliosis is and focus not on specific treatments but on principles to inform choice on best treatment.

This book is an ode to all those who contributed so much of their valuable time to increasing our understanding of a condition that afflicts those who have little or no say in the why, how, and when of treatment.

Colin Nnadi
Oxford, United Kingdom

Acknowledgments

I wish to thank my contributors for sharing their inestimable knowledge in the making of this book. I also wish to thank all of the research team involved in the Magec Study, with special thanks to Andy Miles and David Mayers. Finally, a big thank you to Dr. Jo Richards and Jennifer Thorne for proof reading chapters.

Contributors

Ahmed Abdelaal, MBChB, MRCS, MSc
Oxford University
Horton General Hospital
Oxford University Hospitals NHS Trust
Oxfordshire, United Kingdom

Behrooz A. Akbarnia, MD
Clinical Professor
Department of Orthopaedic Surgery
University of California, San Diego
President and Founder
Growing Spine Foundation
San Diego, California, United States

Ahmet Alanay, Prof. Dr.
Professor of Orthopedics and Traumatology
Acibadem University Faculty of Medicine
Acibadem Comprehensive Spine Centre
Maslak, Istanbul, Turkey

Andrew Baldock, BSc (Hons), FRCA, FFICM
Consultant Paediatric Anaesthetist
Southampton Children's Hospital
University Hospital Southampton
Southampton, United Kingdom

Robert M. Campbell, Jr., MD
Professor of Orthopaedic Surgery
The University of Pennsylvania Perelman School of
  Medicine
Director
The Center for Thoracic Insufficiency Syndrome
Division of Orthopaedics
The Children's Hospital of Philadelphia
Philadelphia, Pennsylvania, United States

Vivienne Campbell
Consultant Paediatrician in Neurodisability
Chailey Heritage Clinical Services
East Sussex, United Kingdom

Federico Canavese, Prof. MD, PhD
Centre Hospitalier Universitaire Estaing
Service de Chirurgie Infantile
Université d'Auvergne
Faculté de Médecine
Clermont-Ferrand, France

Robert Crawford, MBChB, FRCS, ChM
Consultant Orthopaedic Spine Surgeon
Norfolk & Norwich University Hospital
Norwich, United Kingdom

Ozgur Dede, MD
Assistant Professor of Orthopaedic Surgery
Division of Pediatric Orthopaedics
Children's Hospital of Pittsburgh of UPMC
Pittsburgh, Pennsylvania, United States

Evan M. Davies, BM, FRCS Ed (Tr&Orth)
Consultant Orthopaedic Spinal Surgeon
Clinical Lead
Paediatric Spinal Unit
Southampton Children's Hospital
University Hospital Southampton
Southampton, United Kingdom

Alain Dimeglio, Prof. MD
Université de Montpellier
Faculté de Médecine
Montpellier, France

Jean Dubousset, MD
Professor of Pediatric Orthopaedics
Académie Nationale de Médecine
Paris, France

Hazem Elsebaie, FRCS, MD
Professor of Orthopedic Surgery
Department of Orthopedics
Cairo University
Vice President
Egyptian Scoliosis Society
Cairo, Egypt

Jeremy C.T. Fairbank, MA, MD, FRCS
Professor of Spine Surgery
Consultant Orthopaedic Surgeon
Oxford Spinal Unit
Oxford University Hospitals NHS Trust
Spinal Service
Nuffield Orthopaedic Centre
Oxford, United Kingdom

Adrian Gardner, BM, MRCS, FRCS (T&O)
Consultant Spinal Surgeon
The Royal Orthopaedic Hospital
Birmingham, United Kingdom

Arvindera Ghag, MD, FRCS (C)
Pediatric Spine Surgery
BC Children's Hospital
Vancouver, BC, Canada

Matthew J. Goldstein, MD
Clinical Fellow
San Diego Center for Spinal Disorders
La Jolla, California, United States

Jaime A. Gómez, MD
Assistant Professor, Pediatric Orthopedic and Spine
    Surgery
Albert Einstein College of Medicine
Children's Hospital at Montefiore
Bronx, New York, United States
Spine Surgery Fellow
Hospital for Joint Diseases
New York University
New York, New York, United States

Michael Grevitt, MBBS, BSc, FRCS, FRCS (Orth)
Consultant Spinal Surgeon
Centre for Spinal Studies and Surgery
Queen's Medical Centre Campus
Nottingham University Hospitals NHS Trust
Nottingham, United Kingdom

N.S. Harshavardhana, MD
Clinical Fellow
Twin Cities Spine Center
Minneapolis, Minnesota, United States

Jayaratnam Jayamohan, BSc, MBBS, FRCS (SN) (Eng)
Consultant Paediatric Neurosurgeon
Oxford University Hospitals NHS Trust
Honorary Senior Clinical Lecturer
Oxford University
John Radcliffe Hospital
Oxford, United Kingdom

Sandeep Jayawant, MD, FRCPCH
Consultant Paediatric Neurologist
Oxford Children's Hospital
Oxford University Hospitals NHS Trust
Oxford, United Kingdom

Nima Kabirian, MD
Research Fellow
San Diego Center for Spinal Disorders
San Diego, California, United States

David Marks, MBBS, FRCS, FRCS (Orth)
Consultant Spinal Surgeon
The Royal Orthopaedic Hospital
Birmingham, United Kingdom

Richard E. McCarthy, MD
Professor
Departments of Orthopaedics and Neurosurgery
University of Arkansas for Medical Sciences
Arkansas Children's Hospital
Little Rock, Arkansas, United States

S.M.H. Mehdian, MD, MS (Orth), FRCS (Ed)
Centre for Spinal Studies and Surgery
Queen's Medical Centre Campus
Nottingham, United Kingdom

Min Mehta, MD, FRCS
Consultant Orthopaedic Surgeon (retired)
Royal National Orthopaedic Hospital, NHS Trust
London, United Kingdom

Jorge Mineiro, MD, PhD, FRCSEd
Professor of Orthopaedics
Clinical Director
Head, Orthopaedic Department
CUF Descobertas Hospital
Lisbon, Portugal

Ian W. Nelson, MBBS, FRCS, MCh (Orth)
Bristol Orthopaedic Spine Service
Southmead Hospital and Bristol Royal Hospital for
    Children
Bristol, United Kingdom

Colin Nnadi, MBBS, FRCS (ORTH)
Consultant Spine Surgeon
Oxford University Hospitals NHS Trust
Oxford, United Kingdom

M.H. Hilali Noordeen, FRCS
Consultant Spinal Surgeon
Spinal Deformity Unit
Department of Spinal Surgery
Royal National Orthopaedic Hospital NHS Trust
London, United Kingdom

Howard Park, BS
Columbia University Medical Center
Department of Pediatric Orthopaedic Surgery
Morgan Stanley's Children's Hospital of New York
New York, New York, United States

Nasir A. Quraishi, FRCS (Trauma & Orth)
Consultant Spinal Surgeon
Honorary Clinical Associate Professor
Centre for Spinal Studies & Surgery
Queen's Medical Centre
Nottingham University Hospitals NHS Trust
Nottingham, United Kingdom

Harwant Singh, MD, FRCS, PhD
Consultant Orthopaedic Spine Surgeon
Pantai Hospital
Kuala Lumpur, Malaysia

Laura Streeton, BSc (Hons), PG Cert (Paeds), MRes, MCSP
Senior Paediatric Physiotherapist
Nuffield Orthopaedic Centre
Oxford, United Kingdom

Anne H. Thomson, MD, FRCP, FRCPCH
Consultant in Paediatric Respiratory Medicine (retired)
Oxford Children's Hospital
Oxford University Hospitals NHS Trust
Oxford, United Kingdom

Athanasios I. Tsirikos, MD, FRCS, PhD
Consultant Orthopaedic and Spine Surgeon
Honorary Clinical Senior Lecturer
University of Edinburgh
Clinical Lead
Scottish National Spine Deformity Center
Royal Hospital for Sick Children
Edinburgh, United Kingdom

Peter D. Turnpenny, BSc, MBChB, DRCOG, DCH, FRCP, FRCPCH, FRCPath, FHEA
Consultant Clinical Geneticist
Royal Devon and Exeter Hospital
Honorary Associate Professor
Exeter University Medical School
Clinical Genetics Department
Royal Devon and Exeter Hospital
Exeter, United Kingdom

Michael G. Vitale, MD
Ana Lucia Professor of Pediatric Orthopaedic Surgery
MS Children's Hospital of New York
New York, New York, United States

John K. Webb, FRCS
Consultant Spine Surgeon
Centre for Spinal Studies and Surgery
Queen's Medical Centre Campus
Nottingham, United Kingdom

Part 1

The Growth and Development in Mammalian Spine

1 Frontier of the Impossible

Federico Canavese and Alain Dimeglio

When you have excluded the impossible, whatever remains, however improbable, must be the truth.
—*Sir Arthur Conan Doyle*

Early onset scoliosis is one of the most challenging conditions in pediatric orthopedics and an important health issue. It is a condition with the potential to cause severe adverse consequences. The pathologic changes induced on a growing organism by an early onset spinal deformity can be dramatic and can, in the most severe cases, lead to death. A vertebral column that is not permitted to grow normally will affect the growth potential of the whole upper body, resulting in a short trunk, a disproportionate body habitus, and an underdeveloped thoracic cage (▶ Fig. 1.1).

Pediatric orthopedic surgeons, by using the option of surgically managing young and very young children with early onset spinal deformity, have opened up a new perspective for spinal surgery. They have in effect broken down barriers that were previously felt to be insurmountable. Ingenuity has meant that management strategies have changed dramatically, shifting from a defensive attitude toward an offensive one. However, this audacious surgery is not without risk.

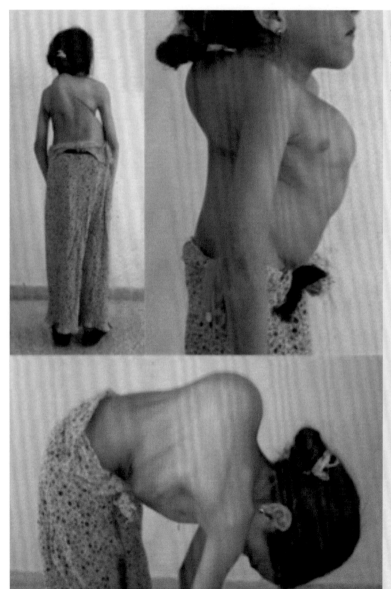

Fig. 1.1 Patients with untreated early onset scoliosis (infantile idiopathic scoliosis). The loss of sitting height is related to the severity of the deformity. A thoracic spine height of at least 18 to 22 cm is necessary to avoid thoracic insufficiency syndrome.

In young children with progressive deformity, there is a decrease of longitudinal growth and a loss of the normal proportionality of trunk growth. Abnormal growth leads to a deficit that sustains the deformity. As the spinal deformity progresses, by a "domino effect," not only spinal growth but also the size and shape of the thoracic cage are modified. This distortion of the thoracic cage ultimately impairs lung development and cardiac function. Over time, the spine disorder changes in nature from a mainly orthopedic issue to a severe, systematic pediatric disease associated with thoracic insufficiency syndrome, cor pulmonale, and, in the most severe cases, death (► Fig. 1.2).

Early spine fusion is not the answer for dealing with progressive, early onset spinal deformities. Arthrodesis in the thoracic spine at an early age does not address the impact of the deformity on the shape of the thoracic cage shape and development of the lung parenchyma, and it does not address the preservation of cardiopulmonary function. Moreover, early spinal fusion, especially in the thoracic region, is a cause of respiratory insufficiency and adds a loss of pulmonary function to the preexisting spinal deformity (► Fig. 1.3).

The ideal treatment of early onset scoliosis has not yet been identified; both clinicians and surgeons still face multiple challenges, including preserving the thoracic

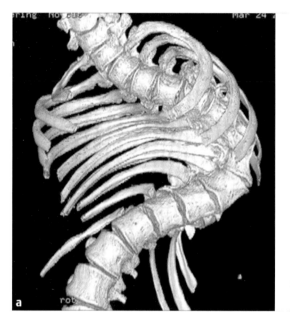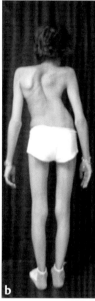

Fig. 1.2 In young children with progressive deformity, distortion of the thoracic cage (a) leads to a decrease of longitudinal growth and (b) a loss of the normal proportionality of trunk growth.

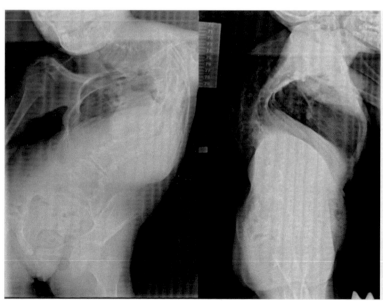

Fig. 1.3 Early fusion is not able to control the progression of the deformity. This patient, an 11-year-old girl with atretic meningocele, diastematomyelia, and tethered cord, had multiple surgeries. The spinal deformity progressed, and the crankshaft phenomenon occurred. Arthrodesis in the thoracic spine at an early age does not address the impact of the deformity on the shape of the thoracic cage and development of the lung parenchyma, and it does not address the preservation of pulmonary function.

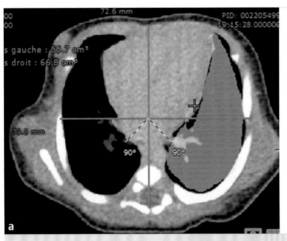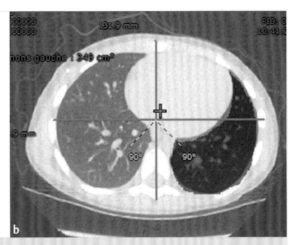

Fig. 1.4 The morphology of the thorax changes with growth, from a cylindrical shape at birth (**a**) to an ovoid shape at the age of 5 years (**b**).

spine, thoracic cage, lung growth, and cardiac function without reducing spinal motion. However, patients with early onset scoliosis are a heterogeneous population, so that it is difficult to compare the outcomes of different management strategies in meaningful numbers of patients; in addition, there is a lack of outcome assessment tools for this complex group of patients.

Management strategies must consider the complete life span of the patient, and the effects of treatment on distorted spinal and chest growth must be considered. Before any treatment is started, a convincing answer to these three questions must be given:

1. What is the functional benefit of the treatment?
2. What is the potential morbidity of the treatment?
3. What quality of life can be anticipated?

1.1 The Rib–Vertebral–Sternal Complex

In the concept of the rib–vertebral–sternal complex, a normal interaction occurs among the organic components of the spine, thoracic cage, and cardiorespiratory system.[1,2,3] This complex encloses the three-dimensional thoracic cavity and tends to be an elastic structural model similar to a cube in shape. However, in the presence of scoliosis, the complex becomes flat, rigid, and elliptical and prevents the lungs from expanding. These deformities can be lethal in the most severe cases as a result of reciprocal interactions and influences among the various skeletal and organic components of the thoracic cage and cavity that are not well understood. The development of the thoracic cage and lungs is a complex process that requires perfect synergy among the various components of the rib–vertebral–sternal complex. Alterations in any of these elements affect and change the development and growth of the others.

It must be remembered that the thoracic cage volume represents about 6% of its definitive volume at birth, about 30% by the age of 5 years, and about 50% by the age of 10 years (▶ Fig. 1.4). Moreover, between the age of 10 years and skeletal maturity, the thoracic cage volume doubles, and its volumetric growth ends on an upward trend.

To preserve thoracic motility and permit normal development of the respiratory tree, treatment should not focus only on the spine but should also consider the rib–vertebral–sternal complex as a whole.

1.2 Growth Holds the Basics

Sitting height correlates strictly with trunk height and is the best indicator for monitoring thoracic cage and spinal growth. In children with severe spinal deformities, the loss of sitting height is related to the severity of the deformity. For this reason, it is important to monitor changes in sitting height rather than in standing height in children with progressive spinal deformities. Standing height does not always exactly correlate with the loss of trunk height in children with severe spinal deformities because it includes subischial height.

It is important to follow the stages of growth. Three periods can be identified: (1) between birth and 5 years of age, characterized by a significant spinal growth; (2) between 5 years of age and the beginning of puberty, characterized by a reduction in spinal growth (also known as the quiescent phase); (3) the pubertal growth spurt, characterized by a new increase of spinal growth (▶ Table 1.1).

Trunk growth is crucial between birth and 5 years of age because sitting height increases by 28 cm, whereas between 5 years of age and skeletal maturity the remaining trunk growth is 30 cm (▶ Fig. 1.5). Moreover, the T1-S1 segment increases by 10 cm between birth and 5 years of age and almost doubles in length between 5 years of age and skeletal maturity (► Table 1.2). It is therefore necessary to act fast, before pulmonary and cardiac alterations induced by a distorted spinal growth become irreversible. It is important to adapt management to growth rates. After the age of 5 years, the growth of the trunk decreases. Height increases by 2.5 cm and weight by 2.5 kg per year. This quiescent phase has to be used to stabilize the clinical situation because at the time of the pubertal growth spurt, the resumption of growth is going to worsen the spinal deformity. It is necessary to get ready for it and possibly to anticipate the need for a definitive surgery.

All growths are interrelated. Any abnormal growth, by a "domino effect," leads to another abnormal growth. The irregular growth of vertebral bodies is the basis of a distorted development. Severe, progressive early onset spinal deformities lead to abnormal spine growth that alters thoracic and lung growth, which finally affects the cardiopulmonary system.[1,4]

Table 1.1 Growth of the T1-S1, T1-T12, and L1-L5 segments

Spinal segment	Age (years)						
	1	3	5	7	9	11	Pubertal spurt
T1-S1	2			1			1.8
T1-T12	1.3			0.7			1.1
L1-L5	0.7			0.3			0.7

Note: Values are expressed in centimeters and are average values. A perivertebral arthrodesis in the T1-S1 segment at 5 years of age results in a sitting height of 15 cm (10 cm in the thoracic spine and 5 cm in the lumbar spine).

Table 1.2 Evaluation of the T1-T12 and L1-L5 spinal segments from birth to skeletal maturity

Developmental stage	Spinal segment			
	Males		Females	
	T1-T12	L1-L5	T1-T12	L1-L5
Newborn	11	7.5	11	7.5
Child	18	10.5	18	10.5
Pre-Adolescent	22	12.5	22	12.5
Adult	28	16	26	15.5

Note: Values are expressed in centimeters and are average values.

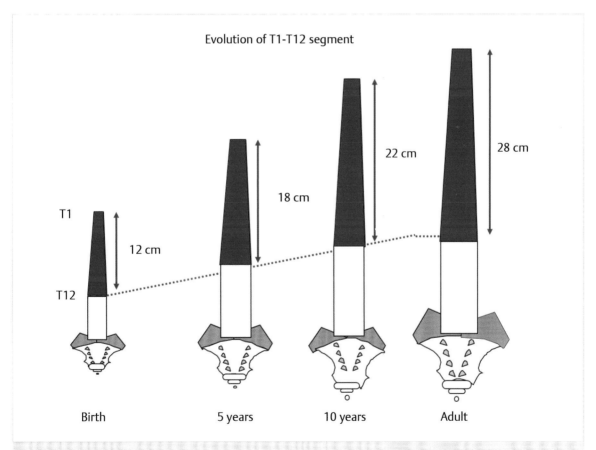

Evolution of T1-T12 segment

T1

T12

12 cm

18 cm

22 cm

28 cm

Birth   5 years   10 years   Adult

Fig. 1.5 Evolution of the T1-T12 segment between birth and adulthood.

The goal of any treatment is to break this vicious cycle; it is necessary to correct all distortions secondary to distorted spinal growth as soon as possible: short height and disproportionate body habitus, underdeveloped thoracic cage and inability to breathe normally, low weight and cardiac dysfunction. Tachypnea, ventricular tachycardia, dyspnea, tracheomalacia, weight loss, and chronic obstructive pulmonary diseases are often more worrisome elements than the distortion of the vertebral column itself.

1.3 Alveolarization: When Is It Complete?

Pediatric respiratory physiology is not well understood. It is difficult to investigate children younger than 5 years of age. Every day, a child exchanges 12,000 L of air. At birth, the lung parenchyma volume is 400 cc^3; it is approximately 900 and 1,500 cc^3 at ages 5 and 10 years, respectively, and about 4,500 cc^3 for boys and 3,500 cc^3 for girls at skeletal maturity.[1,2]

Lung growth is a complex phenomenon in which different pulmonary structures and regions grow at different rates. At birth, the newborn has the same number of conducting airways as an adult. Tracheal caliber increases two- to threefold between birth and skeletal maturity. In contrast, the peripheral regions of the lung containing alveoli and pulmonary capillaries, also known as the acinar regions, undergo substantial postnatal growth and development.

Alveolarization is the process in which lung alveoli develop by multiplication. Once alveolar cell multiplication ceases, lung growth continues by alveolar cell expansion. It is estimated that about 30 to 50% of alveoli are present at birth; from the late fetal stage to 4 years of age, the number of alveoli grows by a factor of 10.

However, there is no agreement on when alveolarization stops. Some studies suggest that alveolar multiplication is completed by age 3 years, whereas others point out that alveolarization stops at age 8 years. Postmortem studies have shown that patients with early-onset deformities have fewer alveoli than expected, and that emphysematous changes in existing alveoli are present. These studies suggest that mechanical compression is not a factor in reducing the number of alveoli, and that this reduction is probably due to a premature cessation of alveolar proliferation. These data are currently being questioned as new findings are discovered with innovative study techniques such as electric impedance tomography, helium magnetic resonance imaging, and high resolution computed tomography.

The average number of alveoli reaches about 90 million at age 3 years and about 300 million during adulthood. These findings suggest that alveolar multiplication continues beyond early childhood. Moreover, experimental studies have shown that alveolarization continues beyond early life and into maturity in some mammals, and that it can be initiated by experimental pneumonectomy in mature animals. In humans, compensatory lung growth has been reported over a 15-year follow-up period after pneumonectomy in a 33-year-old woman for lung cancer. Moreover, it has been shown that Cobb angle correction does not correlate with either an increase in vital capacity or with a decrease in the spinal penetration index.

Evidence is beginning to accumulate that alveolarization may not be confined to early childhood, as previously thought, and may actually continue into maturity and beyond. Therefore, alveolarization during late childhood or adolescence may provide a repair mechanism for early insults to lung growth.[5,6]

1.4 Surgery Is Part of a Programmed Action

Surgical treatment is not for every patient and not for every surgeon, and it should be done in specialized centers only. Surgery should be part of a well-structured multidisciplinary program. The orthopedic surgeon cannot act alone. Orthopedic surgeons experienced in spine disorders, anesthesiologists, pulmonologists, cardiologists, nutritionists, pediatricians, psychologists, physiotherapists, and pain specialists must work together to evaluate and handle these complex patients in order to obtain the best possible outcomes.

Before surgery is undertaken, four "presurgical" stages are needed to bring the surgical project to a favorable outcome.

1. *Pediatric evaluation* is needed to assess the child as a whole in order to identify and to treat, if possible, any comorbidity.
2. *Nutritional evaluation.* Correction of weight deficit is a priority as surgery is inevitably associated with a loss of weight. Classic prescriptions have a very limited effect, and it is necessary to understand that gastrostomy may be needed to improve weight.
3. *Cardiorespiratory evaluation.* Patients with cardiorespiratory deficits may require daily physiotherapy. It is important not to focus too much attention on surgery and not to leave aside respiratory physiotherapy. Physiotherapy plays an important role in stabilizing these patients before and after surgery. It can be compared with the almost daily re-education of a congenital clubfoot.
4. *Orthopedic evaluation* comes last. It is needed to evaluate the thoracic cage and spinal deformities and to choose the best treatment option (e.g., halo traction can improve the morphology of the spine to facilitate material implantation).

The fate of the child relies both on surgery and on pre- and postoperative care—hence the importance of precise evaluation and a multidisciplinary team of care providers.

1.4.1 Surgical Options: There Is No Ideal Instrumentation

The ideal method of treating early onset scoliosis has not yet been identified. Advancements in growth-friendly procedures are providing physicians with multiple treatment options for children with early onset spinal deformities. However, because of the lack of evidence-based research, there is significant variation among surgeons' opinions when treatment options are being considered. The only available study on surgeons' preferences found a correlation between increasing curve size and the choice of growing rods over nonoperative treatment, rib-based distraction (vertically expandable prosthetic titanium rib), growth guidance (Shilla), and primary fusion.[7] Moreover, a classification of growth-friendly procedures based on the mechanism by which they modulate spinal and chest wall growth has been developed in recent years. This classification identifies distraction-based, compression-based, and growth-guided techniques.

Growth-sparing surgery is not an isolated act; it is peppered with numerous faux pas. There is a clear correlation between complication rates and the number of surgical procedures. The amount of distraction-based growth tends to decrease over time, the gain in spinal length is minimal and may not be worth further lengthenings, proximal junctional kyphosis is a severe complication requiring complex revision surgeries, and neither the neurologic nor the infectious risks are negligible.

Modern techniques and instrumentation control only one plane of the deformity because distraction forces are applied either to the spine or to the thoracic cage. Over the past few years, several studies have demonstrated that nearly normal growth can be attained with the vertical expandable prosthetic titanium rib, growing rods, or a Shilla-type procedure. All of these techniques aim to restore normal spinal growth by controlling progression of the deformity. However, no instrumentation is currently available that is able to control the three-dimensional nature of early-onset spinal deformities.

Opening wedge thoracostomy can increase the thoracic volume by "opening" the thoracic cage in the way that a parasol is opened (parasol effect). The procedure avoids the median line, leaving the spine unaltered. It is important that this procedure be undertaken before the end of bronchial tree development. However, the technique has the drawbacks of stiffening the thoracic cage and wrinkling the muscles of the chest, resulting in an increase in the amount of energy needed to breathe.[8]

Growing rods applied on either side of the vertebral column are able to modulate growth and control the deformity in frontal and sagittal planes. However, they are unable to prevent proximal junctional kyphosis, and the gain achieved with repeated lengthening tends to decrease with each subsequent lengthening and over time.[9]

More recently, alternative growth guidance techniques have been developed so that spinal deformities can be treated without the necessity of repeated operative lengthenings. In one of them, two stainless steel rods are fixed to the corrected apex of the curve by pedicle screws. The system guides growth at the ends of dual rods, with the apex of the curve corrected, fused, and fixed to the rods. Vertebral growth occurs cephalad and caudad through extraperiosteal sliding pedicle screws. However, this surgical option remains relatively extensive, involving at least 6 to 8 of 17 vertebrae.[10]

The placement of screws in the neurocentral synchondrosis, vertebral body tethering, and nitinol stapling of the apical vertebrae are other surgical interventions currently under development. The rationale behind these procedures is to limit spine growth asymmetrically, maintain spinal motion, preserve intervertebral disk physiology, and prevent the need for spinal fusion.[11,12]

Magnetically controlled, remotely distractible growing rod systems have been developed to reduce the number of repetitive surgeries under general anesthesia, decrease the number of hospitalizations, facilitate outpatient rod distraction, and reduce the number of wound complications and psychological problems. Moreover, distraction is gradual and performed at regular intervals with the child in a conscious state. Gradual and almost daily distraction is probably the most effective surgical procedure. It is very close to the principles of distraction osteogenesis introduced by Ilizarov about four decades ago.[13,14] This technique still presents some technical imperfections that need to be improved.

1.4.2 The Dark Side of Surgery

Surgery in patients with early onset scoliosis has a high morbidity rate. This is a major concern. Repetitive surgeries worsen the risk of complication, and it has been shown that any additional, unplanned intervention increases the risk for a complication by more than 20%. The structure of the vertebra contributes to the challenge of surgery: reduced size, the presence of osteoporosis, and the presence of cartilage that characterizes the "infantile" vertebra. At the age of 5 years, only one-third of the vertebral volume is ossified.

The rate of complications ranges from 8 to 50%; skin problems, wound and anesthetic complications, device migration, fractures, autofusion, hardware failure, infections, and decompensation have all been reported. Repeated hospitalizations for lengthenings and for unplanned surgical procedures increase the child's time away from school and can have repercussions on the child's psychological well-being.[15]

Overall, the risk of developing a complication is increased by a vital capacity of less than 50%, a Cobb angle of more than 50 degrees, kyphosis of more than 60 degrees, weight less of more than 20 kg, comorbidities, and a higher number of previous surgeries (▶ Table 1.3). Repetitive surgeries can induce spontaneous fusion; autofusion of ribs and vertebral bodies may then make definitive surgery more challenging.[16]

1.4.3 From Minimally to Maximally Invasive Surgery

At first, the goal is to limit surgery as much as possible. Because of repetitive surgical procedures, however, the surgeon gradually operates on almost the whole spine and forgets the need to spare levels as well as spinal motion. From surgical procedure to surgical procedure, from one complication to another, the surgeon stiffens the spine. Obsessed with repeating surgical procedures, the surgeon tends to forget that preservation of the vertebrae is essential for spinal growth. In fact, some procedures do stiffen about one-half of the T1-S1 segment without the surgeon realizing it (▶ Fig. 1.6 and ▶ Fig. 1.7). It is important not to forget that between T1 and S1 there are only 18 vertebrae!

In very young children, surgery should be limited as much as possible, and extensive arthrodesis of the spine should be avoided. Nevertheless, the surgeon can use hybrid constructs, such as growing rods in the back and staples at the apex of the deformity. Moreover, the surgeon can modify the instrumentation depending on the age of the patient, using smaller devices in younger

Table 1.3 Assessment of surgical risk

Surgical risk	Walking ability	Weight	Cardiac function	Respiratory function (VC)	Sleep	Comorbidities
Average	Ambulatory	>40 kg	Normal	Normal	Normal	No
Increased	Ambulatory with aid	20–40 kg	Reduced	Reduced, but > 50%	Hypersomnia	
High	Nonambulatory	<20 kg or obese	Significantly impaired	<50%	Nocturnal hypercapnic hypoventilation, obstructive sleep apnea	Yes

Abbreviation: VC, vital capacity.
Note: Besides neuromuscular pathology, factors such as walking ability, nutritional status, cardiopulmonary function, and the presence of other comorbidities must be taken into account before surgery in order to minimize surgical risk. Morbidity is higher in nonambulatory patients with reduced weight and impaired cardiopulmonary function.

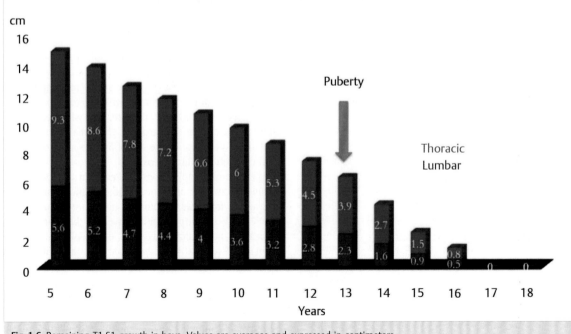

Fig. 1.6 Remaining T1-S1 growth in boys. Values are averages and expressed in centimeters.

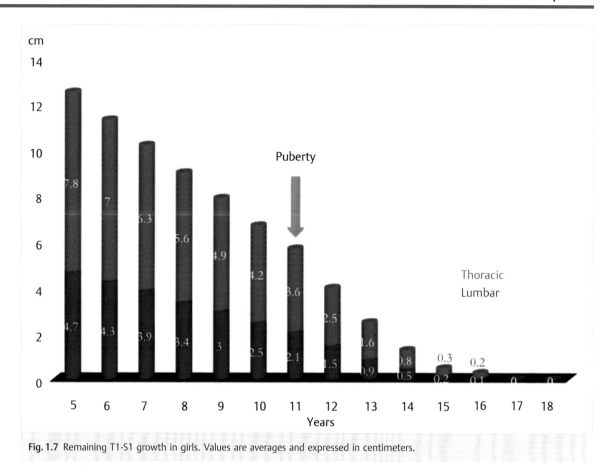

Fig. 1.7 Remaining T1-S1 growth in girls. Values are averages and expressed in centimeters.

children and bulkier instrumentation in older patients. It is fundamental that before any surgical program is started, these principles must be fully understood by everyone, surgeon included.

1.5 Serial Casting: Don't Put the Finger in the Gear

Challenging the growing spine means preserving the thoracic spine, thoracic cage, and lung growth without reducing spinal motion. The morbidity related to surgical procedures has favored the return of conservative treatment—that is, serial casting.

Casting is a nonoperative option that can be considered in the management of the young and very young child with early onset progressive spinal deformity. It can be used either as a *delaying tactic*, in order to prevent progression of the deformity for several years before definitive fusion, or as a *definitive treatment* option. It has been shown that in patients treated aggressively with casting before the age of 20 months for curves averaging 30 degrees, scoliosis was stabilized and/or reduced to 10 degrees or less at skeletal maturity. On the other hand, children undergoing cast treatment after the age of 30 months for curves averaging 50 degrees did not gain

significant correction, although their spinal curvature did not progress.[17] The main advantage of casting is that the spine is left alone. Moreover, it helps the surgeon not to put a finger in the spinal gear! The implantation of growth-sparing devices, near and/or at the level of the spine, affects spinal growth as demonstrated by both experimental and clinical studies.[1,2,3,18] Even if growth-sparing devices are implanted at a reasonable distance from the spine, autofusion of ribs and vertebral bodies may make definitive instrumented fusion more challenging for the surgeon and riskier for the patient, and the end result is less satisfactory for everybody.[16]

Unlike surgery, serial casting is an alternative that does not negatively affect or further alter spinal growth, and it can be used as a "positive" corrective force because it plays an important role in delaying or even eliminating the need for growth-sparing surgery. However, serial casting is not indicated for all types of early onset spinal deformities. At first sight, casting may appear like a constrictive force applied to the thoracic cage, limiting its expansion. Indeed, if well moulded, a cast does not compress the thoracic cage, and respiratory movements are allowed. These data can be considered to promote conservative means of treatment in young and very young patients, to allow expansion of the thoracic cage, lung growth, and cardiac function.

1.6 Crankshaft Phenomenon Is a Constant Enemy

In the crankshaft phenomenon, a spinal deformity progresses when the anterior portion of the spine continues to grow while the posterior portion is restricted by arthrodesis (▸ Fig. 1.3). The best way of controlling a pathologic spinal segment is to control all growth cartilages included in the pathologic zone. Nevertheless, it is very important for a surgeon to consider the state of skeletal maturity and the amount of growth remaining in the spinal segment to be fused. The Crankshaft phenomenon is manifested not only by an increase in the Cobb angle but also by a worsening of spinal imbalance, increased kyphosis, and progression of the *spinal penetration index*, characterized by penetration of the apical portion of the deformity inside the thoracic cage.

1.7 To Distract Kyphosis Is a Paradox

Sagittal plane correction is critical to the long-term success of scoliosis surgery. Proximal junctional kyphosis can occur during the treatment of early onset scoliosis, regardless of the preferred surgical procedure. It can become severe enough to require complex secondary interventions. Today, recognized independent risk factors for proximal junctional kyphosis are preoperative thoracic hyperkyphosis, proximal thoracic kyphosis, and a more proximal level of lower instrumented vertebrae (▸ Table 1.4).

Is it possible to avoid proximal junctional kyphosis? To answer this enigma, we should first understand where proximal junctional kyphosis comes from. Is proximal junctional kyphosis an issue limited to the spine? Or is it favored by underlying medical issues? In other words, despite the presence of early onset spinal deformity, are some patients more at risk for developing proximal junctional kyphosis than others?

Mechanical and genetic factors can be responsible for proximal junctional kyphosis. The restoration of normal sagittal alignment is one of the fundamental goals in scoliosis correction surgery, and rod pre-contouring is a standard procedure in almost all modern correction techniques for sagittal alignment control. However, in patients with early onset spinal deformities, it is not always possible to adapt the instrumentation to the spinal anatomy, in particular in the cervical region. When confronted with kyphosis, surgeons tend to increase the number of proximal and distal anchors.

When dealing with patients who have neurofibromatosis, chondrodystrophy, or spondyloepiphyseal dysplasia, the physician must remember that the cervical spine is pathologic. In those cases, it is wiser to treat the cervical spine first and then focus on the spinal deformity located below. It is necessary to know how to handle the cervical spine before treating the thoracic deformity in order to minimize potential neurologic complications.

Moreover, it is important to note that the surgeon is sometimes in a "biomechanical illegality." Certain kyphoscoliotic deformities are going to deteriorate when distraction is applied to correct the scoliotic portion of the spine; kyphosis does not tolerate distraction! The sagittal profile tends to deteriorate when repetitive distraction surgeries are performed.

1.8 The More You Lengthen, the Less You Lengthen

The economic concept outlined by the *law of diminishing returns* has been transposed to pediatric orthopedics. This law postulates that with constant factors of production, when new employees are hired, the marginal product of an additional employee will at some point be less than the marginal product of the previous employee. Therefore, from this point on, each additional employee will provide less and less return. In early onset spinal deformities treated with growing systems, the picture is similar. The gain achieved by repeated lengthening tends to decrease with each subsequent lengthening and over time. Successful initial lengthening of the spine appears to be a shortcut to unsuccessful subsequent lengthenings. This phenomenon is likely due to progressive stiffness or autofusion of the spine caused by repetitive and sudden distractions.[19]

Each distraction has to have a positive effect on sitting height. Sitting height correlates strictly with trunk height. Therefore, it is a more objective parameter than standing

Table 1.4 How to avoid proximal junctional kyphosis according to published data

Do/do not	Vertical expandable prosthetic titanium rib (VEPTR)	Growing rods
Do	Increase the number of anchors	Contour the proximal portion of the rod
Do	Bypass the apex of the kyphosis	Use gentle dissection
Do not	Apply proximal fixation below T4 (fourth rib)	Apply proximal fixation below T4
Do not	Make distal fixation too proximal; extend to pelvis if needed	Use hypercorrection
	A flexible spine does not predict good outcomes.	

height for the assessment of spinal growth. Standing height is less reliable because lower extremity growth may mask ineffective distractions.

1.9 What about Definitive Fusion?

The heterogeneity that characterizes growth-friendly techniques also applies to the management of children who have reached the end of the expansion phase of their growing instrumentation.[20] Final treatment varies with the underlying diagnosis, the condition of the spine and chest wall, and the instrumentation used.

Definitive fusion stops further spinal growth and achieves definitive correction. It becomes appropriate when patients have achieved sufficient thoracic spine length and thoracic cage volume. The timing of the procedure remains controversial, but in general, patients who are at least 10 years of age have completed the greatest part of their thoracic growth.

At the beginning of puberty, the T1-S1 segment still has to grow about 7 cm, of which approximately 4 cm is at the level of the thoracic spine and 3 cm is at the level of the lumbar spine. It is wiser to lose some growth than to have the deformity progress. Moreover, correction of the deformity compensates for the loss of height due to spinal fusion. Anticipation is sometimes the best strategy.

1.10 Heterogeneity of Etiologies, Diversity of Strategies

Patients who have early onset scoliosis are a heterogeneous population characterized by multiple etiologies. There is no single management strategy. There is no absolute truth. It is necessary to adapt treatment to each patient's need. Children with neuromuscular scoliosis at a young age have a set of challenges and problems, as well as treatment options, different from those of children with infantile idiopathic scoliosis or children with syndromes. All of these children have acquired scoliosis at an early age, but the manifestations, complications, and outcome of treatment vary. Age is another parameter that must be taken into account. Clearly, the 17-month-old child, the 5-year-old child, and the 9-year-old child with a spinal deformity are different facets of the problem and represent different opportunities for care.

Surgery must be finely shaded. In other words, a child with infantile idiopathic scoliosis can be treated by serial casting, a child with thoracic insufficiency syndrome due to congenital scoliosis and fused ribs may mostly benefit from open thoracostomy and rib distraction, and a child with neurologic scoliosis may be treated with dual growing rods. On the other hand, in the case of a child with

cerebral palsy and a collapsing spine, it may be worth waiting until the patient reaches age 10 and then perform a definitive fusion. In patients with low weight (e.g., Rett syndrome), it is not worth waiting for the pubertal growth spurt because their low body weight prevents puberty. On the other hand, patients with one- or two-level congenital malformations can benefit from limited early fusion; in this case, the surgeon is less concerned about definitive and limited surgery.

1.11 Conclusion: Don't Be Obsessed by the Centimeter

Treatment of the growing spine is a unique challenge. Patients with early onset spinal deformities are young, with significant remaining growth. Every failure causes psychological trauma for the family.

Managing the growing spine means preserving the thoracic spine, thoracic cage, and lung growth without reducing spinal motion. Have we the means of our ambitions? Probably not.

Obsession with the centimeter does not have to distract the surgeon from the fundamental priorities:
- What is the clinical picture?
- What is the annual weight gain? As a rule of thumb, annual weight gain should be 2.5 kg between 5 years of age and the beginning of the puberty.
- What is the annual increase in sitting height? In principle, between 5 and 11 years of age, the sitting height should increase annually by 2.5 cm.
- What is the evolution of the vital capacity?

Finally, the objectives to be achieved are the following:
- An improved clinical picture;
- A weight gain of about 2.5 kg per year;
- A thoracic spine height of 18 to 22 cm or more, which is necessary to avoid severe respiratory insufficiency;
- A vital capacity of at least 50%.

The ultimate goal of treatment is to improve the natural history of the patient's spinal deformity as well as the patient's quality of life, and to have these sick children become independent adults. The contract with families must be clear. This is a long-term treatment. It is necessary to explain the obstacles to be overcome and not to underestimate the risks.

It is also important to understand how to prioritize a patient's needs. There is a *short-term priority*, in which the main goal is to stop progression of the spinal deformity. There is a *midterm priority*, in which the primary objective is to improve cardiorespiratory function and weight. There is a *long-term priority*, in which the ultimate goal is to have these patients become independent adults with an acceptable quality of life. We should prevent a child from becoming the end result of a juxtaposition of surgical procedures.

The path that remains to be traveled is still long, but new perspectives in the field of respiratory physiology, pediatric nutrition, and surgery are on the horizon.

Nothing is impossible. We call impossible what human beings take a long time to achieve.
—Albert Camus

References

[1] Dimeglio A, Canavese F. The growing spine: how spinal deformities influence normal spine and thoracic cage growth. Eur Spine J 2012; 21: 64–70

[2] Canavese F, Dimeglio A, Volpatti D et al. Dorsal arthrodesis of thoracic spine and effects on thorax growth in prepubertal New Zealand white rabbits. Spine 2007; 32: E443–E450

[3] Canavese F, Dimeglio A, Granier M et al. Arthrodesis of the first six dorsal vertebrae in prepubertal New Zealand white rabbits and thoracic growth to skeletal maturity: the role of the "rib-vertebral-sternal complex." Minerva Ortop Traumatol 2007; 58: 369–378

[4] Dimeglio A. Growth of the spine before age 5 years. J Pediatr Orthop B 1993; 1: 102–107

[5] Narayanan M, Owers-Bradley J, Beardsmore CS et al. Alveolarization continues during childhood and adolescence: new evidence from helium-3 magnetic resonance. Am J Respir Crit Care Med 2012; 185: 186–191

[6] Butler JP, Loring SH, Patz S, Tsuda A, Yablonskiy DA, Mentzer SJ. Evidence for adult lung growth in humans. N Engl J Med 2012; 367: 244–247

[7] Yang JS, McElroy MJ, Akbarnia BA et al. Growing rods for spinal deformity: characterizing consensus and variation in current use. J Pediatr Orthop 2010; 30: 264–270

[8] Campbell RM Jr Smith MD, Mayes TC et al. The effect of opening wedge thoracostomy on thoracic insufficiency syndrome associated with fused ribs and congenital scoliosis. J Bone Joint Surg Am 2004; 86-A: 1659–1674

[9] Thompson GH, Akbarnia BA, Campbell RM Jr. Growing rod techniques in early-onset scoliosis. J Pediatr Orthop 2007; 27: 354–361

[10] McCarthy RE, Luhmann S, Lenke L, McCullough FL. The Shilla growth guidance technique for early-onset spinal deformities at 2-year follow-up: a preliminary report. J Pediatr Orthop 2014; 34: 1–7

[11] Zhang H, Sucato DJ. Unilateral pedicle screw epiphysiodesis of the neurocentral synchondrosis. Production of idiopathic-like scoliosis in an immature animal model. J Bone Joint Surg Am 2008; 90: 2460–2469

[12] Betz RR, Kim J, D'Andrea LP, Mulcahey MJ, Balsara RK, Clements DH. An innovative technique of vertebral body stapling for the treatment of patients with adolescent idiopathic scoliosis: a feasibility, safety, and utility study. Spine 2003; 28: S255–S265

[13] Cheung KM, Cheung JP, Samartzis D et al. Magnetically controlled growing rods for severe spinal curvature in young children: a prospective case series. Lancet 2012; 379: 1967–1974

[14] Wick JM, Konze J. A magnetic approach to treating progressive early-onset scoliosis. AORN J 2012; 96: 163–173

[15] Bess S, Akbarnia BA, Thompson GH et al. Complications of growing-rod treatment for early-onset scoliosis: analysis of one hundred and forty patients. J Bone Joint Surg Am 2010; 92: 2533–2543

[16] Lattig F, Taurman R, Hell AK. Treatment of early onset spinal deformity (EOSD) with VEPTR: a challenge for the final correction spondylodesis: a case series. J Spinal Disord Tech 2012[Epub ahead of print]

[17] Mehta MH. Growth as a corrective force in the early treatment of progressive infantile scoliosis. J Bone Joint Surg Br 2005; 87: 1237–1247

[18] Karol LA, Johnston C, Mladenov K, Schochet P, Walters P, Browne RH. Pulmonary function following early thoracic fusion in non-neuromuscular scoliosis. J Bone Joint Surg Am 2008; 90: 1272–1281

[19] Sankar WN, Skaggs DL, Yazici M et al. Lengthening of dual growing rods and the law of diminishing returns. Spine 2011; 36: 806–809

[20] Akbarnia BA, Campbell RM, Dimeglio A et al. Fusionless procedures for the management of early-onset spine deformities in 2011: what do we know? J Child Orthop 2011; 5: 159–172

2 Development of the Spine

Alain Dimeglio and Federico Canavese

Only a perfect knowledge of normal growth parameters allows a thorough understanding of the pathologic changes induced in a growing organism by an early onset spinal deformity. As the spinal deformity progresses, not only is spinal growth affected; by a "domino effect," the size and shape of the thoracic cage are modified as well. This distortion of the thorax interferes with lung development. Over time, the spine disorder changes in nature from a mainly orthopedic issue to a severe, systemic pediatric disease causing thoracic insufficiency syndrome, cor pulmonale, and, in the most severe cases, death.

The growing spine is a mosaic of growth plates characterized by changes in rhythm. During growth, complex phenomena follow one another in very rapid succession. These events are well synchronized to maintain harmonious limb and spine relationships, as growth in the various body segments does not occur simultaneously in the same magnitude or at the same rate. The slightest error or modification can lead to a malformation or deformity, with negative effects on standing and sitting height; the shape, volume, and circumference of the thoracic cage; and lung development.[1,2]

2.1 Clinical Examination and Biometric Measurements

Growth holds the basics, and any surgical strategy should be adjusted according to the ratio between remaining growth and elapsed growth (▶ Table 2.1).

A height gauge, scales, a metric tape, and a bone age atlas are required at the time of consultation. All growths

are synchronized, but each one has its own rhythm (▶ Fig. 2.1). A thorough analysis of the standing and sitting height, arm span, weight, thoracic perimeter, T1-S1 spinal segment length, and respiratory function helps the surgeon to plan the best treatment at the right time. Therefore, these measurements should be repeated and carefully recorded at regular intervals to provide a real-time image of growth and charts that facilitate decision making. A clinical examination every 4 to 6 months allows the clinician to assess the growth velocity of the child and the different body segments easily.[1,2]

2.1.1 Standing Height

The gain in standing height is approximately 25 cm during the first year of life and about 12.5 cm during the second year. Between the ages of 2 and 3 years, the gain in standing height is approximately 9 cm annually, and between the ages of 3 and 4 years, the gain in standing height is approximately 7 cm annually. At 5 years of age, the standing height increases by 5 to 5.5 cm each year in both boys and girls. At the beginning of puberty, the average remaining growth in the standing height is about 22.5 cm for boys (13%) and 20.5 cm for girls (11%).

Growth velocity is the best indicator of the beginning of puberty, on which so many decisions rest. The first sign of puberty is an increase in the rate of growth in the standing height to more than 0.5 cm per month or more than 6 to 7 cm per year.[1,2,3,4] Growth charts show that a standing height growth velocity of more than 6 cm per year in girls and more than 7 cm per year in boys is evidence that the patient is within his or her greatest growth spurt.[1,2,3,4] This rapid and significant increase in the growth rate is called peak height velocity or acceleration phase. During this phase, the average remaining growth in the standing height is about 16.5 cm for boys and 15 cm for girls. The first 2 years of puberty, characterized by significant growth, are followed by 3 years of a gradual and steady reduction in the growth rate, the so-called deceleration phase, during which the average remaining growth in the standing height is about 6 cm for boys and 5 cm for girls.[1,2,3]

In 77% of boys, the first physical sign of puberty is testicular growth, which occurs on average 3.5 years before adult height is attained. In 93% of girls, the first physical sign of puberty occurs about 2 years before menarche, and final height is usually achieved 2.5 to 3 years after menarche.[1,2,3,4]

The standing height is a global marker comprising two components: sitting height and subischial height. Because the trunk and the subischial region often grow at different rates and at different times, the standing height does

Table 2.1 Growth is a change in proportion

Developmental stage	Sitting height		Lower extremities
	Head	Trunk	
Fetus (early pregnancy)	50%	32%	18%
Fetus (late pregnancy)	35%	40%	25%
Newborn	25%	40%	35%
Infant	23%	37%	40%
Child	20%	35%	45%
Pre-Adolescent	18%	34%	48%
Adult	13%	40%	47%

Note: The ratio of the sitting height to the length of the lower extremities varies with age; it is 4.5 during early pregnancy, 3 during late pregnancy, 1.9 at birth, 1.3 during childhood, and 1 at skeletal maturity.[1,2,3,4]

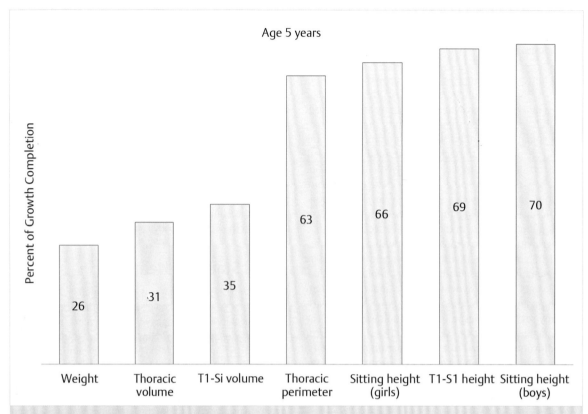

Fig. 2.1 All growths are synchronized, but each one has its own rhythm. Growths do not progress at the same pace. At 5 years of age, the increases in weight and thoracic volume remain limited relative to the other growth indicators. At 5 years of age, children have reached 26% of their final weight but between 66% and 70% of their final sitting height.

not always exactly correlate with a loss of trunk height in children with severe spinal deformities.[1,2,3,4]

2.1.2 Sitting Height

The sitting height correlates strictly with trunk height and is on average about 34 cm at birth; it is 88 cm at the end of growth for girls and 92 cm at the end of growth for boys. In children with severe spinal deformities, the loss of sitting height is related to the severity of the deformity. For this reason, it is important to monitor changes in sitting height rather than in standing height in children with progressive spinal deformities. During the first 3 years of life, or in a child with a neurologic disorder or a collapsing spine, it is recommended to measure the sitting height with the child in a supine position.

Growth is a succession of acceleration and deceleration phases comprising three periods. The first period is from birth to age 5 and is characterized by a gain in sitting height of 27 cm, with a gain of 12 cm occurring during the first year of life. The second period is from age 5 to 10 years and is a quiescent phase in which sitting height increases by 2.5 cm per year. The third period is characterized by a gain in sitting height of about 12 cm and corresponds to puberty.[1,2,3] During peak height velocity or

acceleration phase,[4] the average remaining growth in the sitting height is about 12.5 cm for boys and about 11.5 cm for girls (► Fig. 2.2, ► Fig. 2.3, ► Fig. 2.4). The average remaining growth in the sitting height during the deceleration phase is about 4 cm for boys and 3.5 cm for girls.[1,2,3,4]

2.1.3 Weight

Weight is a useful parameter for evaluating growth and increases 20-fold from birth to skeletal maturity. At 5 years of age, weight is approximately 20 kg; it is 30 kg by 10 years and reaches 60 kg or more by 16 years. In particular, weight usually doubles during the pubertal spurt, and each year of puberty corresponds to a weight increase of about 5 kg. This information should be kept in mind when a child is treated with a brace. Moreover, in a patient whose weight is 10% or more above normal, a scoliosis brace may be less effective than in a patient whose weight is within 10% above normal.[1,2,3,4]

Growth energy requirements during the first 3 years of life are enormous and much greater than those of adults: 110 calories vs. 40 calories per kilogram per day; 2 g vs. 1 g of proteins per kilogram per day; and 150 mL vs. 5 mL of water per kilogram per day. Moreover, skeletal

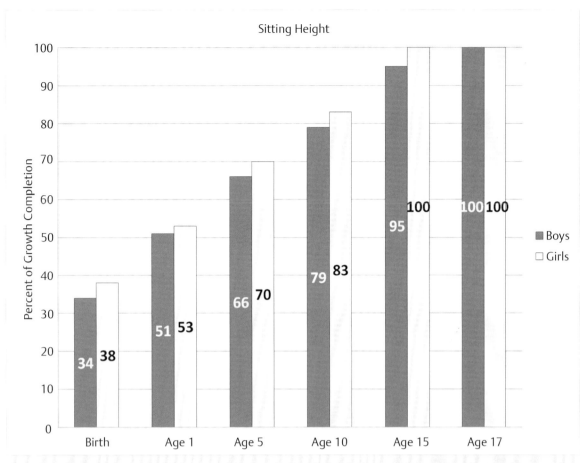

Fig. 2.2 Percentage of remaining sitting height growth in boys (*gray*) and girls (*white*). Sitting height growth is completed 2 years earlier in girls than in boys on average.

mineralization alone requires the storage of 1 kg of calcium between birth and adulthood.

Because most children with severe spinal deformities or neurologic impairment have a low body mass index (BMI) and thus are at a higher risk of surgical morbidity, weight is a valuable indicator. In selected cases, a hypercaloric nutritive protocol should be initiated before surgery. Children with pulmonary insufficiency characteristically have poor nutrition because the energy expenditure for the extra work of breathing approaches the nutritional gain derived from eating. It has been demonstrated that in about two-thirds of children with severe spinal deformities and thoracic insufficiency syndrome treated with expansion thoracoplasty surgery, the nutritional status improves significantly postoperatively.

Of note, the BMI can be misleading. A 9-year-old child with severe scoliosis, a standing height of 110 cm, and a weight of 12 kg can have a BMI that is somewhat reassuring. However, this information does not reflect reality because the standing height is similar to that of a child of 1 to 5 years of age and the weight comparable to that of a 2-year-old child. In children with low weight, the pubertal spurt changes are moderate because the weight must be at least 40 kg for the spurt to be normal.[1,2,3]

The average birth weight is approximately 3 kg, which means that the blood volume is about 0.3 L. Weight plays an essential role in surgical planning, and the surgeon's margin for maneuver is very narrow. Any weight loss, however slight, after spinal surgery before 5 years of age can have serious consequences. A 1-kg postoperative weight loss in an 18-kg patient represents about 6% of the total body weight, and therefore there is a major difference between operating on a 40-kg child and a 20-kg child. For this reason, children with spinal deformities who weigh less than 20 kg should be differentiated from those weighing more than 20 kg. Of note, weight gain in children after spinal surgery is a good indicator that the clinical situation is under control.[1,2,3]

2.1.4 Arm Span

The arm span is an indirect measurement to evaluate standing height and can be used to assess predicted height in nonambulatory children with neuromuscular disorders, cerebral palsy, or myelomeningocele.

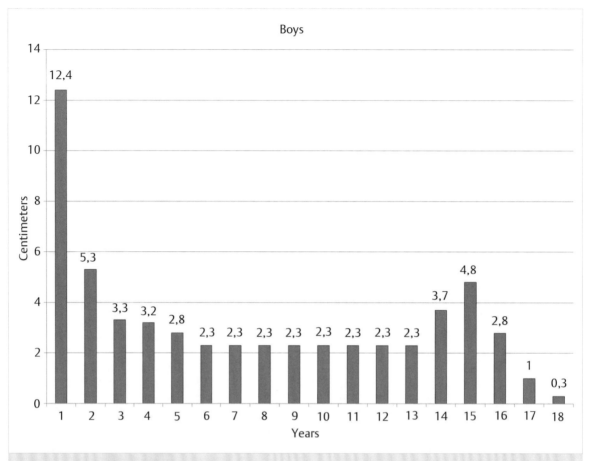

Fig. 2.3 Sitting height gain in boys. Values are expressed in centimeters and are average values.[1,2,3] In boys, the pubertal spurt occurs between 13 and 15 years of age.

The arm span and the standing height have an almost perfect linear correlation. The standing height corresponds to approximately 97% of the arm span, with a small gender difference; the ratio of the arm span to the total standing height is greater in boys than it is in girls. This relationship persists throughout puberty and into adulthood. In 77% of healthy children, the arm span will be 0 to 5 cm greater than the standing height; in 22%, it will be 5 to 10 cm greater; and in 1% it will be greater by 10 cm or more. As a rule of thumb, the arm span divided by 2 is very close to the sitting height, and the arm span divided by 4 is close to the length of the T1-S1 spinal segment.[1,2,3]

2.2 Spine and Thoracic Cage

The action of the spinal growth plates can be defined by four words: harmony, interaction, synchronization, and hierarchy. Symmetric and harmonious growth characterizes normal spines, although spinal growth itself is the product of more than 130 growth plates working at different paces. The development of the spine consists of a complex series of events involving multiple metabolic processes, genes, and signaling pathways.

The first 5 years of life are critical. In severe scoliosis, growth becomes asymmetric as a result of growth plate disorganization. Complex spinal deformities alter the growth of the spinal cartilage; as a result, the vertebral bodies become progressively distorted and can perpetuate the disorder by altering thoracic cage and lung growth (► Fig. 2.5). Therefore, many scoliotic deformities can become growth plate disorders over time.[2,5]

Because of the complexity of the three-dimensional organization of the growth plates, no surgical implant is capable of controlling them in all spatial planes. Attempts have been made with staples, growing rods, vertebral tethering bands, rib expanders, trolley constructs, and apical arthrodesis. However, the results remain controversial.

The crankshaft phenomenon is the progression of a spinal deformity during which the anterior portion of the spine continues to grow while the posterior portion is blocked by arthrodesis. Growth modulation devices should restore normal growth plate development and

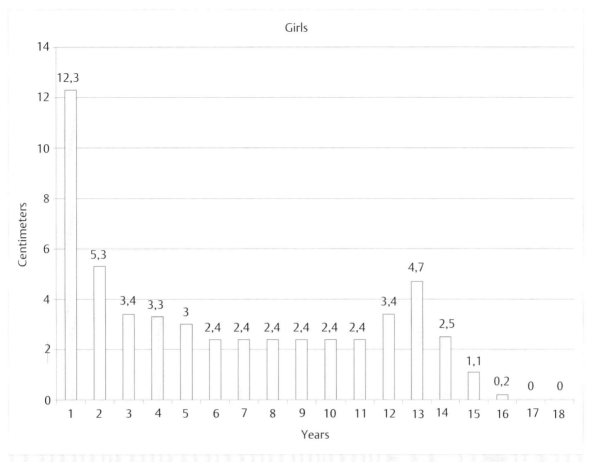

Girls

Fig. 2.4 Sitting height gain in girls. Values are expressed in centimeters and are average values.[1,2,3] In girls, the pubertal spurt occurs between 11 and 13 years of age.

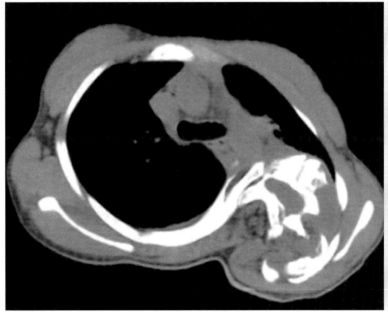

Fig. 2.5 Effects of spinal deformity on chest size and shape. Computed tomographic scan (transverse section) shows severe scoliosis with chest cage deformity.. As a result of severe spinal deformities, the apical portion of the deformity penetrates inside the thoracic cage (endothoracic hump). The "spinal penetration index" measures the amount of endothoracic hump.[1,2,3,4,5]

should control the crankshaft phenomenon.[1,2,3,4] Moreover, growth modulation devices should follow the pace of spinal and thoracic growth by providing about 2.5 cm of sitting height and 2.5 kg of weight per year between ages 5 and 10, and 4 to 5 cm of sitting height and 5 kg of weight per year during the pubertal spurt.[1,2,3,4]

2.2.1 Ossification of the Spine

Ossification of the vertebral bodies starts at the third month of intrauterine life. It begins in the thoracolumbar area and radiates from there both proximally and caudally.

Within the cervical spine, ossification centers appear first in the neural arches and then in the vertebral bodies. Ossification starts in the lower cervical spine and develops proximally.

Moreover, ossification centers in the anterior and posterior portions of the vertebrae do not grow at the same pace. In the thoracic region, posterior growth is faster than anterior growth, resulting in the progressive development of thoracic kyphosis. On the other hand, in the lumbar area, posterior growth is slower than anterior growth, resulting in lumbar lordosis.[1,2,3,4]

2.2.2 Neurocentral Synchondrosis and Spinal Canal

The bilateral neurocentral synchondroses are cartilaginous growth plates located between the neural arch and the centrum of the vertebral body (between the single anterior and the bilateral neural arch ossification centers). These structures play an essential role in the growth of the vertebral body and the posterior arch and are called bipolar growth plates because they contribute to the growth of both structures. Moreover, they allow the vertebral arch to grow in tandem with the spinal cord. Anatomical and radiographic studies have suggested that the neurocentral synchondroses disappear well before adolescence. However, more recent magnetic resonance imaging studies have demonstrated that these structures are still visible, and probably active, until 11 to 16 years of age. After that time, the neurocentral synchondroses have fused and are no longer visible on magnetic resonance images. When present, the synchondroses are visible on both T1- and T2-weighted images.

It has been shown in a growing pig model that unilateral transpedicular screw fixation that traverses a neurocentral synchondrosis can produce asymmetric growth of the synchondrosis, leading to scoliosis in which the convexity is on the side of the screw fixation and the pedicle is small and short on the side of the concavity of the spinal deformity. However, in humans, the neurocentral synchondrosis fuses around age 9, and by 5 years of age the spinal canal has already grown to about 95% of its definitive size. The thoracic spinal canal is narrower than the cervical or lumbar canal. As a rule of thumb, a perivertebral arthrodesis performed after age 5 should have no influence on the size of the spinal canal.[2,5]

2.2.3 C1-C7 Spinal Segment

The cervical spine, from C1 to C7, measures about 3.5 cm at birth, doubles in length by the age of 6 (between 7 and 7.4 cm), and measures 12 to 13 cm at skeletal maturity. The cervical spine represents about one-fifth of the C1-S1 segment and about 15% of the sitting height.[1,2,3,4]

2.2.4 T1-S1 Spinal Segment

Assessment of the T1-S1 spinal segment is important because many spinal deformities originate in this segment. At birth, the T1-S1 segment measures about 20 cm and reaches 45 cm at skeletal maturity. It should be recalled that the height of the spine accounts for 60% of the total sitting height, with the head and the pelvis accounting for the remaining 40%.

The T1-S1 segment (two-thirds of which is the thoracic spine and one-third the lumbar spine) accounts for approximately 50% of the sitting height (▶ Table 2.1). It grows about 10 cm during the first 5 years of life (2 cm per year), about 5 cm between the ages of 5 and 10 (1 cm per year), and about 10 cm between age 10 and skeletal maturity (1.8 cm per year; ▶ Table 2.2). It has been shown that early surgery in patients with scoliosis developing before 4 years of age does not modify the deformation produced by scoliosis or preserve respiratory function, even when the anterior growth of the spine is arrested. Therefore, it is very important for the surgeon to consider the state of skeletal maturity and the amount of growth remaining in the segment of the spine that is to be fused.[1,2,3,5,6]

2.2.5 T1-T12 Spinal Segment

T1-T12 is the posterior pillar of the thoracic cage and a strategic segment. It measures about 12 cm at birth,

Table 2.2 Evaluation of the T1-T12 and L1-L5 spinal segments from birth to skeletal maturity

Developmental stage	Spinal segment			
	Males		Females	
	T1-T12	L1-L5	T1-T12	L1-L5
Newborn	11	7.5	11	7.5
Child	18	10.5	18	10.5
Pre-Adolescent	22	12.5	22	12.5
Adult	28	16	26	15.5

Note: Values are expressed in centimeters and are average values.[1,2,3,4]

Table 2.3 Growth of the T1-S1, T1-T12, and L1-L5 segments

Spinal segment	Age (years)						
	1	3	5	7	9	11	Pubertal spurt
T1-S1	2			1			1.8
T1-T12	1.3			0.7			1.1
L1-L5	0.7			0.3			0.7

Note: Values are expressed in centimeters and are average values.[1,2,3,4]

18 cm at 5 years of age, and about 27 cm on average at skeletal maturity. The thoracic spine makes up 30% of the sitting height, and a single thoracic vertebra with its disk represents about 2.5% of sitting height. In normal children, the longitudinal growth of the thoracic spine is approximately 1.3 cm per year between birth and 5 years, 0.7 cm per year between the ages of 5 and 10, and 1.1 cm per year during puberty (▶ Table 2.3). A precocious arthrodesis of this segment has effects on thoracic growth and lung development. In young children with progressive deformity, there is a decrease of longitudinal growth and a loss of the normal proportionality of trunk growth (▶ Table 2.1 and ▶ Table 2.2). Without treatment, progressive early onset spinal deformity has been associated with short trunk, short stature, and often respiratory insufficiency. The loss of vital capacity in patients with untreated early onset scoliosis has been shown to be 15% greater than the loss in those with adolescent idiopathic scoliosis. Emans et al showed that pelvic inlet width, measured by computed tomography or plain radiography, is an age-independent predictor of the expected thoracic dimensions in unaffected children and adolescents. This study also established normal-range standards of the chest and spine dimensions to help in the assessment of treatment outcomes.[2,7] The thoracic spine is connected to the rib cage by the costovertebral articulations, which consist of the costal head joint and the costotransverse joint. The 12 thoracic vertebral bodies have costal facets, which articulate with two costal heads, and two transverse processes, each of which articulates with the tubercle of one of these ribs per side. Altogether, these synovial articulations, which constitute the costovertebral joints, play an essential role in elevating and depressing the ribs so as to increase the anteroposterior and transverse diameters of the thoracic cavity during respiration. Moreover, the costovertebral junction plays an important role in stabilizing the thoracic spine in the sagittal, coronal, and transverse planes.

Respiratory problems can develop after an early vertebral arthrodesis or as a consequence of preexisting severe vertebral deformities, and they can vary in pattern and timing according to the existing degree of deformity. The varying extent of an experimental arthrodesis also affects both growth and thoracopulmonary function differently.

Early spinal fusion for progressive scoliosis limits further spinal growth and results in diminished thoracic height, and therefore a long-term loss of vital capacity. It must be borne in mind that early spinal fusion, especially in the thoracic region,[8,9] is a cause of respiratory insufficiency and adds a loss of pulmonary function to the spinal deformity. Karol et al reported that a thoracic spinal height of 18 cm or more is necessary to avoid severe respiratory insufficiency.[8] In addition, they showed that children undergoing early spinal fusion have a reduction of thoracic depth and a shorter T1-T12 segment compared with normal subjects (▶ Table 2.2). The forced vital capacity may decrease to 50% of the predicted volume if more than 60% of the thoracic spine (i.e., eight thoracic vertebrae) is fused before the age of 8 years. Karol et al confirmed with their clinical work some of the experimental findings previously published by Canavese et al.[9]

2.2.6 L1-L5 Spinal Segment

The lumbar vertebrae have well-developed vertebral bodies, in addition to spinous, transverse, and superior articular processes that provide attachment sites for ligaments and muscles (erector spinae and transversospinales muscles).

At birth, the lumbar vertebrae are relatively smaller than the cervical and thoracic vertebrae. During growth, the lumbar vertebrae and disks increase in size about 2 mm per year, while in the thoracic spine, the average increase is only 1 mm per year.

The L1-L5 length is approximately 7.5 cm at birth and 16 cm on average at skeletal maturity. The lumbar spine makes up about 18% of the sitting height, and a single lumbar vertebra and its disk represent 3.5% of sitting height. At age 10 years, the lumbar spine has reached about 90% of its final height, but only 60% of its definitive volume (▶ Table 2.2). The volume of the lumbar vertebrae increases sixfold from the age of 5 years to skeletal maturity. A perivertebral arthrodesis of the lumbar spine after the age of 10 years results in minimal loss of sitting height.[1,2,3,5]

2.2.7 Intervertebral Disks

At birth, the intervertebral disks account for about one-third of the C1-S1 length. At skeletal maturity, the intervertebral disks account for 22% of the cervical spine, 18% of the thoracic spine, and 25% of the lumbar spine length.[1,2,3,4]

2.2.8 Thoracic Cage Volume, Circumference, and Shape

The thoracic cage is the fourth dimension of the spine. The thoracic cage volume is about 6% of its definitive size at birth, 30% by age 5, and about 50% by age 10. Moreover,

Table 2.4 Modification of chest shape during growth

Developmental stage	Chest dimensions			Chest shape
	Chest depth	Chest width	Ratio of depth to width	
Birth	79	72	1.1	Round–ovoid
5 years	132	150	0.9	Ovoid
10 years	160	220	0.7	Elliptical
Skeletal maturity	210	280	0.7	Elliptical

Note: The overall shape of the thoracic cage evolves from ovoid at birth to elliptical at skeletal maturity. Values are expressed in millimeters and are average values.[1,2,3,4]

between age 10 and skeletal maturity, the thoracic cage volume doubles and its volumetric growth stops. All types of growth do not progress at the same speed. At 5 years of age, the trunk has reached between 66% and 70% of its final height, whereas the thoracic volume is only 31% of its definitive size (▶ Fig. 2.1).

The thoracic circumference corresponds to 95% of the sitting height and increases both during the first 5 years of life and puberty. On average, the newborn thoracic perimeter is 32.3 cm in boys and 31.5 cm in girls, and it will attain a mean value of 89.2 cm in boys and 85.4 cm in girls.

The shape of the thoracic cage shape varies with age. At birth, the difference between thoracic depth and width is minimal, and the ratio of thoracic depth to thoracic width is very close to 1. Conversely, at skeletal maturity, the ratio of thoracic depth to thoracic width is lower than 1 because the width has increased more than the depth. For this reason, the overall shape of the thoracic cage evolves from ovoid at birth to elliptical at skeletal maturity (▶ Table 2.4). At the end of growth, the thorax has an average depth of 21 cm in boys and 17.7 cm in girls, with an average width of 28 cm in boys and 24.7 cm in girls. At skeletal maturity, the thoracic depth and width represent about 20% and 30% of sitting height, respectively.[1,2,3,5]

An opening wedge thoracostomy can increase the thoracic volume (parasol effect). It is important to perform such a procedure before the development of the bronchial tree ends at 8 years of age. However, a disadvantage of this procedure is that it increases the stiffness of the thoracic cage and thus the amount of energy needed to breathe.[2,4]

2.3 Growth of the Lungs and Chest Cage

The "golden" period for growth of both the thoracic spine and thoracic cage occurs between birth and 4 years of age and coincides with lung development. Lung and thoracic cage volumes increase in a nonlinear fashion over the first 20 years of life, with rapid growth occurring before 4 years of age and during the pubertal growth spurt. The volumes of both structures are proportional to the standing height when spinal disease is absent. Normal values for lung function and volume in children are based primarily on the standing height. The source of potential respiratory failure is the sum of extrinsic disturbances of the chest wall functions and intrinsic alveolar hypoplasia. Thoracic cage deformities prevent the lungs from expanding, thus preventing lung tissue hyperplasia. Moreover, intrinsic alveolar hypoplasia is often associated with severe spinal and chest wall deformities, such as spondylocostal dysplasia, Jeune syndrome, and Jarcho-Levin syndrome. It is therefore important to preserve both thoracic growth and lung volume during this critical period of life. Postmortem studies have shown that individuals with early onset deformities have fewer alveoli than expected and emphysematous changes in existing alveoli. These studies suggest that mechanical compression is not a factor in reducing the number of alveoli, and that this reduction is probably due to a premature cessation of alveolar proliferation. Indeed, from the late fetal stage to 4 years of age, the number of alveoli grows by a factor of 10, and the development of the bronchial tree ends around 8 to 9 years of age.

In a review of 1,050 normal computed tomographic scans of the chest with three-dimensional volumetric reconstruction of the pulmonary system, Gollogly et al showed that lung parenchyma volume is a function of age. The volume of the lung parenchyma at birth is 400 cc, It is approximately 900 cc and 1,500 cc at ages 5 and 10 years, respectively, and about 4,500 cc for boys and 3,500 cc for girls at skeletal maturity. From birth to skeletal maturity, lung weight increases from 60 to 750 g. Lung growth is complex because different pulmonary structures and regions grow at different rates.

A newborn has the same number of conducting airways as an adult. Tracheal caliber increases two- to threefold between birth and skeletal maturity. In contrast, the peripheral regions of the lung, which contain alveoli and pulmonary capillaries (acinar regions), undergo substantial postnatal growth and development. From infancy to adulthood, the alveolar number increases up to 6-fold, and the alveolar–capillary surface area increases more than 10-fold as a result of increases in alveolar number, complexity, and septa and of capillary development. Early onset scoliosis therefore adversely affects thoracic growth in the critical period of maximum respiratory growth and induces irreversible changes in the thoracopulmonary structure.[8,9,10] Early onset and progressive spinal deformities tend to increase mortality in early adulthood. In particular, it has been shown patients with a vital capacity below 45% of predicted or scoliosis of 110 degrees or more are at high risk for respiratory failure.[1,2,3,4,5,6,7,8,9,10]

2.3.1 Rib–Vertebral–Sternal Complex

The concept of the rib–vertebral–sternal complex was introduced in 2007.[9,10] It is now known that spinal deformations adversely affect development of the thorax by changing its shape and reducing its normal motility. The rib–vertebral–sternal complex, which fits the thoracic cavity in three dimensions, tends to constitute an elastic structural model similar to a cube in shape. However, in the presence of scoliosis, it becomes flat, rigid, and elliptical, thus preventing the lungs from expanding. These deformations, which can be lethal in the most severe cases, result from mutual interactions and influences among the various skeletal and organic components of the thoracic cage and cavity that are still not well understood. Several studies have focused on the anatomical influences of experimental arthrodesis on spinal growth, chest development, and thoracopulmonary function.[9,10] These reports have demonstrated that early arthrodesis, as well as severe spinal deformities, can adversely affect the development of the spine and thorax by changing their shape and reducing normal mobility (▶ Fig. 2.6). Canavese et al evaluated the consequences of disturbed growth of vertebral bodies on the development of the ribs, sternum, and lungs, which form part of the rib–vertebral–sternal complex.[10] These influences are much more evident when the arthrodesis is carried out in the critical portion of the thoracic spine (i.e., the T1-T6 segment). The development of the thoracic cage and lungs is a complex process that requires perfect synergy among the various components of the rib–vertebral–sternal complex. Alterations in any of these elements affect and change the development and growth of the others. To preserve thoracic motility and permit a normal development of the respiratory tree, treatment should not focus only on the spine but should consider the rib–vertebral–sternal complex as a whole.[9]

Maximal compensatory lung growth may well be limited to a specific time after birth and diminish after the period of alveolar multiplication is complete. Published estimates of this period of alveolar multiplication vary from 1 to 8 years of age. The optimal timing of surgical interventions to expand the thoracic cage so as to both minimize progressive postnatal pulmonary hypoplasia and maximize compensatory lung growth still needs to be determined but is likely to be early rather than late in childhood.[10]

2.4 Early Onset Scoliosis Is a Pediatric Disease

Truth is behind a critical analysis of the growth charts. The numbers from growth charts are to be interpreted in the dynamics. Only a critical analysis of all growth parameters over time unmasks and allows an understanding of the magnitude of the deficits induced by an early onset spinal deformity.

2.4.1 A Vital Capacity of 50% at Age 8 Years Will Be Less at Age 16 Years

Spinal growth and thoracic growth follow strict rules and can be controlled only by following the requirements of the process. Four different scenarios can be identified: (1) The clinical picture worsens. Abnormal growth leads to a deficit that sustains the deformity in the same way that a rolling snowball enlarges ("snowball effect"). Reduced body mass index (BMI) due to weight loss weakens, among other structures, the respiratory muscles and thus makes breathing more difficult. (2) The clinical picture is stable. (3) The clinical picture gets slightly better, with improvement of the various clinical parameters, such as weight, vital capacity, and sitting height. (4) The clinical

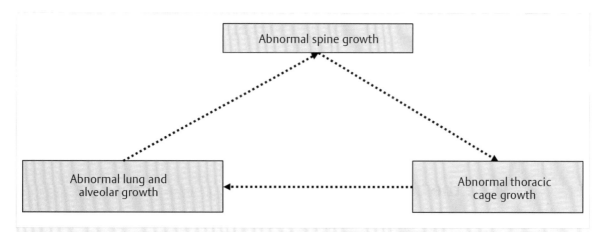

Fig. 2.6 Distorted growth of the spine induces alterations in the growth of the thoracic cage that lead to a reduction of lung and alveolar growth. Complex spinal deformities alter the growth of the spinal cartilage, and progressive distortion of the vertebral bodies can perpetuate the disorder by altering growth of the thoracic cage and lungs.

picture returns to normal. In this ideal scenario, all the clinical parameters recover from the deficits induced by the deformity. Unfortunately, this is unlikely to happen because most children with severe spinal deformities end up at skeletal maturity with a short trunk, a significant loss of vital capacity, and a disproportionate body habitus.

Surgical strategies must consider the complete life span of the patient and should aim to obtain 40 kg of weight, 50% of the vital capacity, a T1-S1 segment of about 30 cm, and a T1-T12 segment of at least 20 cm in order to prevent the most severe clinical pictures. However, two basic questions needs to be answered before any surgical treatment is considered: What is the functional benefit, and what is the morbidity risk? It must be remembered that the thoracic cage is part of the deformity (rib–vertebral–sternal complex). There are normal interactions among the organic components of the spine, the thoracic cage, and the lungs. Both early onset spinal deformities and early spinal arthrodesis alter spinal growth and affect thoracic development by changing the shape of the thorax and reducing its normal mobility. Treatment of the growing spine poses unique challenges involving preservation of the thoracic spine, thoracic cage, and lung growth without a reduction of spinal motion. The principle that a short, straight spine, produced by an early fusion, is better than a long, curved spine is no longer generally accepted.[1,2,3,4,5,6,7,8,9,10]

References

[1] Dimeglio A, Bonnel F. Le Rachis en Croissance. Paris, France: Springer; 1990

[2] Dimeglio A, Canavese F. The growing spine: how spinal deformities influence normal spine and thoracic cage growth. Eur Spine J 2012; 21: 64–70

[3] Dimeglio A, Canavese F, Charles YP. Growth and adolescent idiopathic scoliosis: when and how much? J Pediatr Orthop 2011; 31 Suppl: S28–S36

[4] Akbarnia BA, Campbell RM, Dimeglio A et al. Fusionless procedures for the management of early-onset spine deformities in 2011: what do we know? J Child Orthop 2011; 5: 159–172

[5] Dimeglio A. Growth of the spine before age 5 years. J Pediatr Orthop B 1993; 1: 102–107

[6] Goldberg CJ, Gillic I, Connaughton O et al. Respiratory function and cosmesis at maturity in infantile-onset scoliosis. Spine 2003; 28: 2397–2406

[7] Emans JB, Ciarlo M, Callahan M, Zurakowski D. Prediction of thoracic dimensions and spine length based on individual pelvic dimensions in children and adolescents: an age-independent, individualized standard for evaluation of outcome in early onset spinal deformity. Spine 2005; 30: 2824–2829

[8] Karol LA, Johnston C, Mladenov K, Schochet P, Walters P, Browne RH. Pulmonary function following early thoracic fusion in non-neuromuscular scoliosis. J Bone Joint Surg Am 2008; 90: 1272–1281

[9] Canavese F, Dimeglio A, Volpatti D et al. Dorsal arthrodesis of thoracic spine and effects on thorax growth in prepubertal New Zealand white rabbits. Spine 2007; 32: E443–E450

[10] Canavese F, Dimeglio A, Granier M et al. Arthrodesis of the first six dorsal vertebrae in prepubertal New Zealand white rabbits and thoracic growth to skeletal maturity: the role of the "rib-vertebral-sternal complex." Minerva Ortop Traumatol 2007; 58: 369–378

3 The Genetics of Congenital Scoliosis and Abnormal Vertebral Segmentation

Peter D. Turnpenny

Before the modern molecular era, genetic analyses were often undertaken as epidemiologic studies, leading to the detailed assembly of empiric data that would allow analysis of possible inheritance patterns and recurrence risks for the purpose of genetic counseling. In the field of infantile idiopathic scoliosis, Wynne-Davies examined 134 infants and their first-degree relatives and found that approximately 3% of parents and 3% of siblings had the same, or a similar, deformity.[1] Congenital heart disease was present in 2.5% (the general population incidence is ~6 per 1,000 live births) and mental retardation in 13%, suggesting that a significant proportion of children had a syndromic form of congenital scoliosis (CS). Erol et al studied 81 patients with different forms of CS and segmentation defects of the vertebrae (SDV); of 39 patients prospectively recruited into study, 15 (38%) were found to have multiple-organ/syndromic associations, many of which fit into the oculo-auriculo-vertebral (OAV) (or Goldenhar) spectrum.[2] Purkiss et al studied 237 patients with CS and identified 49 patients who had two or more family members with congenital or idiopathic scoliosis, suggesting a much higher recurrence rate of 20.7%.[3] There was also a history of idiopathic scoliosis in 17.3% of the families. Maisenbacher et al reported that 10% of patients with CS reported having first-degree relatives with idiopathic scoliosis.[4] These risk data are diverse, and there is a need for more studies with clearer phenotypic stratification.

▶ Table 3.1 lists rare syndromes that may include CS and/or SDV, along with the genetic basis, if known. Most are very rare, and those most commonly encountered in clinical practice are OAV/Goldenhar spectrum, VATER or VACTERL (*v*ertebral, *a*nal, *c*ardiac, *t*racheo-*e*sophageal, *r*enal, and *l*imb) association, MURCS (*m*üllerian duct, *r*enal aplasia, *c*ervicothoracic *s*omite dysplasia) association, and maternal diabetes syndrome. The pathogenesis of these broad clinical groups is poorly understood. Any case series presenting to the spinal surgeon, pediatrician, or geneticist will demonstrate enormous radiologic and structural heterogeneity, and a syndromic or genetic diagnosis will be at best vague (including the OAV/VACTERL/MURCS associations because the cause[s] of these groups is unknown) and at worst completely elusive. ▶ Table 3.1 is a reminder that young (and not so young) patients presenting with CS/SDV should be examined and investigated very thoroughly for additional anomalies and a syndrome diagnosis considered. Referral to a clinical geneticist should therefore be part of the patient care pathway.

Although CS is frequently associated with SDV, this is not always so, and it may occur in severe forms of some syndromes in which segmentation anomalies are absent, although abnormalities of vertebral *formation* may be present. A presentation of this kind should prompt consideration of a diagnosis of one of the skeletal dysplasias, although a precise radiologic diagnosis may require follow-up skeletal surveys as the child grows and generalized bone growth evolves. A clinical genetics opinion with a view to genetic testing may be very helpful, and examples include the following: congenital contractural arachnodactyly (Beals syndrome), which is autosomal dominant and due to mutations in *FBN2*; chondrodysplasia punctata, Conradi–Hünermann type (Happle syndrome), which is X-linked and due to mutations in the *EBP* gene; diastrophic dysplasia, which is autosomal recessive and due to mutations in the sulfate transporter gene *SLC26A2* (also known as *DTDST*); and spondylometaphyseal dysplasia, Kozlowski type, which is autosomal dominant and due to mutations in *TRPV4*.

3.1 The Spondylocostal Dysostoses and Somitogenesis

The main progress in understanding the genetic basis of SDV has come through the study of somitogenesis in animal models, particularly the mouse but also chick. Animals with specific gene knockouts are generated and multiple gene expression assays undertaken to help elucidate the developmental pathways. Somitogenesis is the sequential process whereby paired blocks of paraxial mesoderm are patterned from the presomitic mesoderm to form somites. It takes place between 20 and 32 days of human embryonic development, and in this process, pairs of somites are laid down on either side of the midline in a rostrocaudal direction. In mice, a pair of somites is formed every 1 to 3 hours, whereas in humans, the process is estimated to have a periodicity of 6 to 12 hours based on cell culture models and analysis of staged anatomical collections.[5,6] Somites ultimately give rise to four substructures: sclerotome, which forms the axial skeleton and ribs; dermotome, which forms the dermis; myotome, which forms the axial musculature; and syndetome, which forms the tendons.[7,8] Somitogenesis begins shortly after gastrulation and continues until the pre-programmed number of somite blocks is formed. In humans, 31 blocks of paired tissue are formed, but the number is specific for each species. The formation of somite boundaries is precisely timed and begins with the most rostral (head) somite, with the progressive laying down of more caudal somites. The establishment of boundaries takes

Table 3.1 Some syndromes and disorders that include segmentation defects of the vertebrae

Syndrome/disorder	OMIM	Gene
Acrofacial dysostosis	263750	*DHODH*
Alagille syndrome	118450	*JAG1, NOTCH2*
Anhalt syndrome*	601344	
Atelosteogenesis type III	108721	*FLNB*
Campomelic dysplasia	211970	*SOX9*
Casamassima–Morton–Nance syndrome*	271520	
Caudal regression*	182940	
Cerebro-facio-thoracic dysplasia*	213980	*TMC01*
CHARGE syndrome	214800	*CHD7*
"Chromosomal"		
Currarino syndrome	176450	*HLXB9*
Atelosteogenesis type II (de la Chapelle syndrome)	256050	*SLC26A2*
DiGeorge syndrome / deletion 22q11.2 / velocardiofacial syndrome	188400	
Dysspondylochondromatosis*		
Femoral hypoplasia–unusual facies*	134780	
Fibrodysplasia ossificans progressiva	135100	*ACVR1*
Fryns–Moerman syndrome*		
Goldenhar / OAV spectrum*	164210	
Holmes–Schimke*		
Incontinentia pigmenti	308310	*IKBKG*
Kabuki syndrome*	147920	*MLL2*
McKusick–Kaufman syndrome	236700	*MKKS*
KBG syndrome*	148050	*ANKRD11*
Klippel–Feil anomaly*	148900	*GDF6, PAX1†*
Larsen syndrome	150250	*FLNB*
Lower mesodermal agenesis*		
Maternal diabetes mellitus*		
MURCS association*	601076	
Multiple pterygium syndrome	265000	*CHRNG*
OEIS syndrome*	258040	
PHAVER syndrome*	261575	
RAPADILINO syndrome (*RECQL4*-related disorders)	266280	*RECQL4*
Robinow syndrome (*ROR2*-related disorders)	180700	*ROR2*

Table 3.1 continued

Syndrome/disorder	OMIM	Gene
Rolland–Desbuquois type*	224400	
Rokitansky sequence*	277000	*WNT4†*
Silverman–Handmaker type of dyssegmental dysplasia (DDSH)	224410	*HSPG2*
Simpson–Golabi–Behmel syndrome	312870	*GPC3*
Sirenomelia*	182940	
Spondylo-carpo-tarsal synostosis	272460	*FLNB*
Thakker–Donnai syndrome*	227255	
Toriello syndrome*		
Urioste syndrome*		
VATER / VACTERL association*	192350	
Verloove–Vanhorick syndrome*	215850	
Wildervanck syndrome*	314600	
Zimmer syndrome*	301090	

Abbreviations: CHARGE, coloboma, heart disease, atresia choanae, retarded growth, genital hypoplasia, ear anomalies; MURCS, müllerian duct, renal aplasia, cervicothoracic somite dysplasia; OAV, oculo-auriculo-vertebral; OEIS, omphalocele, exstrophy, imperforate anus, spinal defects; OMIM, Online Mendelian Inheritance in Man; PHAVER, pterygia, heart defects, autosomal recessive inheritance, vertebral defects, ear anomalies, radial defects; RAPADILINO, radial ray defect, patellae hypoplasia or aplasia and cleft or highly arched palate, diarrhea and dislocated joints, little size and limb malformations, long slender nose and normal intelligence; VACTERL, vertebral, anal, cardiac, tracheoesophageal, renal, and limb.
* Underlying cause not known.
† Possible associations reported: PAX1[73] and WNT4.[74]

place as a result of very finely tuned molecular processes determined by activation and negative feedback interactions between components of the Notch, Wnt and FGF signaling pathways.[9,10] In the rostral third of the presomitic mesoderm, the formation of segmental boundaries is subject to levels of the factor FGF8; this is produced in the caudal region of the embryo[11] and probably maintains cells in an immature state until levels fall below a threshold, allowing boundary formation. Somites already harbor specification toward their eventual vertebral identity, a process regulated by the Hox family of transcription factors,[12] which also display oscillatory expression in the mouse during somitogenesis.[13]

The Wnt signaling pathway also displays oscillatory expression in a temporal phase different from that of Notch pathway genes, and it plays a key role in the segmentation clock.[14,15,16] The mediators of the determination front and the segmentation clock (Notch, FGF, Wnt) are required for forming the somite boundary and specify

Table 3.2 Proposed definitions for the terms *spondylocostal dysostosis* and *spondylothoracic dysostosis*[72]

Features	Spondylocostal dysostosis	Spondylothoracic dysostosis
General	No major asymmetry to chest shape Mild, nonprogressive scoliosis Multiple SDV (M-SDV; > 10 contiguous segments) Absence of a bar Malaligned ribs with intercostal points of fusion	Chest shape symmetric, with ribs fanning out in a "crablike" appearance Mild, nonprogressive scoliosis or no scoliosis Generalized SDV (G-SDV) Regularly aligned ribs, fused posteriorly at the costovertebral origins, but no points of intercostal fusion
Specific, descriptive	"Pebble beach" appearance of the vertebrae in early childhood radiographs (▶ Fig. 3.1)	"Tramline" appearance of prominent vertebral pedicles in early childhood radiographs, not seen in SCD (▶ Fig. 3.2) "Sickle cell" appearance of vertebrae on transverse imaging[40]

Abbreviations: SCD, spondylocostal dysostosis; SDV, segmentation defects of the vertebrae.

the rostrocaudal patterning of presumptive somites, for which *Mesp2* is crucial.[17] *Mesp2* is expressed caudal to the somite that is in the process of forming, and this domain is set where Notch signaling is active, FGF signaling is absent, and the transcription factor Tbx6 is expressed. Precise periodicity in the establishment of somite blocks is mediated by several so-called cycling, or oscillatory, genes, two of which, *LFNG* and *HES7*, have been implicated in humans as well as animals.

Somites themselves, having formed, are subsequently partitioned into rostral and caudal compartments, with vertebrae formed from the caudal compartment of one somite and the adjacent rostral compartment of the next, a phenomenon known as resegmentation.[18,19,20,21] An understanding of the molecular biology of somitogenesis in animal models, in combination with finding patients and families with specific forms, or patterns, of segmentation anomalies, has led to the most definitive progress in understanding the causes of CS/SDV, albeit in a rare group of disorders. Ongoing research is identifying more cycling genes and pathways involved in the regulation of somitogenesis.

3.2 Terminology

At this point, it is necessary to explain the use of terms, which in clinical practice is very inconsistent and confusing. The term *spondylocostal dysostosis* (SCD) has been, and continues to be, applied to a wide variety of radiologic phenotypes in which abnormal segmentation is evident, together with rib involvement. For the purposes of this review, however, the definition given in ▶ Table 3.2 is used. A number of attempts have been made to classify SDV. The scheme proposed by Mortier et al combines phenotype and inheritance pattern (▶ Table 3.3).[22] The scheme proposed by Takikawa et al allows a very broad definition of SCD (▶ Table 3.4),[23] but both these schemes identify Jarcho–Levin syndrome[24] with a crablike chest, which on more detailed scrutiny is misapplied. The surgical approach to classification of McMaster and Singh distinguishes between formation and segmentation errors

Table 3.3 Previously proposed classification of segmentation defects of the vertebrae according to Mortier et al[22]

Nomenclature	Definition
Jarcho–Levin syndrome	Autosomal recessive Symmetric crablike chest Lethal
Spondylothoracic dysostosis	Autosomal recessive Intrafamilial variability, severe/lethal Associated anomalies uncommon
Spondylocostal dysostosis	Autosomal dominant Benign
Heterogeneous group	Sporadic Associated anomalies common

Table 3.4 Previously proposed classification / definition of segmentation defects of the vertebrae according to Takikawa et al[23]

Nomenclature	Definition
Jarcho–Levin syndrome	Symmetric crablike chest
Spondylocostal dysostosis	More than two vertebral anomalies associated with rib anomalies (fusion and/or absence)

(▶ Table 3.5).[25] Like the scheme of McMaster and Singh, the classification scheme for vertebral abnormalities of Aburakawa et al,[23,26] which includes vertebral morphology (▶ Table 3.6), does not attempt to identify phenotypic patterns of malformation based on assessment of the spine as a whole. Vertebral fusion or segmentation errors involving the cervical region, Klippel–Feil anomaly, has been subclassified (▶ Table 3.7),[27,28] and Clarke et al (▶ Table 3.8) proposed a further, detailed classification combining modes of inheritance.[29] The use of a limited number of terms in these classification schemes fails to reflect the great diversity of radiologic SDV phenotypes seen in clinical practice, and the schemes do not incorporate knowledge from molecular genetics. Furthermore,

Table 3.5 Classification (surgical/anatomical) of vertebral segmentation abnormalities causing congenital kyphosis/kyphoscoliosis according to McMaster and Singh[25]

Type	Anatomical deformity	Anomalies
I	Anterior failure of vertebral body formation	Posterolateral quadrant vertebrae • Single vertebra • Two adjacent vertebrae Posterior hemivertebrae • Single vertebra • Two adjacent vertebrae Butterfly (sagittal cleft) vertebrae Anterior or anterolateral wedged vertebrae • Single vertebra • Two adjacent vertebrae
II	Anterior failure of vertebral body segmentation	Anterior unsegmented bar Anterolateral unsegmented bar
III	Mixed	Anterolateral unsegmented bar Contralateral posterolateral quadrant vertebrae
IV	Unclassifiable	

Table 3.6 Classification of vertebral segmentation abnormalities[23,26] (modified North American classification)

Failure of formation
Type I
A. Double pedicle
B. Semisegmented
C. Incarcerated
Type II
D. Not incarcerated, no lateral shift
E. Not incarcerated, plus lateral shift
Type III
F. Multiple
Type IV
G. Wedge
H. Butterfly
Failure of segmentation
I. Unilateral bar
J. Complete block
K. Wedge (plus narrow disk)
Mixed
L. Unilateral bar plus hemivertebra
M. Unclassifiable
Note: Hemivertebrae are seen in types B through F and in type L.

Table 3.7 Classification of Klippel–Feil anomaly, referring to segmentation defects or fusion of the cervical vertebrae, according to Feil and Thomsen[27,28]

Type	Site	Anomaly
I	Cervical and upper thoracic vertebrae	Massive fusion with synostosis
II	Cervical vertebrae	One or two interspaces only, hemivertebrae, occipito-atlantoid fusion
III	Cervical and lower thoracic or lumbar vertebrae	Fusion

Table 3.8 Classification of Klippel–Feil anomaly according to Clarke et al[29] (adapted from original publication)

Class	Vertebral fusions	Inheritance	Possible anomalies
KF1	Only class with C1 fusions C1 fusion not dominant Variable expression of other fusions	Recessive	Very short neck; heart, urogenital, craniofacial, hearing, limb, digital, ocular defects Variable expression
KF2	C2-C3 fusion dominant C2-C3 most rostral fusion Cervical, thoracic, and lumbar fusion variable within a family	Dominant	Craniofacial, hearing, otolaryngeal, skeletal, and limb defects Variable expression
KF3	Isolated cervical fusions Variable position Any cervical fusion except C1	Recessive or reduced penetrance	Craniofacial, facial dysmorphology Variable expression
KF4	Fusion of cervical vertebrae, data limited	Possibly X-linked Predominantly females affected	Hearing and ocular anomalies: abducens palsy with retraction bulbi, also called Wildervanck syndrome

Table 3.9 Genes causing generalized segmentation defects of the vertebrae (i.e., "spondylocostal dysostosis") according to the definition proposed in ▶ Table 3.2

Gene symbol	Chromosomal locus	Protein name
DLL3	19q13.1	Delta-like protein 3
MESP2	15q26.1	Mesoderm posterior protein 2
LFNG	7p22	Beta-1,3-N-acetylglucosaminyl-transferase lunatic fringe
HES7	17p13.2	Transcription factor HES-7
TBX6	16p11.2	DNA-binding protein T-BOX-6

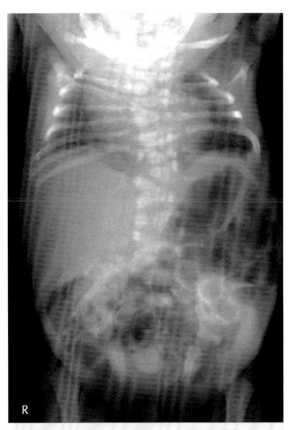

Fig. 3.1 The radiologic phenotype of spondylocostal dysostosis type 1, due to mutated *DLL3*. This shows segmentation abnormalities throughout the vertebral column and the variable ovoid appearance of multiple vertebrae—the "pebble beach" sign. The ribs are malaligned, with points of fusion along their length.

the diversity of SDV is not captured within the classification of osteochondrodysplasias.[30,31] A new scheme for classification and reporting from the International Consortium for Vertebral Anomalies and Scoliosis (ICVAS) is described later.

According to the definition used here, SCD is a condition characterized by a short trunk and short stature due to multiple or generalized SDV (M-SDV or G-SDV), usually accompanied by rib fusions and/or malalignment. A mild, nonprogressive kyphoscoliosis is present, usually without additional organ abnormalities. Five Notch signaling pathway genes are now linked to this group, four demonstrating autosomal recessive inheritance and one autosomal dominant inheritance. These are now described in more detail, and ▶ Table 3.9 summarizes the conditions and their genes.

In clinical practice, patients with abnormal vertebral segmentation, usually with only regional or very limited involvement of the spine, are much more commonly seen than patients with the rare monogenic forms, which perhaps affect 1 in 1,000 newborns. They are likely to occur sporadically, demonstrate more asymmetry, and be associated with other organ malformations.

3.3 Clinical Description and Genetics of the Subtypes of Spondylocostal Dysostosis

3.3.1 Spondylocostal Dysostosis Type 1 (SCD1)

More than 30 *DLL3* mutations have now been identified and most of these published.[32,33] All cases follow autosomal recessive inheritance. The majority of these mutations give rise to a consistent radiologic and clinical phenotype. G-SDV (including hemivertebrae) is present (i. e., the entire spine is involved), and there is a general consistency in the abnormal form and shape of the vertebrae in the different regions, from cervical to lumbar, although

in some cases the thoracic region is more severely disrupted. The radiologic appearances in childhood are of vertebrae that are circular or ovoid on anteroposterior projection, and they have smooth outlines (▶ Fig. 3.1). To this appearance the term *pebble beach sign* has been applied.[33] Stature is affected to a variable degree, with those mildly affected having approximately 15 cm less than their predicted height on the basis of arm span measurements (assuming arm length is unaffected). Variability in stature can be marked within families.[34]

We know of two patients with slightly milder phenotypes due to mutated *DLL3*, both with less dramatic vertebral segmentation abnormalities, even though the whole spine was involved (unpublished data). Both these patients had missense, rather than protein truncation, mutations. Some missense mutations, although not all, appear give rise to milder phenotypes.

The trunk is shortened to a variable degree, the abdomen protrudes, and life-threatening complications are rare, although one of the affected patients in the family reported by Turnpenny et al. (1991) succumbed at age 7 months with a large patent ductus arteriosus and a hypoplastic diaphragm at necropsy.[34] Some other reports have also highlighted persistent foramen ovale. There appears to be an increased risk of inguinal hernias in men with SCD1,[34,35] which may be due to increased intra-abdominal pressure secondary to a shortened trunk. Usually, however, the spinal malformation in SCD1 is isolated. Learning difficulties or intellectual disability is not a feature of SCD1. Although affected individuals have mild scoliotic curves from an early stage, these appear to remain stable throughout life in the majority of cases, and spinal surgery is usually not required.

The Genetics of SCD1

Genetic mapping by autozygosity was used to identify a locus for autosomal recessive SCD at chromosome 19q13.1[36] in an extensive Arab–Israeli kindred first reported in 1991.[34] This region is syntenic with the murine chromosome 7 region harboring the *Dll3* gene, which is truncated in the pudgy mouse,[37] in which the vertebral malformation is strikingly similar to that in patients with SCD1. Mutations were found in *DLL3* in three consanguineous families.[38] The organization of human *DLL3* is almost identical to mouse *Dll3*, excepting the terminal exon, which corresponds to a fusion of mouse exons 9 and 10, resulting in a human protein of 32 additional amino acids. There is variability in the size of the mouse and human introns. The gene is sequentially ordered with a signal sequence (SS), the delta-serrate-lag (DSL) domain, six highly conserved epidermal growth factor (EGF) repeats, and a transmembrane (TM) region. Approximately 75% of positive cases have protein truncation nonsense mutations (the rest being missense), and parental consanguinity is seen in the same proportion of cases. Two missense mutations, C309 R and G404C, have been seen in association with slightly milder radiologic phenotypes, possibly because of the position of these residues within the EGF domains.

3.3.2 Spondylocostal Dysostosis Type 2 (SCD2)

Only one family with SCD due to a mutation in *MESP2*, demonstrating autosomal recessive inheritance, has been published,[39] but a second affected family with the same mutation and similar radiologic phenotype was presented at an international meeting in 2005. Subsequent haplotype analysis failed to show evidence of a common ancestry for the two families (unpublished data), so the particular 4-base pair (bp) duplication mutation is recurrent. A further case of SCD2 was a compound heterozygote for *MESP2* mutations identified in a service laboratory (unpublished data). In SCD2, the radiologic phenotype is similar to, but distinguishable from, that of SCD1, and the ribs are more normally aligned.

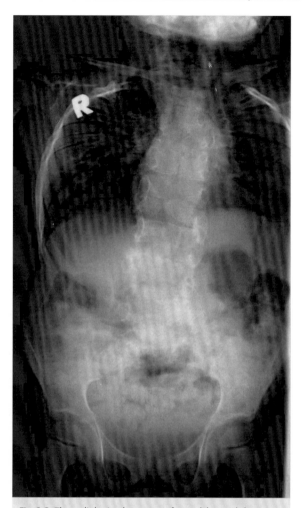

Fig. 3.2 The radiologic phenotype of spondylocostal dysostosis type 2, due to mutated *MESP2*. This shows segmentation abnormalities throughout the vertebral column, with the thoracic region most severely disrupted. (Reproduced from Turnpenny et al. (2009). © University of Washington.)

Segmentation defects appear more severe in the thoracic vertebrae than in the lumbar vertebrae, which are relatively spared (► Fig. 3.2). Stature is affected to a small degree. As with SCD1, no additional organ abnormalities have been reported.

The Genetics of SCD2

A genome-wide scanning strategy was used to demonstrate linkage to 15q21.3–15q26.1 in a consanguineous family in which results of testing for *DLL3* were negative. Within this region lies the somitogenesis gene *MESP2*, and sequencing identified a 4-bp (AGGC) duplication, a frameshift mutation for which the affected subjects were homozygous and the parents heterozygous.[39] The mutation was not found in 68 normal ethnically matched control chromosomes.

The *MESP2* gene codes for a basic helix–loop–helix (bHLH) transcription factor and encodes a protein of 397 amino acids; the human MESP2 protein has 58.1% identity with mouse Mesp2. The human MESP2 amino-terminus contains a bHLH region encompassing 51 amino acids, which is divided into an 11-residue basic domain, a 13-residue helix I domain, an 11-residue loop domain, and a 16-residue helix II domain. The loop region is conserved between mouse and human *Mesp1* and *Mesp2*. In addition, both *Mesp1* and *Mesp2* contain a unique CPXCP motif immediately carboxy-terminal to the bHLH domain. The amino- and carboxy-terminal domains are separated in human *MESP2* by a GQ repeat region, which is also present in human *MESP1* (2 repeats) but have expanded in human *MESP2* (13 repeats). Mouse *Mesp1* and *Mesp2* do not contain any GQ repeats, but they do contain a couple of QX repeats in the same region. In cases designated SCD2, the mutations identified do not appear to give rise to nonsense-mediated decay of the derivative protein, in contrast to the effect of mutations in STD, the more severe phenotype due to mutated *MESP2*.

3.4 Spondylothoracic Dysostosis (STD)

In SCD, points of fusion along the length of the ribs are usually apparent, whereas in STD the ribs are fused *posteriorly* and fan out laterally (crablike appearance) without points of fusion along their length. In early life, multiple rounded hemivertebrae (pebble beach sign[33]) characterize SCD1 (*DLL3* gene), and the vertebral pedicles are poorly visualized. By contrast, in *MESP2*-associated SCD and STD, the vertebral pedicles are well formed and prominent in fetal life and early childhood (▶ Fig. 3.3), for which we suggest the term *tramline sign*. STD, in its most severe form, carries a significant risk of life-threatening respiratory insufficiency in infancy, and the condition has been well delineated and described by Cornier et al.[40] The patients in most reported cases are Puerto Rican, but the condition has been seen globally. Mutations in *MESP2* are of the type that give rise to nonsense-medicated decay.

3.4.1 Spondylocostal Dysostosis Type 3 (SCD3)

Only one family with SCD due to a mutation in *LFNG* has been reported and, to our knowledge, remains unique.[41] The family was of Lebanese Arab extraction and the parents consanguineous. In this case, segmentation disruption was more severe than in SCD1 and SCD2, giving rise to marked truncal shortening and apparently normal limb length (▶ Fig. 3.4). Multiple vertebral ossification centers in the thoracic spine, with very angular shapes, were apparent. The severe foreshortening of the spine was emphasized by the comparison of the patient's arm

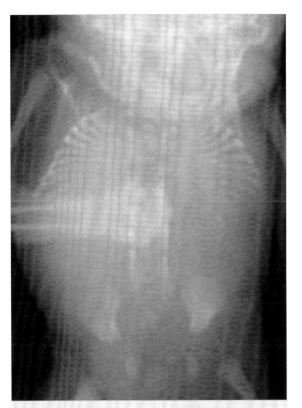

Fig. 3.3 The radiologic phenotype of spondylothoracic dysostosis, due to mutated *MESP2*. This shows severe shortening of the spine, generalized segmentation defects, a crablike fanning out of the ribs from their posterior costovertebral origins, and well-aligned ribs. The vertebral pedicles are ossified at this early stage (in contrast to spondylocostal dysostosis type 1), which we have called the tramline sign. (Reproduced courtesy of eLS.)

span (186.5 cm) with the patient's adult height (155 cm; lower segment, 92.5 cm). The patient also demonstrated a minor form of distal arthrogryposis in the upper limbs, although it is not known whether this feature is integral to the condition or secondary to peripheral nerve entrapment.

The Genetics of SCD3

A candidate gene approach was used to identify the genetic cause of SCD in an individual in whom no mutation could be found in *DLL3* or *MESP2*. Lunatic fringe, *LFNG*, encodes a glycosyltransferase (fucose-specific β1,3 N-acetylglucosamine) that post-translationally modifies the Notch family of cell surface receptors, a key step in the regulation of this signaling pathway,[42] and *LFNG* is one of the "cycling" genes whose wave of expression in the presomitic mesoderm, in a caudal–rostral direction, is crucial to the establishment of the next somite boundary. *LFNG* was sequenced because its expression is severely dysregulated in mouse embryos that lack *Dll3* (the phenotypes of *Dll3* and *Lfng* null mutant mice are

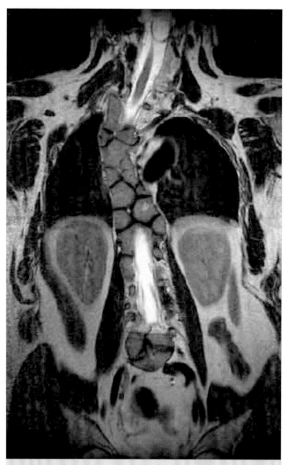

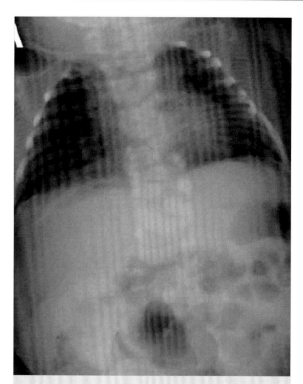

Fig. 3.5 The radiologic phenotype of spondylocostal dysostosis type 4, due to mutated *HES7*. This shows segmentation abnormalities throughout the vertebral column, and the appearance resembles that of spondylocostal dysostosis type 2 / spondylothoracic dysostosis. (Reproduced with permission from Sparrow et al. (2008). © Oxford University Press.)

Fig. 3.4 The radiologic phenotype of spondylocostal dysostosis type 3, due to mutated *LFNG*. This shows severe shortening of the thoracic spine in particular. (Reproduced from Sparrow et al. (2006). © Elsevier.)

virtually identical), and it is associated with the Notch signaling pathway (like *DLL3* and *MESP2*). In the affected case, homozygosity for a missense mutation (c.564C→A) was detected that resulted in the substitution of leucine for phenylalanine (F188L); the unaffected parents were heterozygous for the mutation. Further evidence that this missense mutation in *LFNG* was causative of SCD was provided by a number of assays undertaken to assess the function of F188 L. It was shown that F188 L did not localize to the Golgi apparatus, as in the wild-type LFNG protein, and that F188 L lacked transferase activity. It was therefore concluded that c.564C→A was pathogenic in homozygous individuals.

3.4.2 Spondylocostal Dysostosis Type 4 (SCD4)

To date, two reports describe SCD in association with mutations in *HES7*.[43,44] In the first of these cases, the affected subject had G-SDV in a pattern not dissimilar to that seen in mild STD, with ribs appearing to show fusion posteriorly and fanning out in a crablike fashion (► Fig. 3.5). The patient was homozygous for a *HES7* mutation and also had a lumbar myelomeningocele neural tube defect; there were no associated malformations in the second reported family, in which SCD occurred only in subjects who were compound heterozygotes for *HES7* mutations.[44] The possible association of SCD4 with neural tube defect, and other midline defects, remains to be elucidated.

The Genetics of SCD4

HES7 encodes a bHLH-Orange domain transcriptional repressor protein that is both a direct target of the Notch signaling pathway and part of a negative feedback mechanism required to attenuate Notch signaling. Like *LFNG*, *HES7* is one of the cycling genes of the Notch pathway.[45,46] As such, it is expressed in the presomitic mesoderm in an oscillatory pattern, which is achieved by an autoregulatory loop. Once translated, HES proteins act on their own promoters to repress transcription, and because of the short half-life of HES proteins, autorepression is relieved, which allows a new wave of transcription and translation every 90 to 120 minutes in the mouse.

3.4.3 Spondylocostal Dysostosis Type 5 (SCD5)—Autosomal Dominant

Only one genetic cause of autosomal dominant SCD has thus far been identified—namely, mutated *TBX6*.[47] The mutation segregated with the condition over two generations in a Macedonian family that appeared to be affected over three generations. They were previously shown not have a mutation in *DLL3*, *MESP2*, *LFNG*, or *HES7*,[48] and the family demonstrated a generalized pattern of SDV without any additional malformations (▸ Fig. 3.6).

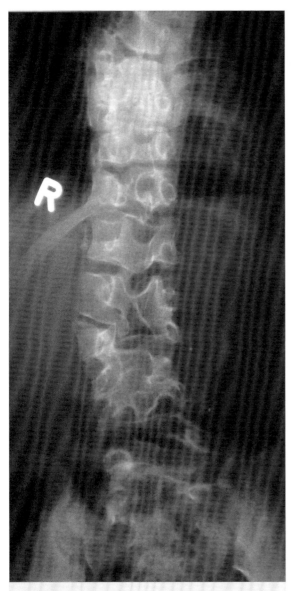

Fig. 3.6 The radiologic phenotype of spondylocostal dysostosis type 5, due to mutated *TBX6*. This shows segmentation abnormalities throughout the vertebral column in an adult. The pattern is similar to that seen in an adult with spondylocostal dysostosis type 1. (Reproduced courtesy of Dr. Zoran Gucev.)

The Genetics of SCD5

The *TBX6*, or T-box6, gene codes for a putative DNA-binding protein that is expressed in somite precursor cells, indicating that it is implicated in the specification of the paraxial mesoderm. Studies in the mouse have shown that the Tbx6 protein is directly bound to the *Mesp2* gene and that it mediates Notch signaling and subsequent *Mesp2* transcription in the presomitic mesoderm. In this one reported family, exome capture and next-generation sequencing were used to identify a stop loss mutation in *TBX6* that segregated with the phenotype in two generations (Sparrow et al 2013), and the mutation was shown by functional studies to have a deleterious effect on the transcriptional activation activity of the TBX6 protein, probably secondary to haploinsufficiency.

3.5 A New Classification and Radiologic Reporting System for Segmentation Defects of the Vertebrae

Currently, the use of nomenclature to describe CS / SDV is very inconsistent and confusing, even though some authors have recognized the existence of different entities and applied a rational distinction in the use of terms.[49,50] This applies to the eponym *Jarcho–Levin* syndrome, which we propose should be discontinued. *Klippel–Feil* anomaly, as a term, is long established and used more specifically in relation to fusion anomalies of the cervical vertebrae (▸ Table 3.7, ▸ Table 3.8). Discontinued use of Klippel–Feil is probably unrealistic despite a wide range of phenotypes. We recommend that the terms *spondylocostal dysostosis* and *spondylothoracic dysostosis* be reserved for specific phenotypes (▸ Table 3.2). Strictly speaking, these conditions are dysostoses, not dysplasias, because they are due to errors of segmentation or formation early in morphogenesis rather than to an ongoing abnormality of chondro-osseous tissues during pre- and postnatal life.

Experience indicates that the widely used terms *Jarcho–Levin syndrome*,[51,52,53,54,55,56] *costovertebral syndrome*,[57,58,59] *spondylocostal dysostosis* (SCD, or SCDO according to OMIM [Online Mendelian Inheritance in Man] nomenclature),[60,61] and *spondylothoracic dysplasia*[62,63,64] are used interchangeably and indiscriminately.[23,65,66] In 1938, Jarcho and Levin reported two siblings with short trunks, M-SDV, and abnormally aligned ribs with points of fusion. Since this initial report, *Jarcho–Levin syndrome* has been applied as an umbrella term covering a wide range of radiologic phenotypes with different patterns of SDV. However, many reports have equated Jarcho–Levin syndrome with the distinctive phenotype of a severely shortened spine and a crablike appearance of the ribs as they fan out from their posterior

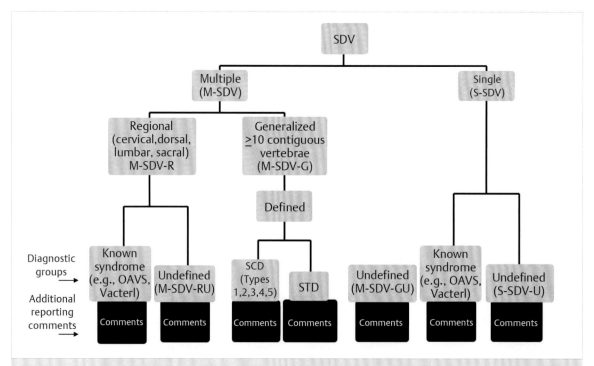

Fig. 3.7 The classification algorithm for segmentation defects of the vertebrae proposed by ICVAS, the International Consortium for Vertebral Anomalies and Scoliosis. It is suggested that each patient can be placed within one of seven basic categories, with provision for further description of the specific findings in any individual. Abbreviations: SCD, spondylocostal dysostosis; SDV, segmentation defects of the vertebrae; STD, spondylothoracic dysostosis; OAVS, oculo-auriculo-vertebral spectrum; Vacterl, vertebral, anal, cardiac, tracheoesophageal, renal, and limb.

origins, for which the preferred term today is *spondylo-thoracic dysostosis*,[40,56] first suggested by Moseley and Bonforte.[62] Berdon et al have clarified the historical record.[67] The incidence of STD is relatively high in Puerto Ricans compared with others because of a founder effect *MESP2* mutation.[68] The ethnicity of the siblings reported by Jarcho and Levin was "colored," the siblings did not manifest the distinctive crablike appearance of the ribs, and their phenotype was closer to that of either SCD2 or SCD4, as described above.[24] A further example illustrating inconsistency is a rare eponymous entity with marked diversity in the few reported cases—namely, Casamassima–Morton–Nance syndrome.[69] This combines SDV with urogenital anomalies and apparently follows autosomal recessive inheritance. However, subsequent reports[70,71] demonstrate a different SDV phenotype from the cases of Casamassima et al,[69] and consistency across all three reports, based on the SDV phenotype, is lacking.

The newly proposed classification and reporting system for SDV conditions is illustrated in ▶ Fig. 3.7 and was developed by a working group of the International Consortium for Vertebral Anomalies and Scoliosis (ICVAS). The goal of ICVAS was to produce a classification system for SDV that provides simple, uniform terminology and can be applied both to human and animal models. The system takes into account that these conditions can be either syndromic or nonsyndromic. The numerous examples of syndromes and associations are outlined in ▶ Table 3.1. Nonsyndromic conditions include most cases of mendelian SCD and STD (as defined in this chapter), in which the malformation is usually restricted to the spine. There are many examples of cases of single or multiple SDV with limited regional involvement and associated kyphoscoliosis, and of cases classified as Klippel–Feil anomaly (without other associations). As a generalization, these conditions are caused by a defective genetic determination of somitogenesis with or without nonintrinsic disruption of normal segmentation and/or formation of vertebrae. In the proposed scheme (▶ Fig. 3.7), conditions essentially fall into one of seven categories. This simplification allows for uniformity between observers. For example, a case with limited thoracic spine involvement that might previously have been diagnosed as Jarcho–Levin syndrome or SCD would now be classified and reported as a case of undefined regional (thoracic) M-SDV. Once any particular case has been placed within one of the seven categories, further detailed descriptions of the position and effects of the segmentation anomalies can be added. Where appropriate, therefore, the ICVAS scheme incorporates existing terminology. This greatly reduces confusion that might be generated by use of the terms *Jarcho–Levin syndrome* and *spondylocostal dysostosis*. We suggest that cases in which at least 10 vertebral segments are affected, but noncontiguously, be designated as a "multiregional" form of M-SDV rather than as G-SDV. This group of phenotypes appears to be diverse, and further delineation will be possible only with advances in our understanding of causation.

The usefulness of correlating a detailed clinical examination with radiologic findings has been well described previously.[2] The system has been tried out[72] and allows a more precise characterization of radiologic phenotypes than does the indiscriminate use of a small number of terms, including eponyms. Furthermore, the system incorporates assessment of the radiographic patterns of the spine as a whole, in addition to the malformations of individual vertebrae. A consistent use of terminology with this system will improve diagnostic consensus and the stratification of patient cohorts for the testing of novel gene candidates and evaluation of the natural history. Adoption of the ICVAS classification system in clinical practice is recommended here, although it is recognized that patient management often depends on additional assessments (e.g., of respiratory function, in cases with restricted lung capacity and/or associated kyphoscoliosis), as well as the monitoring of changes over time. It is also recognized that the system will evolve over time as the identification of new genes brings clarity to the causation of different conditions, and groups of conditions, associated with CS and SDV.

3.6 Acknowledgments

I am indebted to those scientific colleagues in Exeter, United Kingdom, with whom I have had the pleasure of working, particularly Sian Ellard but also Neil Whittock and Beth Young. Our Exeter-based research has been supported by grants from Action Research and the British Scoliosis Research Foundation. I am equally in debt to my colleagues in ICVAS, particularly Olivier Pourquié, Sally Dunwoodie, Kenro Kusumi, Phil Giampietro, Alberto Santiago-Cornier, Amaka Offiah, and Ben Alman. The support of all, in particular the superb molecular and cell biology research of the scientists in this group, has been crucial to the development of this manuscript.

3.7 References

[1] Wynne-Davies R. Infantile idiopathic scoliosis. Causative factors, particularly in the first six months of life. J Bone Joint Surg Br 1975; 57: 138–141

[2] Erol B, Tracy MR, Dormans JP et al. Congenital scoliosis and vertebral malformations: characterization of segmental defects for genetic analysis. J Pediatr Orthop 2004; 24: 674–682

[3] Purkiss SB, Driscoll B, Cole WG, Alman B. Idiopathic scoliosis in families of children with congenital scoliosis. Clin Orthop Relat Res 2002: 27–31

[4] Maisenbacher MK, Han JS, O'brien ML et al. Molecular analysis of congenital scoliosis: a candidate gene approach. Hum Genet 2005; 116: 416–419

[5] William DA, Saitta B, Gibson JD et al. Identification of oscillatory genes in somitogenesis from functional genomic analysis of a human mesenchymal stem cell model. Dev Biol 2007; 305: 172–186

[6] Eckalbar WL, Fisher RE, Rawls A, Kusumi K. Scoliosis and segmentation defects of the vertebrae. Wiley Interdiscip Rev Dev Biol 2012; 1: 401–423

[7] Keynes RJ, Stern CD. Mechanisms of vertebrate segmentation. Development 1988; 103: 413–429

[8] Brent AE, Schweitzer R, Tabin CJ. A somitic compartment of tendon progenitors. Cell 2003; 113: 235–248

[9] Dequéant M-L, Pourquié O. Segmental patterning of the vertebrate embryonic axis. Nat Rev Genet 2008; 9: 370–382

[10] Gibb S, Maroto M, Dale JK. The segmentation clock mechanism moves up a notch. Trends Cell Biol 2010; 20: 593–600

[11] Dubrulle J, McGrew MJ, Pourquié O. FGF signaling controls somite boundary position and regulates segmentation clock control of spatiotemporal Hox gene activation. Cell 2001; 106: 219–232

[12] Krumlauf R. Hox genes in vertebrate development. Cell 1994; 78: 191–201

[13] Zákány J, Kmita M, Alarcon P, de la Pompa JL, Duboule D. Localized and transient transcription of Hox genes suggests a link between patterning and the segmentation clock. Cell 2001; 106: 207–217

[14] Aulehla A, Wehrle C, Brand-Saberi B et al. Wnt3a plays a major role in the segmentation clock controlling somitogenesis. Dev Cell 2003; 4: 395–406

[15] Aulehla A, Herrmann BG. Segmentation in vertebrates: clock and gradient finally joined. Genes Dev 2004; 18: 2060–2067

[16] Hofmann M, Schuster-Gossler K, Watabe-Rudolph M, Aulehla A, Herrmann BG, Gossler A. WNT signaling, in synergy with T/TBX6, controls Notch signaling by regulating Dll1 expression in the presomitic mesoderm of mouse embryos. Genes Dev 2004; 18: 2712–2717

[17] Saga Y. The mechanism of somite formation in mice. Curr Opin Genet Dev 2012; 22: 331–338

[18] Remak R. Untersuchungen über die entwicklung der Wirbeltiere. Berlin, Germany: Reimer;

[19] Bagnall KM, Higgins SJ, Sanders EJ. The contribution made by cells from a single somite to tissues within a body segment and assessment of their integration with similar cells from adjacent segments. Development 1989; 107: 931–943

[20] Ewan KB, Everett AW. Evidence for resegmentation in the formation of the vertebral column using the novel approach of retroviral-mediated gene transfer. Exp Cell Res 1992; 198: 315–320

[21] Goldstein RS, Kalcheim C. Determination of epithelial half-somites in skeletal morphogenesis. Development 1992; 116: 441–445

[22] Mortier GR, Lachman RS, Bocian M, Rimoin DL. Multiple vertebral segmentation defects: analysis of 26 new patients and review of the literature. Am J Med Genet 1996; 61: 310–319

[23] Takikawa K, Haga N, Maruyama T et al. Spine and rib abnormalities and stature in spondylocostal dysostosis. Spine 2006; 31: E192–E197

[24] Jarcho S, Levin PM. Hereditary malformation of the vertebral bodies. Bull Johns Hopkins Hosp 1938; 62: 216–226

[25] McMaster MJ, Singh H. Natural history of congenital kyphosis and kyphoscoliosis. A study of one hundred and twelve patients. J Bone Joint Surg Am 1999; 81: 1367–1383

[26] Aburakawa K, Harada M, Otake S. Clinical evaluations of the treatment of congenital scoliosis. Orthop Surg Trauma 1996; 39: 55–62

[27] Feil A. L'absence et la diminution des vertebres cervicales [thesis]. Paris, France: Libraire Litteraire et Medicale; 1919

[28] Thomsen MN, Schneider U, Weber M, Johannisson R, Niethard FU. Scoliosis and congenital anomalies associated with Klippel-Feil syndrome types I-III. Spine 1997; 22: 396–401

[29] Clarke RA, Catalan G, Diwan AD, Kearsley JH. Heterogeneity in Klippel-Feil syndrome: a new classification. Pediatr Radiol 1998; 28: 967–974

[30] Offiah AC, Hall CM. Radiological diagnosis of the constitutional disorders of bone. As easy as A, B, C? Pediatr Radiol 2003; 33: 153–161

[31] Superti-Furga A, Unger S. Nosology and classification of genetic skeletal disorders: 2006 revision. Am J Med Genet A 2007; 143: 1–18

[32] Bonafé L, Giunta C, Gassner M, Steinmann B, Superti-Furga A. A cluster of autosomal recessive spondylocostal dysostosis caused by three newly identified DLL3 mutations segregating in a small village. Clin Genet 2003; 64: 28–35

[33] Turnpenny PD, Whittock N, Duncan J, Dunwoodie S, Kusumi K, Ellard S. Novel mutations in DLL3, a somitogenesis gene encoding a ligand for the Notch signalling pathway, cause a consistent pattern of abnormal vertebral segmentation in spondylocostal dysostosis. J Med Genet 2003; 40: 333–339

[34] Turnpenny PD, Thwaites RJ, Boulos FN. Evidence for variable gene expression in a large inbred kindred with autosomal recessive spondylocostal dysostosis. J Med Genet 1991; 28: 27–33

[35] Bonaime JL, Bonne B, Joannard A et al. Spondylo-vertebral and spondylo-thoracic dysostosis. Clinical, radiological and genetic study, apropos of 7 observations [in French] Pediatrie 1978; 33: 173–188

[36] Turnpenny PD, Bulman MP, Frayling TM et al. A gene for autosomal recessive spondylocostal dysostosis maps to 19q13.1-q13.3. Am J Hum Genet 1999; 65: 175–182

[37] Kusumi K, Sun ES, Kerrebrock AW et al. The mouse pudgy mutation disrupts Delta homologue Dll3 and initiation of early somite boundaries. Nat Genet 1998; 19: 274–278

[38] Bulman MP, Kusumi K, Frayling TM et al. Mutations in the human delta homologue, DLL3, cause axial skeletal defects in spondylocostal dysostosis. Nat Genet 2000; 24: 438–441

[39] Whittock NV, Sparrow DB, Wouters MA et al. Mutated MESP2 causes spondylocostal dysostosis in humans. Am J Hum Genet 2004; 74: 1249–1254

[40] Cornier AS, Ramírez N, Arroyo S et al. Phenotype characterization and natural history of spondylothoracic dysplasia syndrome: a series of 27 new cases. Am J Med Genet A 2004; 128A: 120–126

[41] Sparrow DB, Chapman G, Wouters MA et al. Mutation of the LUNATIC FRINGE gene in humans causes spondylocostal dysostosis with a severe vertebral phenotype. Am J Hum Genet 2006; 78: 28–37

[42] Haines N, Irvine KD. Glycosylation regulates Notch signalling. Nat Rev Mol Cell Biol 2003; 4: 786–797

[43] Sparrow DB, Guillén-Navarro E, Fatkin D, Dunwoodie SL. Mutation of Hairy-and-Enhancer-of-Split-7 in humans causes spondylocostal dysostosis. Hum Mol Genet 2008; 17: 3761–3766

[44] Sparrow DB, Sillence D, Wouters MA, Turnpenny PD, Dunwoodie SL. Two novel missense mutations in HAIRY-AND-ENHANCER-OF-SPLIT-7 in a family with spondylocostal dysostosis. Eur J Hum Genet 2010; 18: 674–679

[45] Bessho Y, Miyoshi G, Sakata R, Kageyama R. Hes7: a bHLH-type repressor gene regulated by Notch and expressed in the presomitic mesoderm. Genes Cells 2001; 6: 175–185

[46] Bessho Y, Sakata R, Komatsu S, Shiota K, Yamada S, Kageyama R. Dynamic expression and essential functions of Hes7 in somite segmentation. Genes Dev 2001b; 15: 2642–2647

[47] Sparrow DB, McInerney-Leo A, Gucev ZS et al. Autosomal dominant spondylocostal dysostosis is caused by mutation in TBX6. Hum Mol Genet 2013; 22: 1625–1631

[48] Gucev ZS, Tasic V, Pop-Jordanova N et al. Autosomal dominant spondylocostal dysostosis in three generations of a Macedonian family: negative mutation analysis of DLL3, MESP2, HES7, and LFNG. Am J Med Genet A 2010; 152A: 1378–1382

[49] Aymé S, Preus M. Spondylocostal/spondylothoracic dysostosis: the clinical basis for prognosticating and genetic counseling. Am J Med Genet 1986; 24: 599–606

[50] Roberts AP, Conner AN, Tolmie JL, Connor JM. Spondylothoracic and spondylocostal dysostosis. Hereditary forms of spinal deformity. J Bone Joint Surg Br 1988; 70: 123–126

[51] Perez-Comas A, Garcia-Castro JM. Occipito-facial-cervicothoracic-abdomino-digital dysplasia: Jarcho Levin syndrome of vertebral anomalies. Report of six cases and review of the literature. J Pediatr 1974; 85: 388–391

[52] Karnes PS, Day D, Berry SA, Pierpont ME. Jarcho-Levin syndrome: four new cases and classification of subtypes. Am J Med Genet 1991; 40: 264–270

[53] Martínez-Frías ML, Urioste M. Segmentation anomalies of the vertebras and ribs: a developmental field defect: epidemiologic evidence. Am J Med Genet 1994; 49: 36–44

[54] Rastogi D, Rosenzweig EB, Koumbourlis A. Pulmonary hypertension in Jarcho-Levin syndrome. Am J Med Genet 2002; 107: 250–252

[55] Bannykh SI, Emery SC, Gerber J-K, Jones KL, Benirschke K, Masliah E. Aberrant Pax1 and Pax9 expression in Jarcho-Levin syndrome: report of two Caucasian siblings and literature review. Am J Med Genet A 2003; 120A: 241–246

[56] Cornier AS, Ramirez N, Carlo S, Reiss A. Controversies surrounding Jarcho-Levin syndrome. Curr Opin Pediatr 2003; 15: 614–620

[57] Cantú JM, Urrusti J, Rosales G, Rojas A. Evidence for autosomal recessive inheritance of costovertebral dysplasia. Clin Genet 1971; 2: 149–154

[58] Bartsocas CS, Kiossoglou KA, Papas CV, Xanthou-Tsingoglou M, Anagnostakis DE, Daskalopoulou HD. Costovertebral dysplasia. Birth Defects Orig Artic Ser 1974; 10: 221–226

[59] David TJ, Glass A. Hereditary costovertebral dysplasia with malignant cerebral tumour. J Med Genet 1983; 20: 441–444

[60] Rimoin DL, Fletcher BD, McKusick VA. Spondylocostal dysplasia. A dominantly inherited form of short-trunked dwarfism. Am J Med 1968; 45: 948–953

[61] Silengo MC, Cavallaro S, Franceschini P. Recessive spondylocostal dysostosis: two new cases. Clin Genet 1978; 13: 289–294

[62] Moseley JE, Bonforte RJ. Spondylothoracic dysplasia—a syndrome of congenital anomalies. Am J Roentgenol Radium Ther Nucl Med 1969; 106: 166–169

[63] Pochaczevsky R, Ratner H, Perles D, Kassner G, Naysan P. Spondylothoracic dysplasia. Radiology 1971; 98: 53–58

[64] Solomon L, Jimenez RB, Reiner L. Spondylothoracic dysostosis: report of two cases and review of the literature. Arch Pathol Lab Med 1978; 102: 201–205

[65] Kozlowski K. Spondylo-costal dysplasia. A further report—review of 14 cases. Rofo 1984; 140: 204–209

[66] Ohashi H, Sugio Y, Kajii T. Spondylocostal dysostosis: report of three patients. Jinrui Idengaku Zasshi 1987; 32: 299–303

[67] Berdon WE, Lampl BS, Cornier AS et al. Clinical and radiological distinction between spondylothoracic dysostosis (Lavy-Moseley syndrome) and spondylocostal dysostosis (Jarcho-Levin syndrome). Pediatr Radiol 2011; 41: 384–388

[68] Cornier AS, Staehling-Hampton K, Delventhal KM et al. Mutations in the MESP2 gene cause spondylothoracic dysostosis/Jarcho-Levin syndrome. Am J Hum Genet 2008; 82: 1334–1341

[69] Casamassima AC, Morton CC, Nance WE et al. Spondylocostal dysostosis associated with anal and urogenital anomalies in a Mennonite sibship. Am J Med Genet 1981; 8: 117–127

[70] Daïkha-Dahmane F, Huten Y, Morvan J, Szpiro-Tapia S, Nessmann C, Eydoux P. Fetus with Casamassima-Morton-Nance syndrome and an inherited (6;9) balanced translocation. Am J Med Genet 1998; 80: 514–517

[71] Poor MA, Alberti O Jr Griscom NT, Driscoll SG, Holmes LB. Nonskeletal malformations in one of three siblings with Jarcho-Levin syndrome of vertebral anomalies. J Pediatr 1983; 103: 270–272

[72] Offiah A, Alman B, Cornier AS et al. ICVAS (International Consortium for Vertebral Anomalies and Scoliosis). Pilot assessment of a radiologic classification system for segmentation defects of the vertebrae. Am J Med Genet A 2010; 152A: 1357–1371

[73] McGaughran JM, Oates A, Donnai D, Read AP, Tassabehji M. Mutations in PAX1 may be associated with Klippel-Feil syndrome. Eur J Hum Genet 2003; 11: 468–474

[74] Philibert P, Biason-Lauber A, Rouzier R et al. Identification and functional analysis of a new WNT4 gene mutation among 28 adolescent girls with primary amenorrhea and müllerian duct abnormalities: a French collaborative study. J Clin Endocrinol Metab 2008; 93: 895–900

4 Respiratory Implications of Abnormal Development of the Spine

Robert M. Campbell, Jr.

Abnormal development of the spine can cause significant scoliosis, kyphosis, or lordosis, resulting in body deformities that can be distressing to patients and their families. The more serious threat to long-term health is the adverse effect of abnormal development of the spine on pulmonary function. This is well documented for curves exceeding 90 degrees, which cause severe restrictive lung disease, but not well understood for lesser curves; knowledge regarding their long-term effect on pulmonary health, whether they are treated or untreated, is almost completely lacking. Pulmonary function is an important determinant of long-term survival. Increased rates of mortality, mostly resulting from pulmonary failure, have been seen in patients with untreated infantile scoliosis beginning at the age of 20 years, with a rise in mortality rates to fourfold above normal by the age of 60 years.[1] The purpose of this chapter is to outline the biomechanical principles of respiration, which are related to the spine and its normal development; to discuss and critique the available metrics for the clinical and imaging assessment of pulmonary function and spine deformity; and to summarize the known effects of abnormal development of the spine on respiratory biomechanics and function.

4.1 Normal Pulmonary and Thoracic Function

The normal spine is the posterior pillar of support for the thorax, which is the anatomical combination of the rib cage and the thoracic spine, with the diaphragm as its base. The thorax provides structural protection for the vital organs of the chest, including the heart, lungs, and great vessels, and the rib cage provides stabilization for the thoracic spine. However, the most important role of the thorax is its role as the *engine of respiration*, in which it generates a rhythmic expansion of both lungs during breathing through the downward contraction of the diaphragm and posterior lateral expansion of the rib cage by intercostal muscle action.

The volume and flow rate of the air moved during the respiratory cycle by the efforts of the thoracic respiratory engine are easily measured in a cooperative individual through spirometry, and pulmonologists collectively term the multiple values obtained by complex analysis of these two variables *pulmonary function*. One could argue that this term is a misnomer because the act of respiration is totally dependent on the biomechanical expansion of the thorax during inspiration and expiration. So, one is actually measuring for the most part *thoracic function* with spirometry, but it is doubtful that this long-standing misconception will ever be changed.

Pulmonary function testing produces dozens of test values, but the result that most orthopedists focus on is the forced vital capacity (FVC), expressed both as a raw score, liters of air exhaled with maximum effort after deep inspiration, and as FVC percent predicted, a percentage value derived by comparison with normal values of FVC as a function of height. The latter value is usually most emphasized in the surgical literature, and most surgeons assume the FVC percent predicted "score" reflects comprehensive pulmonary function, with an FVC percent predicted of 100% graded as normal. Statistical increases in FVC percent predicted after surgery are usually interpreted as indicators of success. Unfortunately, pulmonary function testing is complex and inherently subject to variability, and it should be used as a metric, especially in children, with caution.

The standards for pulmonary function testing results and the methodology of testing are governed by the American Thoracic Society, and a normal FVC percent predicted can vary from 80% to 100% predicted. This variability is mostly due to testing methodology and the ability of the patient to cooperate consistently with performing the maximum inhale / maximum exhale spirometry maneuver needed to produce the flow / volume curve for FVC. Mild to moderate restrictive lung disease has values varying from 80% to 50% predicted, and restrictive lung disease is considered severe when the FVC is less than 50% predicted. Testing methodology requires three FVC maneuvers, with the average of these used for the final result. Patient cooperation and motivation are critical for the successful reproduction of these FVC maneuvers. Routine spirometry is not recommended for patients younger than 6 years of age because of the inability of young children to cooperate with the maximum inhale / maximum exhale maneuver. These younger children, however, can be assessed with passive approaches, such as infant pulmonary function testing, although such techniques require special equipment and are generally not available at most institutions. For those patients older than 6 years of age, motivation may become an issue for accuracy of the test, with highly motivated children using hyperkinetic "trick maneuvers" to maximize their results, while those with less motivation may have low scores as a result of their half-hearted efforts. With children, the respiratory therapist who is a charismatic coach tends to get the best efforts from patients, whereas others may be unable to coax maximum cooperation from children. Awareness of this inherent variability of the results of pulmonary function testing in children should provide a basis for caution in the interpretation of pulmonary function test differences that may be statistically valid but in fact may be influenced by the "cooperation factor."

Conceptually, the FVC is a measure of the "emergency reserves" an individual can bring to bear when maximum respiration needed, such as in running a race or surviving an episode of acute pneumonia. In the act of maximum respiration, both the primary and accessory muscles of respiration are fully engaged in taking the deepest breath possible followed by maximum expiration, raising the respiratory rate to the highest sustainable level. In contrast, regular quiet breathing is an almost effortless act, very energy efficient, usually not even noticeable to the individual. The volume of air exhaled during normal, quiet breathing is termed *tidal volume*. Restrictive lung disease is present when the FVC is significantly decreased, with almost all authors agreeing that an increased risk of mortality from multiple causes long term is associated with restrictive lung disease, but the issue is not quite entirely clear. Numerous adult survivors of Jarcho–Levin syndrome, despite extremely severe restrictive lung disease in childhood, have been reported,[2] and is unclear what protective mechanism lets them survive with such a low vital capacity.

Physiologically, maximum respiration requires a lot of energy, and alveoli in the superior areas of the lung are recruited, increasing blood flow to the capillary beds, in order to provide maximum oxygenation. Excursion of the regular muscles of respiration is augmented by recruitment of the accessory muscles, including the scalene muscles and sternocleidomastoid muscles. In the FVC maneuver in adults, the diaphragm produces 80% of the total volume exhaled and the rib cage expansion provides the remaining 20%; the diaphragm / rib cage FVC ratio for children is unknown. Maximum respiration depends on maximum expansion and compression of the appropriate thoracic volume for the underlying lungs, appropriate for age. The diaphragm attaches posteriorly just inferior to T12, and the posterior aspect of the diaphragm provides most of the excursion distally to expand the lungs during inspiration. The additional expansion of the lungs provided by the rib cage is an extremely complicated and poorly understood process. It is generally accepted that the most proximal ribs are relatively fixed in position, but the ribs distal to them in the middle of the chest rotate outward anteriorly through the costovertebral joints; this motion is mediated by the contraction of the intercostal muscles. The more distal ribs rotate outward anterior laterally. This rotatory motion is made possible by the flexibility of the chondral ribs centrally. The average man by the age of 60 years has lost 700 mL of vital capacity as a consequence of normal aging,[3] most likely as the result of loss of muscle tone and stiffening of the chondral cartilages from calcification.

In summary, normal respiration depends on a complex sequence of biomechanical events in the thorax; these range from the low energy demands of quiet breathing, producing tidal volume, up to the maximum capacity efforts associated with maximum breathing, producing FVC. Optimal thoracic volume and normal alignment of the ribs, coupled with normal excursion of the costovertebral joints and contraction of the diaphragm, produce respiration that is clinically normal. However, any pathologic process, such as abnormal development of the spine, can introduce complex deformity that degrades the biomechanical efficiency of the thoracic engine of respiration and produces significant restrictive lung disease.

4.2 Assessing the Effects of Abnormal Spinal Development on Respiration

4.2.1 Clinical Presentation

In the child with early onset scoliosis, the first step is to determine the time of onset of the deformity and also define the baseline respiratory status. Can the child keep up with the activities of his or her peer group? Does the child participate in all activities at recess, or are sedentary activities preferred? Does the child participate in active sports? On shopping trips, is the child able to walk unlimited distances without fatigue or breathlessness? It is also important to determine the frequency and type of respiratory illnesses that the child is experiencing, including upper respiratory infections, episodes of respiratory syncytial virus (RSV) bronchiolitis, and frank bacterial or viral pneumonia, and also to note if hospitalization was necessary and whether respiratory support such as oxygen or even intubation was needed. The pattern of frequency of illness should be noted, with increasing bouts of respiratory illness a negative factor. Any need for chronic dependency on respiratory aids, such as continuous positive airway pressure (CPAP), bi-level positive airway pressure (BiPAP), nasal oxygen, or ventilator dependency, should be noted, along with a time line of use. The goal of the respiratory history in children with early onset scoliosis is to establish either that there are no clinical sequelae of the spinal deformity or that there are early signs of respiratory dysfunction, and efforts should be made to establish whether there is progression of the respiratory dysfunction.

4.2.2 Physical Examination of the Patient with Early Onset Scoliosis

The child is evaluated for deformity. The examiner notes the apex of the curve, curve flexibility, unequal shoulder heights, and truncal shift, as well as head balance over the pelvis. In addition, the respiratory status needs to be determined. Check for clubbing of the digits, flaring of the nostrils with breathing, and cyanosis of the lips and nail beds. The resting respiratory rate should be recorded because this reflects the ability of the thoracic engine of respiration to oxygenate the body. Elevation of the respiratory rate above normal means that thoracic function is inadequate to maintain oxygenation with normal rates of respiration, so the mechanism has to be put into "overdrive" with a higher respiratory rate per minute. This raises caloric expenditure, making weight gain more difficult for the growing child, and very rapid rates of respiration interfere with the acts of eating and speaking. A normal respiratory rate is 30 to 80 per minute for a newborn, 20 to 40 per minute for ages 2 to 5 years, and 15 to 25 per minute after the age of 6 years.[4] A brief "challenge test" is helpful in borderline cases. The child is asked to run back and forth a short distance in the halls of the clinic, and the normal child usually does this with ease, but the child on the edge of clinical respiratory insufficiency will become uncomfortable after a short while, complain about breathing hard, and stop running.

4.2.3 Physical Examination of the Patient with Thoracic Insufficiency Syndrome in Early Onset Scoliosis

It is important to determine whether the child with early onset scoliosis has thoracic insufficiency syndrome.[4] This is defined as an inability of the thorax to support normal respiration or lung growth. Significant, progressive thoracic insufficiency syndrome can lead to early mortality from restrictive lung disease. Respiration is abnormal when on physical examination anomalies of the thorax are seen during respiration, such as areas of paradoxical respiration (the chest wall segment collapses inward during inspiration) or an absence of chest wall motion over areas of fused ribs associated with congenital anomalies of the spine. There should also be a general evaluation of the symmetry and size of the thorax. The chest circumference can be measured at the nipple line and compared with normative values to derive a percent predicted value. Low values suggest hypoplastic thorax and probable restrictive lung disease due to reduced volume of the lungs. One important test during the physical examination of these children is an assessment for the marionette sign (▶ Fig. 4.1), in which the patient's head bobs with respiration. When the base of the thorax is too close to the pelvis, in conditions such as lumbar gibbus in patients with myelomeningocele, diaphragm excursion is blocked distally by the abdominal organs, increasing the work of breathing and limiting lung expansion by the diaphragm. This is termed *secondary thoracic insufficiency syndrome.* The same phenomenon is seen unilaterally in pelvic obliquity in neuromuscular scoliosis. As the patient inhales, the diaphragm contracts and encounters resistance from the abdominal organs, which are pushed proximally by the spine deformity, so the diaphragm, in

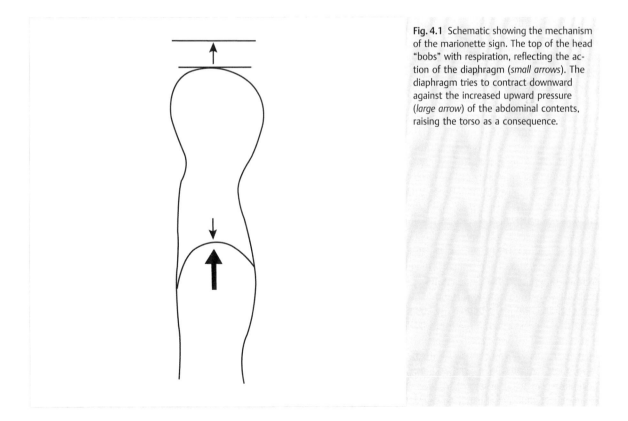

Fig. 4.1 Schematic showing the mechanism of the marionette sign. The top of the head "bobs" with respiration, reflecting the action of the diaphragm (*small arrows*). The diaphragm tries to contract downward against the increased upward pressure (*large arrow*) of the abdominal contents, raising the torso as a consequence.

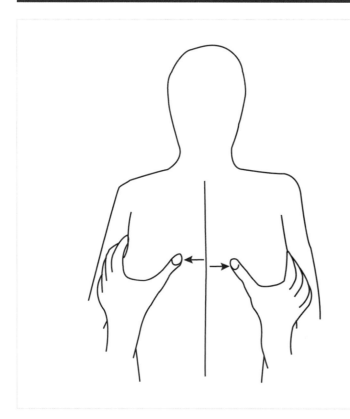

Fig. 4.2 The "thumb excursion" test. The hands are placed lightly on the surface of the thorax with the thumbs equidistant from the spine, and the patient is instructed to take a deep breath. The thumbs move outward with rib cage expansion during inspiration.

essence, is doing a push-up against the body weight, raising the torso a few centimeters and straining to expand the lungs. This is not sustainable, and any condition that further increases the abdominal volume in these children, such as constipation, can tip them over the edge with the development of respiratory failure.

Both the rib cage expansion and diaphragmatic excursion of thoracic function can be assessed clinically to some degree. Rotation of the thoracic spine commonly results in a rib hump on the convex side in early onset scoliosis, and rib cage expansion is commonly hampered in this situation. This can be assessed with the "thumb excursion" test (▶ Fig. 4.2). The examiner places his or her hands at the base of the thorax with the thumbs extended medially to be equidistant from the spine; the hands are held lightly on the surface of the chest, with the metacarpal phalangeal joints of the hands in the midaxillary line. The child is instructed to take a deep breath, and there should be symmetric motion of the thumbs greater than 1 cm away from the midline of the spine resulting from the outward motion of hemithorax expansion. This is graded + 3. If hemithorax motion is limited by deformity, the movement of the chest outward with inspiration is limited, and if the distance is only 0.5 to 1 cm, the grade is + 2. With further stiffness of the chest wall, the distance the thumb moves with respiration may be slight, less than 0.5 cm. Complete absence of motion is graded as + 0. In segments of the chest that are affected by fused ribs in congenital

scoliosis, and on the side of the rib hump in infantile scoliosis, the thumb excursion test grade is usually + 0. Absent careful evaluation, these children may be assumed to have "normal respiration," but the presence of such abnormalities on physical examination clearly defines their respiration as abnormal. They may have normal activity levels, but commonly the respiratory rate is elevated at rest. This can be described as occult respiratory insufficiency, in which the respiratory mechanism compensates by increasing the rate of breathing, with more energy expended to maintain normal body oxygenation.

Once the physical examination points out specific deformities of the spine and rib cage in early onset scoliosis, imaging techniques are the next step in further defining the abnormalities.

4.2.4 Radiographic Evaluation of the Patient with Early Onset Scoliosis for Respiratory Implications

To define deformities of abnormal spinal development that have respiratory implications, the first step is always to obtain weight-bearing anteroposterior (AP) and lateral radiographs of the entire spine. It must be emphasized that it is important to include a full view of the chest and pelvis on both radiographs to help understand the thoracic deformity. The Cobb angle is the long-standing gold standard for measuring the severity of scoliosis, but other forms of thoracic asymmetry, as well as transverse plane abnormalities, also impact respiratory function. A combination of both radiographs and computed tomographic (CT) scans can usually fully visualize the specific abnormalities of the abnormal spine and rib cage. These abnormalities can negatively affect thoracic size, shape, and function and disable the engine of respiration through numerous pathologic mechanisms. The respiratory determinants of spinal development include the following:

- Spinal height;
- Spinal rotation;
- Coronal curve;
- Sagittal curve;
- Thoracic volume;
- Thoracic symmetry;
- Thoracic function.

Although the primary emphasis in an assessment of scoliosis is on measurement of the Cobb angle, the *thoracic spinal height* is equally important and can be assessed by the radiographic height of the thoracic spine, which may be shortened by angular deformity in scoliosis and also by congenital anomalies in congenital scoliosis. The radiographic height can be compared with the values for thoracic spinal height based on chronologic age in tables published by Dimeglio et al,[5] and a value for the thoracic height as a percentage of normal thoracic spinal height can be derived. The thoracic spine grows from birth to 5 years of age at a rate of 1.4 cm per year, from ages 5 to 10 years at 0.6 cm per year, and from ages 10 to 15 years at 1.2 cm per year.[5] This measurement at presentation provides a baseline value indicating the degree of inhibition of growth of the height of the thorax. Subsequent follow-up radiographs similarly analyzed can help one determine if the patient is catching up with normal growth or falling further behind in regard to growth of the height of the thorax. The height of the normal thorax at skeletal maturity is 26.5 cm for females and 28 cm for males. A shortened thorax at skeletal maturity is associated with a high risk of severe restrictive lung disease, reflecting a probable loss of thoracic volume for the underlying lungs due to shortening from vertebral anomaly or early posterior spine fusion.[6]

The degree of *spinal rotation* can be estimated on the AP radiograph but is best viewed on CT transverse sections. These often will show a windswept deformity of the thorax resulting from rotation of the spine into the convexity of the curve, diminishing the volume of the convex lung and distorting the ribs on both sides. Such deformity likely diminishes the ability of the rib cage to expand during respiration on the convex side early and its ability to expand on the concave side late. Lordosis further diminishes the volume of the thorax by reducing the

AP diameter of the chest, and this can be assessed by the posterior penetration index of Dubousset et al.[7]

The *coronal curve* of scoliosis is best assessed on the weight-bearing AP radiograph. It is also important to assess for pelvic obliquity and the relative proximity of the iliac crest to the hemidiaphragm to see if the child is at risk for secondary thoracic insufficiency syndrome. In addition to spinal deformity, thoracic asymmetry can be determined on this radiograph. The concave hemithorax in early onset scoliosis can be assessed by the ratio of the radiographic height of the concave lung to the height of the convex lung as measured from the middle of the first rib down to the midportion of the hemidiaphragm. This is termed *space available for lung* (SAL) and correlates well with vital capacity, much more so than the Cobb angle. Except in very severe scoliosis, the Cobb angle does not correlate well with pulmonary function values.

On the AP radiograph, complex thoracic deformities can be classified into three categories of what are termed *volume depletion deformities of the thorax* (VDDs; ▸ Fig. 4.3). Type I VDD is scoliosis with a chest wall defect on the concave side, clinically resulting in a flail chest. This can be seen in conditions such as spondylocostal dysostosis. Type II VDD is scoliosis with fused ribs on the concavity, a deformity that usually restricts the growth of the concave lung; this can be seen in VATER (*v*ertebral, *a*nal, *t*racheo-*e*sophageal, *r*enal) syndrome. In early onset scoliosis, the ribs may not be fused but are closely apposed on the concave side, which can result in a type II VDD deformity.[8] Type III VDD is a global reduction in the thorax, with type IIIA having a decrease in the height of the thorax, such as is seen in Jarcho–Levin syndrome, and type IIIB having a narrowing of the thorax, such as is seen in Jeune asphyxiating thoracic dystrophy. In both variants of type III VDD, there is severe restrictive lung disease resulting from the loss of thoracic volume and a very high mortality rate with natural history.

Kyphosis is defined on the lateral radiograph. In severe kyphosis, the upper spine "falls forward" into the chest, reducing its height, with the increased AP diameter only partially compensating for the volume loss. Excessive lordosis seen on the lateral radiograph decreases the AP distance of the thorax and so decreases lung volume. Abnormal proximity of the diaphragm to the pelvis in secondary thoracic insufficiency syndrome is also best seen on a weight-bearing lateral radiograph.

Rib cage volume and symmetry are best seen on unenhanced CT scans obtained at 0.5-cm intervals. Lung volumes in children too young for pulmonary function studies can be calculated from CT scans of the thorax obtained during spontaneous breathing with approximately a 10% error rate. CT scans obtained during directed inspiration are more accurate but technically more complex to perform. The results of either study can be compared with normative values[9] to gain insight

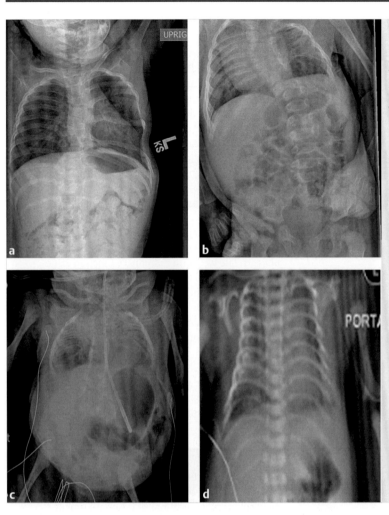

Fig. 4.3 (a) Type I volume depletion deformity (VDD) of the thorax. Rib absence and congenital scoliosis. (b) Type II VDD of the thorax. Fused ribs and congenital scoliosis. (c) Type IIIA VDD of the thorax. Spondylothoracic dysplasia. (d) Type IIIB VDD of the thorax. Jeune syndrome.

into the size of lungs affected by deformity of the thorax, but in very young normal children, the percentile spread of lung volumes as a function of age is extremely small, and only very severe hypoplasia of the lungs can be appreciated.

Thoracic function in respiration can be estimated based on the results of the physical examination—in particular, the thumb excursion test and the marionette sign—but it is impossible to assess the function of the thorax directly based solely on radiographs or CT scans. One reason why the concept of thoracic insufficiency syndrome in early onset scoliosis is unpopular with surgeons is that it is not easily measured on the AP radiograph, in contrast to the Cobb angle for the assessment of scoliosis. At the present time, thoracic function is estimated by a careful clinical history and physical examination, with indirect evidence of dysfunction based on static radiographs and CT scans. For example, a child with VATER syndrome may have a stiff, shortened hemithorax from fused ribs based on examination and AP radiographs, and diminished transverse volume for the lungs based on rotation of the spine into the convexity; however, there is no readily available technology to define the specific segmental deficits in thoracic function. Pulmonary function testing in children age 6 years or older can define changes in the flow and volume of air through the trachea during respiration maneuvers, approximating total thoracic function, but the results are a summation of segmental defects in thoracic function and cannot pinpoint specific biomechanical deficits.

One new approach to this problem, however, is *dynamic lung magnetic resonance imaging* (dMRI), which can allow a specific study of the thoracic performance of each hemithorax (▶ Fig. 4.4), including the change in volume during respiration due to the rib cage as well as the contribution of the change in volume due to diaphragmatic excursion. dMRI can also be used to study obstruction of the diaphragm in secondary thoracic insufficiency syndrome. Campbell et al[10] have presented data to suggest that this syndrome is fairly common in complex early onset scoliosis, and the method has great potential to become a new metric for the dynamic assessment of thoracic function in children with abnormal development of the spine and rib cage.

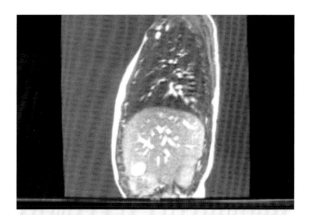

Fig. 4.4 Sagittal section of a dynamic magnetic resonance imaging lung study.

4.3 Treatment Pathways for Abnormal Development of the Spine Based on Respiratory Implications

Multiple pathways now exist for the treatment of early onset scoliosis, but the goals of treatment vary widely. Historically, the treatment of an abnormally developing spine centered strictly on effective correction of the deformity, with only minor attention paid to the issues of growth and respiratory outcomes. Over the past 50 years, marked advances have been made in the design of surgical instrumentation for scoliosis, enhancing the strength of rods and their fixation to the spine, so that greater correction of the Cobb angle is possible; however, little work has been done to advance our understanding of the true health effects of correcting spinal deformity. Indications for treatment are still based solely on the size of the Cobb angle: 10 to 20 degrees, observe; 20 to 40 degrees, brace in the growing child; and for progressive curves that are greater, growing rods or spine fusion in children aged 10 years or older. None of these Cobb angle indications are evidence-based with regard to either the long-term outcomes of deformity correction or their respiratory implications. The biomechanical dysfunction that can explain the anatomical basis for restrictive lung disease in these patients has not been clearly defined. Radiographic correction of the Cobb angle probably improves the health of the patient with scoliosis; however, without a clear understanding of the dynamic respiratory nature of the thorax, including its decline with progressive spinal deformity or improvement with treatment, it is difficult to establish valid indications and effective timing for intervention. Some clear concepts have recently emerged that can aid the surgeon in recognizing the respiratory consequences of the treatment of spinal deformity and its timing.

4.3.1 Effect of Early Spine Fusion on Abnormal Development of the Spine with Its Respiratory Implications

In the past, spine fusion was the most popular treatment for spine deformity, regardless of the patient's age. Over the past 10 years, however, reports have been published challenging the long-held view that early spine fusion is the optimal treatment approach for spine deformity in early onset scoliosis. Goldberg et al in 2003 noted that children with infantile scoliosis who underwent early spine fusion had a low vital capacity at follow-up.[11] Emans et al found a similar effect in patients who had four or more thoracic spinal vertebrae fused before the age of 5 years,[12] and Karol et al, who in 2008[6] reported on 28 patients who underwent fusion early in life, found a strong correlation between restrictive lung disease and height of the thoracic spine at skeletal maturity. Patients with a thoracic spinal height of less than 18 cm at skeletal maturity had a 63% incidence of severe restrictive lung disease (FVC < 50% predicted), and those with a thoracic spinal height of 18 to 22 cm had an incidence of 25%. Patients with a thoracic spinal height of 22 cm to normal had no severe restrictive lung disease. These findings suggest that the thoracic volume (and indirectly the lung volume) are influenced by the final thoracic spinal height at maturity, and when this is diminished, either by early surgery or by congenital deformity, severe restrictive lung disease is a distinct risk. The practice of using spine fusion as the primary treatment for spine deformity in the very young child has diminished considerably over the past 10 years, likely because of the new awareness of the respiratory implications of fusion treatment.

4.3.2 The Timing of Treatment with Growth-Sparing Techniques

Initiating treatment for scoliosis in a young child is always difficult for both the family and the surgeon. The long-term duration of treatment, either by bracing, casting, or growth-sparing instrumentation, tends to make treatment a challenge for most families. Radiographic observation of their spinal deformities is likely to be prolonged for these children because of such issues, but once progression is clearly recognized, then treatment must begin.

Conservative care with either bracing or casting should be considered first for every patient with early onset scoliosis. Bracing is clearly a challenge in infantile scoliosis because of the small size of the patient, but an experienced brace maker can fit such patients, and although it is seldom considered definitive treatment, this pathway can "buy time" by slowing down curve progression. The popularity of casting for scoliosis has increased recently, and its advocates believe that even fairly severe curves can be addressed by this approach. There are considerable data regarding curve correction with conservative care in early onset scoliosis, but a paucity of data regarding respiratory outcome. Anecdotally, narrowing of the thorax has been associated with bracing in some patients, but to our knowledge, no study has been published about the long-term effects of brace or cast pressure on pulmonary function. Mild to moderate curves with some flexibility are the best ones to treat conservatively, but very rigid curves, especially those associated with chest wall anomalies, such as fused ribs or absent ribs, may be better treated by growth-sparing surgery that can address the thoracic deformity. Once progression of a deformity has been demonstrated despite conservative care, then surgery should be considered, but even this concept has become controversial, with some emphasizing delaying surgery at all costs because of the high rate of surgical complications, whereas others emphasize the importance of early surgery to the maximize respiratory outcome.

The Delayed Surgery for Early Onset Scoliosis Group

This group argues that because patients undergoing growing rod and vertical expandable prosthetic titanium rib (VEPTR) growth-sparing surgery for early onset scoliosis require repetitive surgeries and have relatively high surgical complication rates, including wound infection, dislodgment, migration, and breakage, the initiation of these techniques should be delayed as much as possible to shorten the time line of surgical intervention and risk of complications. Furthermore, regarding the use of growing rods, these authors argue that treatment becomes ineffective with the passage of time because it becomes more difficult to expand the rods during lengthening procedures; they use the phrase "law of diminishing returns" to popularize their belief.[13] It must be mentioned that the resistance to growing rod lengthening can be explained biomechanically; the straightened spine is better able to resist the rods trying to stretch it. Furthermore, clinically, these patients have exhibited excellent curve correction and spinal growth, so it is difficult to understand what the authors mean by "diminished returns." It is also not clear what alternative to surgery the authors offer, especially if conservative measures fail. They have not discussed the respiratory implications of delayed surgery.

The Early Surgery for Early Onset Scoliosis Group

This group recommends early surgical intervention, in patients as young as 6 months of age, for spinal and chest wall deformities causing thoracic insufficiency syndrome because of the significant respiratory implications of thoracic inhibition of lung growth by deformity. Lung growth and thoracic growth are interdependent. It is obvious that a thorax too small for normal lung growth will result in extrinsic restrictive lung growth, with the development of restrictive lung disease later in life. Lung growth by alveolar cell multiplication is considered to be maximal during the first 2 years of life and is felt by many to peak by the age of 8 years in normal children. This view has been recently challenged by lung MRI studies,[14] which suggest that lung growth continues throughout young adulthood; however, this new viewpoint will need further verification. At birth, the volume of the thorax is 6.7% of its volume in adulthood; by age 5 it is 30%, and by age 10 it is 50%. Any abnormality of the spine or rib cage has the potential to distort or reduce thoracic volume and function, resulting in less than optimal growth of the underlying lungs. VEPTR treatment of fused ribs and scoliosis resulted in a better postoperative vital capacity of patients undergoing surgery while younger than 2 years of age, when lung growth is rapid, compared with those well past the age of 2 years.[15]

4.4 Conclusion

It must be emphasized that the respiratory consequences of abnormal spinal development are due to complex reasons, and reducing the situation to a simple correction of angular measurement on the AP radiograph neglects the basic premise of treating disease: to have the course of the treated patient be clearly superior to that of the untreated patient. Although mortality is a clear outcome measure for surgical treatment, it is more important to appreciate quality-of-life issues for these children and, it is hoped, maintain a quality of life that will allow them to survive into adulthood. Numerous quality-of-life instruments are used in adults, but the inherent disadvantage of this approach in children is that their parents are filling out the questionnaires and guessing about their children's feelings about life.

The only practical way to evaluate and treat the spinal deformities of young children comprehensively is through a *principle-based* approach, in contrast to a *rules-based* approach. The latter is a reasonable pathway when the patient population is relatively homogeneous, the clinical problem is straightforward and well understood, and the diseases are easily addressed with standardized approaches, but early onset scoliosis is a different animal. Children with spinal deformities are rare, and although pediatric populations with similar degrees of scoliosis are reported, the underlying diseases causing the scoliosis are often widely divergent, making valid comparisons difficult because of the heterogeneity of the subjects. In a principle-based approach to spinal deformity in children, the focus is on the simple.

For example, consider an 18-month-old girl with VATER syndrome. She has a 55-degree congenital curve that is progressive. What principles need to be considered? The first is the baseline position for growth and what treatment would influence growth, as well as the baseline for respiratory implications. History reveals that the child has had several episodes of pneumonia, requiring oxygen support and hospitalization. She also is not keeping up well with her peer group at day care, sitting down frequently and resting. This suggests that her pulmonary reserves are not clinically optimal. Although the child appears pink and well oxygenated, her resting respiratory rate is 60 breaths per minute, well above normal for her age. Her pulmonary function is adequate only with excessive cycles of respiration per minute, and this is not sustainable. The next step is to investigate the possible causes of the thoracic insufficiency syndrome contributing to this clinical picture. Physical examination shows marked stiffness of the left side of the chest during respiration, with shortness of the chest. Radiographs show fused ribs on the left, reducing the ability of the rib cage to expand the left lung. The height of the thoracic spine is only 8 cm, well below the average height of 13 cm in newborns. So not only is the left lung compromised in respiration; both lung volumes are probably reduced by the decreased height of the thorax. CT shows the spine rotated into the convex hemithorax, with probable loss of volume of the right lung. The CT lung volumes are very low when compared with normative data. Physical examination also shows moderate pelvic obliquity due to the congenital curve. Although a marionette sign is absent on physical examination, lung dMRI reveals that the iliac crest is intruding into the upper abdomen and obstructing the hemidiaphragm.

Based on a principle-based approach, we can infer that there is a significant deficit in the volume and expandability of the thorax, affecting the mechanism of respiration and likely the long-term ability of the thorax to grow. This is thoracic insufficiency syndrome. VEPTR expansion thoracoplasty can lengthen the constricted hemithorax and the thoracic reconstruction can be stabilized by a rib-to-rib VEPTR, while the iliac crest obstructing the hemidiaphragm can be moved out of harm's way by a hybrid VEPTR from the proximal ribs to an S-hook on the iliac crest. The principal assumption is that the hemidiaphragm, relieved of obstruction, will improve in performance and "pump" the lung above it, which, it is hoped, will grow because of the expanded volume made available to it by the thoracoplasty. The expanded, fused chest wall certainly cannot move with respiration after surgery—that is impossible—but it is hoped that the diaphragm can take up the slack. With constant distraction by the VEPTRs, it is possible that the thoracic spine will increase in height with growth, further contributing to the volume of both lungs.

Although surgical complications in this patient are possible in the long term, this principle-based approach also provides distinct long-term benefits. The goal is to have the largest, most symmetric, most functional thorax possible by skeletal maturity, and if this is achieved, it is likely that the patient will experience a better quality of life from a respiratory viewpoint and a better survival rate than are likely with the natural history of

this disease or alternative treatments. As a better understanding of these complex diseases evolves, more sophisticated metrics for assessment will be developed to verify these suggested improvements, so that even better treatment approaches can be developed. As Ralph Waldo Emerson said, "To know even one life has breathed easier because you have lived. This is to have succeeded!"

References

[1] Pehrsson K, Larsson S, Oden A, Nachemson A. Long-term follow-up of patients with untreated scoliosis. A study of mortality, causes of death, and symptoms. Spine 1992; 17: 1091–1096

[2] Ramirez N, Santiago-Cornier A, Arroyo S, Acevedo J. The natural history of spondylothoracic dysplasia. Paper presented at: Annual Meeting of the Pediatric Orthopaedic Society of North America; May 2–6, 2001; Cancun, Mexico

[3] Kory RC, Callahan R, Boren HG, Syner JC. The Veterans Administration-Army cooperative study of pulmonary function. I. Clinical spirometry in normal men. Am J Med 1961; 30: 243–258

[4] Campbell RM Jr Smith MD, Mayes TC et al. The characteristics of thoracic insufficiency syndrome associated with fused ribs and congenital scoliosis. J Bone Joint Surg Am 2003; 85-A: 399–408

[5] Dimeglio A, Bonnel F. Le Rachis en Croissance. Paris, France: Springer; 1990

[6] Karol LA, Johnston C, Mladenov K, Schochet P, Walters P, Browne RH. Pulmonary function following early thoracic fusion in non-neuromuscular scoliosis. J Bone Joint Surg Am 2008; 90: 1272–1281

[7] Dubousset J, Wicart P, Pomero V, Barois A, Estournet B. Thoracic scoliosis: exothoracic and endothoracic deformations and the spinal penetration index [in French] Rev Chir Orthop Repar Appar Mot 2002; 88: 9–18

[8] Campbell RM Jr, Smith MD. Thoracic insufficiency syndrome and exotic scoliosis. J Bone Joint Surg 2007; 89-A: 108–122

[9] Gollogly S, Smith JT, White SK, Firth S, White K. The volume of lung parenchyma as a function of age: a review of 1050 normal CT scans of the chest with three-dimensional volumetric reconstruction of the pulmonary system. Spine 2004; 29: 2061–2066

[10] Campbell R, Epelman M, Flynn J, et al. Thoracic function: a new thoracic performance classification based on dynamic lung MRI with identification of a new mechanism for restrictive lung disease in early onset scoliosis, termed posterior obstructive blockade. Paper presented at: 12th International Phillip Zorab Symposium; March 2011; London, UK

[11] Goldberg CJ, Gillic I, Connaughton O et al. Respiratory function and cosmesis at maturity in infantile-onset scoliosis. Spine 2003; 28: 2397–2406

[12] Emans JB, Kassab F, Caubet JF, Hedequist D, Wohl ME, Campbell RM Jr. Earlier and more extensive thoracic fusion is associated with diminished pulmonary function. Outcomes after spinal fusion of 4 or more thoracic spinal segments before age 5. Poster presented at:11th International Meeting on Advanced Spinal Techniques; July 1–3, 2004; Southampton, Bermuda

[13] Sankar WN, Skaggs DL, Yazici M, Johnston CE, Shah SA, Javidan P, Kadakia RV, Day TF, Akbarnia BA. Lengthening of dual growing rods and the law of diminishing returns. Spine 2001; 36: 806–809

[14] Narayanan M, Owers-Bradley J, Beardsmore CS, Mada M, Bell I, Garipov R, Panesar KS, Kuehni CE, Spycher BD, Williams SE, Silverman M. Alveolarization continues during childhood and adolescence: new evidence from helium-3 magnetic resonance. Am J Respir Crit Care Med 2012; 185: 186–191

[15] Campbell RM Jr Smith MD, Mayes TC et al. The effect of opening wedge thoracostomy on thoracic insufficiency syndrome associated with fused ribs and congenital scoliosis. J Bone Joint Surg Am 2004; 86-A: 1659–1674

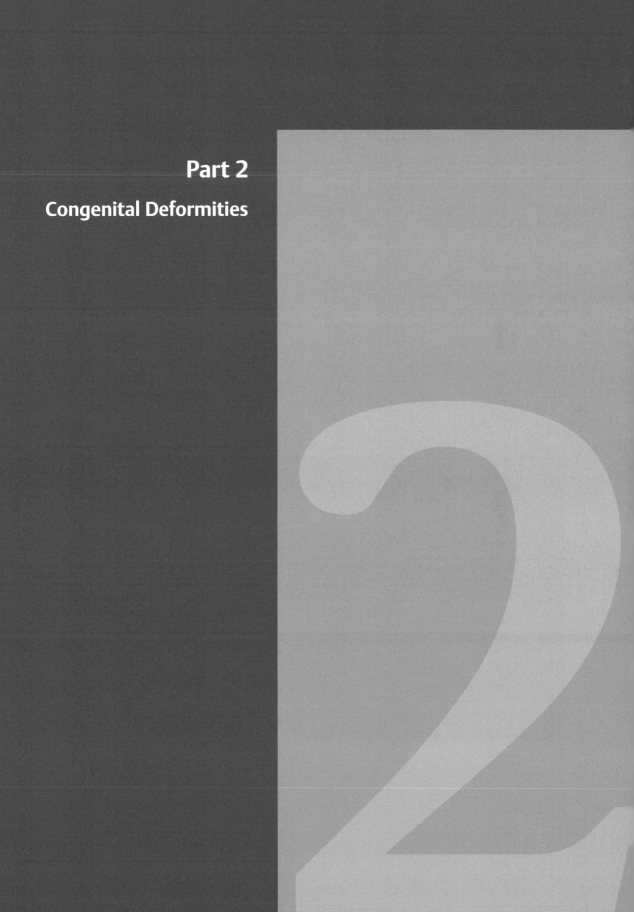

Part 2
Congenital Deformities

5 Neuroaxial Anomalies

Jayaratnam Jayamohan

The relationship between abnormalities of the brain and spinal cord and early onset scoliosis is not fully understood. Most neuroaxial anomalies are congenital or perinatal in origin.

5.1 Congenital Brain Disorders and Craniocervical Junction Anomalies

The developing brain is at risk for injury from conditions like ischemia, hemorrhage, infection, and rarely tumors. If a pregnancy is able to continue despite such insults, the child is frequently born with hemiparesis or hemiplegia and a consequent risk for the development of scoliosis. These cases are relatively uncommon, however, and most of the neuroaxial anomalies causing scoliosis occur within the spinal cord. They are all variations of or related to spinal dysraphism or other developmental anomalies, such as Chiari malformation and diastematomyelia. Anomalies can also be caused by acquired conditions, such as trauma, ischemia, and in particular tumors of the spinal cord. Abnormalities of the craniocervical junction are frequently seen in conjunction with early onset scoliosis (▶ Fig. 5.1).

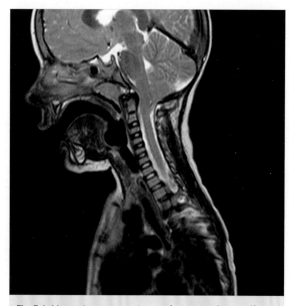

Fig. 5.1 Magnetic resonance image showing a Chiari malformation in a child presenting with scoliosis. Note the intraspinal location of the cerebellar tonsils and the low-lying medulla, causing compression and distortion of the brainstem and cervical cord.

5.2 History

In addition to the standard history taken for any patient with scoliosis, questions regarding developmental milestones should be specifically asked. It is important to discuss antenatal factors, including the method of conception, any ultrasound examinations or measurements done while the baby was in utero, the mother's drug history, and of course any relevant family history.

The birth itself needs to be explored, and it is important to review the initial examination of the child that was performed after delivery. A developmental assessment should be undertaken, based on both the history and the information in any charts that the parents can provide. In the United Kingdom, there is a "Red Book" that contains all the routine developmental assessments that health professionals have performed on babies, and this can often provide significant information if the parents are not able to provide such. Important milestones to assess in regard to neuroaxial anomalies include the time when the child was able to fix and focus (to detect diplopia associated with Chiari malformation) and to swallow. It should be determined whether the child has had repeated chest infections or aspiration-type symptoms. More standard developmental milestones should also be assessed, including sitting, crawling, walking, and hand function. Continence issues may be relevant depending on the age of the child, and it is important to determine not only when continence was achieved but also its nature. For example, daytime urinary incontinence is of greater significance than nighttime wetting in a child aged 4 years.

5.3 Physical Examination

In addition to a standard examination of the patient, particular care should be given to a full neurologic examination of both the peripheral and central nervous system. Any limb discrepancy, including discrepancies in the length and size of the hands and feet, should be noted carefully. The neurologic development of those patients who are to undergo conservative or nonoperative treatment should be monitored regularly. During the physical examination, the entire midline region should be carefully examined from the palate and face all the way down to the anus. Particular care should be taken to look for any associated conditions affecting the scalp, including encephaloceles, dermoids, hairy patches, Mongolian blue spots, and pits. If any pits are found, they should not be probed, and irritant dye should not be injected into them. If the end cannot be clearly seen, the pits are better investigated rather than examined. If an underlying syndrome,

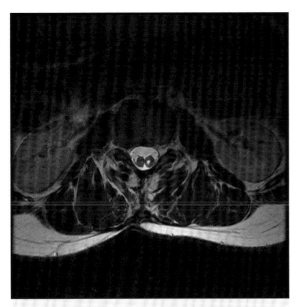

Fig. 5.2 Magnetic resonance image showing a split thoracic cord. This child had two cords within one dural tube.

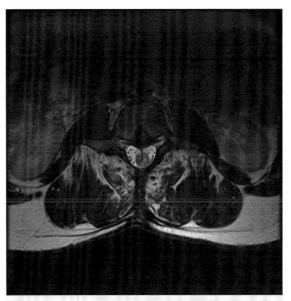

Fig. 5.3 Magnetic resonance image of the same child showing the area where the spilt "originated," with an obvious spur projecting into the cord.

such as the VACTERL (*v*ertebral, *a*nal, *c*ardiac, *t*racheo-*e*sophageal, *r*enal, and *l*imb) association, is suspected, an examination of the full anogenital system may be indicated. It may be best to have a pediatric general surgeon conduct this examination, depending on availability.

5.4 Radiologic Investigation

The investigations for neuroaxial causes of early onset scoliosis will overlap with those for all other causes of the disease. The orthopedic surgeon will often request plain films to assess and document the actual bony anatomy. If a neuroaxial cause is being sought, then magnetic resonance (MR) imaging of the entire brain and spinal cord is indicated. This will enable any associated anomalies to be identified. In particular, MR imaging is helpful for assessing the craniocervical junction, any split cord malformations, and tethering of the cord, and it may also identify some brain anomalies, such as tumors and infarction. It is important to discuss such a request with the radiologist so that the correct sequences are performed and detailed investigations of any areas that may appear to be abnormal are obtained, in particular when split cord malformations are suspected.

Computed tomography (CT) is often needed when a split cord is suspected. Although MR imaging may show the split and suggest the presence of a disruptive structure, CT will be better placed to show whether a bony spur, cartilaginous strut, or fibrous brand is involved in the split. CT should be undertaken in conjunction with MR imaging, which may help identify a split cord or a split dura (▶ Fig. 5.2 and ▶ Fig. 5.3). In cases in which such

an anomaly is noted, CT angiography may be helpful, in particular to identify major spinal arteries, such as the artery of Adamkiewicz. However, the level of information that can be ascertained from such an investigation will vary according to the child's size and renal function (which may limit the amount of contrast that can be administered) and by the abilities of both the scanner and the radiologist. Again, close coordination with the radiologist is necessary to ensure that these tests are performed only if necessary.

Urologic investigations will often be required. Although they are not directly related to the scoliosis, they will be important to make sure that the patient does not have any neuropathic disorders of the bladder and renal system. Patients with scoliosis may also require a respiratory assessment, in particular before the administration of a general anesthetic or major surgery.

5.5 Management

The two basic arms of the management of neuroaxial anomalies are conservative and surgical. Some patients may well be managed with conservative treatments, including, of course, physiotherapy, but also orthotic assistance. This can vary from a relatively minor device, such as a foot raise or an ankle–foot orthosis (AFO), to a brace or other aid for standing and mobility.

Surgical treatment is clearly aimed at one of the underlying causes. Some brain disorders can be treated by surgical methods. If not treatable with medication, dystonia may be mitigated by deep brain stimulation.

Chiari malformations are treated surgically with a foramen magnum decompression. This involves a posterior suboccipital approach to expose the occiput and usually the arch of the first cervical vertebra. Bone is removed from the foramen magnum region of the occipital bone and the arch of C1. There can then be further progressive intervention, including opening of the dura, opening of the arachnoid membrane, separation of the cerebellar tonsils, and finally resection of the tonsils. There is still no clear indication regarding when each of these increasingly more aggressive surgical options should be used, and debate continues as to whether the choice makes a difference. Generally, most neurosurgeons would agree that all of the surgical options have their place, depending on the specific anatomy and symptomatology of the specific patient.

Syrinx formation may often be an indication for more aggressive surgery. Surgery for diastematomyelia can take place anywhere along the cord. The precise surgery that is required will very much depend on the anatomical configuration of the split. In general terms, the cause of the split will need to be removed to prevent further trauma to the spinal cord during growth of the spine. If the cord is split along with the dura, then frequently both dural tubes can be left intact during removal of the spur or band, and provided that no cerebrospinal fluid (CSF) is encountered, the operation can cease at this point. However, if the spur is intradural, then the dura will have to be opened to enable removal. Closure of the dura can be difficult, in particular if there is a ventral defect in the dura. However, with careful planning, closure can be achieved, and such surgery may be performed at the same time as bony surgery on the spine, given that the levels of the apex of the curve and the diastematomyelia are frequently the same. The risks of such complex combination surgery need to be considered, however, in particular if the dura must be opened. If this is the case, the role of lumbar CSF drainage should be assessed. Frequently, this can facilitate dural closure and skin closure with less risk of CSF leak. If revision surgery is needed, then a pseudomeningocele can be a significant problem, and all efforts should be made to avoid this occurrence.

Open myelomeningoceles clearly require early closure after birth. Closed myelomeningoceles and encephaloceles may be watched and treated conservatively or may be treated surgically. The indications for surgery with closed defects are not fully clear. Some neurosurgeons believe that prophylactic surgery is indicated to prevent neurologic deterioration. Others believe that because of the risks of surgical intervention, surgery is required only after neurologic deterioration has been shown to be ongoing. The latter is the author's view, but this is a live issue.

If there are signs of tethering and either scoliosis is progressing or the orthopedic treatment will involve increasing tension on the cord, then untethering is indicated. It is important that any diastematomyelia be attended to before untethering because once the cord is untethered, the symptoms caused by the diastematomyelia may worsen. The surgery will depend on the exact anatomy but will consist of cutting of the filum terminale if this is the cause of the tethering, disconnection of a fatty filum from any subcutaneous fat, and removal of any associated lesion, such as a dermoid. If an open myelomeningocele has been closed, an attempt should be made to ensure that as many layers similar to the normal layers around the spinal cord, conus, and cauda equina as possible are approximated. Ideally, at least three layers will involve dura, fascia, and skin. Many textbooks describe seven layers, but in reality this is very hard to achieve. Separation of the nervous tissue from superficial tissue, to reduce potential scarring and retethering, as well as to exclude the external world and its infective risks, is the real aim of these layer closures.

The treatment of spasticity can consist of oral medication such as baclofen, diazepam, gabapentin, and others. If this is not sufficient, then surgical treatment may consist of placement of an intrathecal baclofen pump to deliver drug directly to the CSF or selective dorsal rhizotomy. There is little evidence that dorsal rhizotomy relieves scoliosis, but it may reduce limb spasticity. There is some conflicting evidence about the effects of oral antispasmodics or intrathecal baclofen on scoliosis. If the scoliosis is due to overactivity of one of the extensor muscle groups, then intrathecal baclofen may be effective; however, if the scoliosis is due to weakness, then the intrathecal baclofen may relax muscle tone further and exacerbate the scoliosis. Therefore, whenever a patient with a condition like diplegic cerebral palsy is treated with a muscle relaxant, it is important to gauge the effects on any scoliosis.

If an intrathecal pump is present, then the catheter must be carefully looked after during any spinal surgery. It will travel from the pump (usually placed anteriorly in the abdominal wall) around the side of the abdomen to enter the intrathecal space via the interlaminar space in the midline (like a lumbar drain). Thus, it can easily be cut by a misplaced surgical incision during spinal surgery. This will, of course, cause increased spasticity postoperatively. However, the risks are much higher than just this; in an acute baclofen withdrawal, patients are at risk for major systemic complications that may be life-threatening, including hyperthermia and rhabdomyolysis caused by excessive muscle tone, seizures, multi-system organ failure, cardiac arrest, coma, and death. Urgent expert help is required in such circumstances.

If a tumor or other space-occupying lesion is found, some thought must be given to the possible pathology and the risk-to-benefit ratio of surgery. In the presence of worsening scoliosis, there will almost always be an indication sufficient to warrant surgery. The decision of whether to try to obtain a complete excision will depend

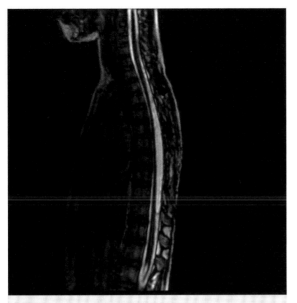

Fig. 5.4 Magnetic resonance image showing a dorsal arachnoid cyst. This child had previously undergone surgery for the cyst (presenting with scoliosis). After 5 years, the scoliosis again began to progress, and imaging shows a clear recurrence of the cyst, requiring further surgery.

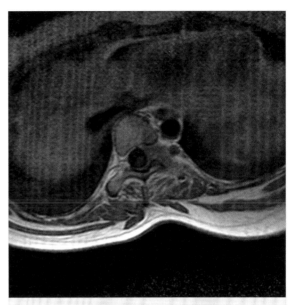

Fig. 5.5 Axial MRI showing a left sided neurofibroma. Note the expansion of the nerve root foramen.

on the relationship between the lesion and the cord, the risks of damage, and the need to remove the lesion completely. Arachnoid cysts (▶ Fig. 5.4) and benign lesions (▶ Fig. 5.5) may be completely cured by surgery. However, malignant tumors, in particular intraparenchymal cord tumors, may be best managed with a combination of surgery and adjuvant treatment. A detailed discussion is outside the scope of this book, but the treatment of such lesions is well documented in the neurosurgical literature.

6 Congenital Deformities of the Spine

Athanasios I. Tsirikos

The spectrum of congenital deformities of the spine includes a range of conditions that blend gradually from scoliosis through kyphoscoliosis to pure kyphosis. These deformities occur when an asymmetric failure of development of one or more vertebrae results in a localized imbalance in the longitudinal growth of the spine and an increasing curvature affecting the coronal and/or sagittal plane, with a risk for progression during skeletal growth. The consequence of unbalanced growth of the spine can be the development of a benign curve with slow or no progression, in which case observation may be the only treatment required. In contrast, there are types of vertebral abnormalities that can produce considerable asymmetry in spinal growth and the development of very aggressive deformities with consequent functional, cosmetic, respiratory, and neurologic complications. Understanding the anatomical features of the individual vertebral anomalies and their relation to the remainder of the spine makes it possible to predict those abnormalities that are likely to produce a severe curve. Recognizing the natural history of the deformity at an early stage can in turn allow appropriate surgical treatment, with the aim of preventing the development of severe spinal curvature and trunk decompensation that would require much more complex and dangerous treatment with a suboptimal clinical outcome.

6.1 Incidence

Congenital scoliosis is the most common type of deformity; it had a prevalence of nearly 80% among more than 1,000 patients with congenital deformities of the spine followed as part of the Scottish National Spine Deformity Service. Congenital kyphoscoliosis is the second most common type of deformity, affecting 14% of patients, while congenital kyphosis has developed in 6% of our patients. Congenital scoliosis has a prevalence of 1 in 1,000 live births, with a reported familial incidence of 1 to 5%. Girls are affected more often than boys.

6.2 Etiology

The causes of congenital vertebral anomalies are likely to be genetic factors, including defects in the Notch signaling pathways. The Notch 1 gene has been shown to coordinate the process of somitogenesis by regulating the development of vertebral precursors in mice. Chromosome 13 and 17 translocations have been associated with the development of hemivertebrae. Genetic theories are supported by molecular, animal, and twin population studies, including several demonstrations of abnormal HOX gene expression. Environmental factors have also been suggested, and these include exposure to toxins including carbon monoxide, the use of antiepileptic medication, and maternal diabetes.

6.3 Embryologic Development

The embryologic development of the spine and that of the ribs are closely interrelated, and the complete anatomical mold is formed in mesenchyme during the first 6 weeks of intrauterine life. Mesodermally derived adjacent somites coalesce during this period of development and yield vertebral bodies ventrally and neural arches dorsally; these ossify during organogenesis through a single primary center in the centrum for the body and two centers dorsally for the arches. Anomalies of the spine and ribs may occur during this period of fetal development, and once the mesenchymal mold is established, the cartilaginous and bony stages follow that pattern. Five secondary ossification centers ossify the vertebral end plates, as well as the spinous and transverse processes after birth.

Vertebral anomalies occurring during the mesenchymal stage may be due either to a unilateral defect of formation or to segmentation of the primitive vertebrae, resulting in a unilateral imbalance in the longitudinal growth of the spine that produces a congenital scoliosis. Vertebral anomalies may also occur during the subsequent chondrification stage and are thought to be due to a localized failure of vascularization of the developing cartilaginous centrum. This results in varying degrees of failure of vertebral formation, producing a congenital kyphosis or kyphoscoliosis. In the late chondrification and ossification stages, bony metaplasia may occur in the anterior part of the anulus fibrosus and ring apophysis, producing an anterior or anterolateral unsegmented bar that can also result in a congenital kyphosis or kyphoscoliosis.

The ribs form from costal processes, which are small, lateral mesenchymal condensations of the developing thoracic somites and contribute cells to all parts of the developing ribs. The distal tips of the costal processes elongate to form ribs only in the thoracic spine. The ribs develop from cartilaginous precursors that ossify during the fetal period. Rib anomalies (fused ribs, bifid ribs, chest wall defects) probably form during the process of segmentation and resegmentation of the developing somites, after which the ribs come to articulate between the definitive thoracic vertebrae.

The scapula develops along with the arm. The arm bud appears in the third week of embryonic life as a small swelling opposite the vertebral segments from C5 to T1.

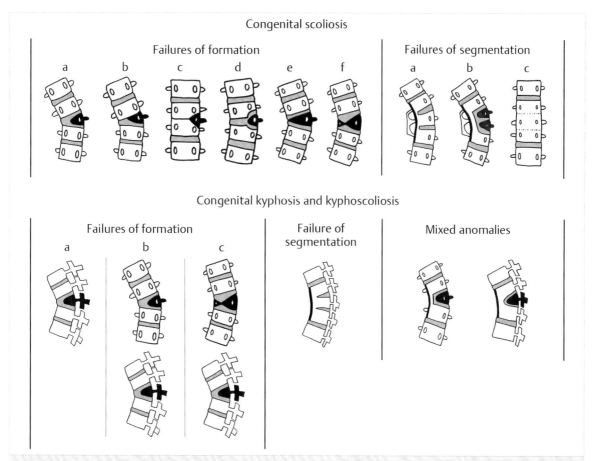

Fig. 6.1 Classification of congenital scoliosis, kyphoscoliosis, and kyphosis. Congenital scoliosis is classified into failures of formation (*a*, fully segmented hemivertebra; *b*, semisegmented hemivertebra; *c*, unsegmented hemivertebra; *d*, incarcerated hemivertebra; *e*, wedge vertebra; *f*, asymmetric butterfly vertebra) and failures of segmentation (*a*, unilateral unsegmented bar; *b*, unilateral unsegmented bar with contralateral hemivertebra; *c*, block vertebra). Congenital kyphosis or kyphoscoliosis is classified into failures of formation (*a*, posterior hemivertebra; *b*, posterolateral quadrant vertebra; *c*, posterior asymmetric butterfly vertebra), failures of segmentation (anterior unsegmented bar), and mixed anomalies (anterolateral unsegmented bar with posterolateral quadrant vertebra).

The scapula appears in mesenchyme during the fifth week and gradually migrates caudally. By the end of the third fetal month, it reaches its final anatomical position lateral to the spine and extending from T2 to T7-T8. Occasionally, the scapula may fail to descend fully to its normal position and remains in a permanently elevated location, a condition known as a Sprengel deformity.

6.4 Classification

Congenital deformities of the spine are classified by their anatomical location, as well as by the pathologic anatomy of the anomalous vertebrae (▶ Fig. 6.1). Congenital vertebral abnormalities producing a scoliosis, kyphosis, or kyphoscoliosis can be due mainly to a *failure of vertebral formation* or a *failure of vertebral segmentation*. *Mixed anomalies* are less common, and these are often unclassifiable and difficult to define at birth, when the spine is only 30% ossified.

6.4.1 Congenital Scoliosis

Failures of vertebral formation causing a scoliosis can be complete or incomplete. *Complete failures* include four types of hemivertebra, in which one-half of the vertebral body has failed to form. A hemivertebra can be fully segmented, semisegmented, unsegmented, or incarcerated. A fully segmented hemivertebra has cephalic and caudal end plates and is separated from the vertebrae above and below by normal disk spaces. A semisegmented hemivertebra has only one end plate and is congenitally fused to either the vertebra above or the vertebra below, with one remaining disk space. The space contralateral to the hemivertebra where the vertebral body has not formed is occupied by disk. An unsegmented hemivertebra is fused to both the cephalic and caudal vertebrae, with no contralateral disk space and no growth potential. An incarcerated hemivertebra is a small, ovoid vertebral segment that sits within a niche formed between the vertebrae above and below. It also has very limited growth potential and limited ability to produce a deformity. The presence of a fully segmented or semisegmented hemivertebra with normal growth plates causes an asymmetric development of the spine because the opposite side is deficient and lacks growth; therefore, a scoliosis develops. *Incomplete failures* of vertebral formation include a wedge vertebra and an asymmetric butterfly vertebra. A wedge vertebra has bilateral pedicles, but the concave pedicle is hypoplastic. This produces height asymmetry on the concave side and the development of a curvature. An asymmetric butterfly vertebra can cause a scoliosis if there is a localized imbalance of vertebral body growth.

Failures of vertebral segmentation can be unilateral or bilateral. Unilateral failures of segmentation include an unsegmented bar with or without contralateral hemivertebrae at the same level. The bar can extend across two or more segments and constitutes a unilateral tether of vertebral growth, which in the presence of normal contralateral end plates (as demonstrated by open disk spaces opposite the bar on plain radiographs) produces a rapidly progressive scoliosis. Scoliosis develops as a consequence of a combination of inhibition of growth caused by the unsegmented bar and the preservation of contralateral growth, which is more accelerated in the presence of one or more hemivertebrae at the same level. A bilateral failure of segmentation produces a block vertebral segment, which does not have growth potential and does not carry a risk for the development of a significant deformity.

6.4.2 Congenital Kyphosis and Kyphoscoliosis

Failures of vertebral formation can also cause a congenital kyphosis or kyphoscoliosis. These include a posterior hemivertebra and a posterolateral quadrant vertebra, which are due to anterior and anterolateral aplasia of the developing vertebral body, respectively. A posterior hemivertebra produces a pure kyphosis, whereas a posterolateral quadrant vertebra causes a kyphoscoliosis. Congenital kyphoscoliosis can also develop in the presence of an asymmetric butterfly vertebra (sagittal cleft vertebra due to anteromedial aplasia) or a wedge vertebra (due to anterolateral hypoplasia).

Failures of vertebral segmentation include an anterior unsegmented bar, which can produce a congenital kyphosis with slow progression and a limited need for treatment. In contrast, an anterolateral unsegmented bar with or without a contralateral hemivertebra at the same level leads to severe growth imbalance and the development of a congenital kyphoscoliosis with a high risk for progression.

Congenital kyphosis due to either failure of formation or failure of segmentation can be associated with an *aligned* or a *displaced spinal canal* (▶ Fig. 6.2). If the spinal canal alignment is normal, there is good continuity of the line across the posterior aspect of the vertebral bodies at the levels of the kyphosis. In contrast, a displaced spinal

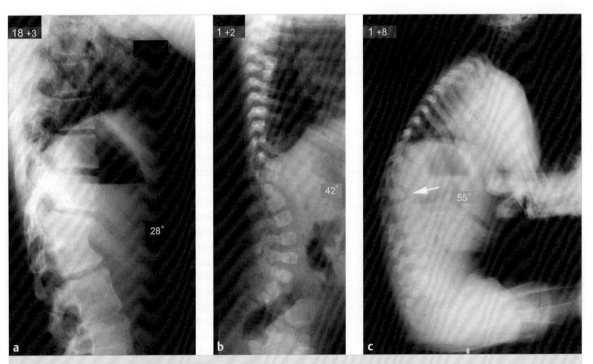

Fig. 6.2 (a) Lateral radiograph of a skeletally mature patient with a small congenital kyphosis due to an anterior unsegmented bar between T12 and L1 and an aligned spinal canal. (b) Lateral radiograph of a young child with a congenital kyphosis due to a posterior hemivertebra at L1 and an aligned canal. (c) Lateral radiograph of a young child with a congenital kyphosis due to a posterior hemivertebra at L1 (*white arrow*) and a subluxed spinal canal at the T12-L1 segment with a localized step-off deformity and segmental instability.

canal occurs as a step-off deformity at the level of a sub-luxed or dislocated vertebral segment due to the presence of a hypoplastic vertebra. This type of deformity is progressive, and the spine is highly unstable in the sagittal and axial planes; therefore, it carries a significant risk for neurologic complications.

Mixed anomalies can affect large segments and different areas of the spine and comprise a combination of failures of vertebral formation and segmentation. Advances in imaging techniques have allowed a better definition of the anatomy of these vertebral defects, which are often very difficult to categorize. They are commonly associated with rib and chest wall abnormalities, so that both spinal growth and thoracic growth are tethered.

Recent classification schemes have been developed to include the posterior element anatomy based on the assessment of three-dimensional images obtained with computed tomography. The congenital vertebral anomalies have been classified into solitary simple, multiple simple, complex, and segmentation failures. The posterior vertebral arch can be intact or abnormally formed. This includes bifid areas with open access to the spinal canal or laminae, which are partially or fully fused, often on the opposite side of a hemivertebra between the vertebrae above and below. Abnormalities affecting the posterior bony structures may not correspond to the level of the vertebral body defect. Current limitations of the three-dimensional classification system include uncertainty of intra- and interobserver reliability, additional exposure of children to radiation, and an increase in cost. Surgical planning requires a detailed understanding of the anatomy of the affected vertebrae. Therefore, despite these limitations, preoperative computed tomography with three-dimensional reconstruction can provide useful information and reduce the risk for neurologic damage during surgery.

6.5 Natural History

The natural history of a spinal deformity depends on the type, number, and location of congenital vertebral anomalies, as well as their relationship to the adjacent segments of the spine. Maximal progression of a deformity is expected during the first 3 years of life and during the pubertal growth spurt, which are the stages when skeletal growth is accelerated. Curves due to a failure of vertebral formation or segmentation follow a predictable pattern of development, whereas predicting the deterioration of curves due to mixed anomalies may be challenging. Close monitoring of congenital curves is required at puberty because progression can be observed even in previously stable deformities. Curves that affect transitional areas of the spine, especially the thoracolumbar or lumbosacral region, carry the greatest risk for deterioration.

6.5.1 Congenital Scoliosis

The prognosis of a congenital scoliosis due to a fully segmented hemivertebra is often difficult to determine. Surgical treatment is indicated in patients who present with severe curves or with documented progression of a minimum of 5 degrees within 6 months of observation. Curve deterioration is generally slow, at mean rate of 1 to 2 degrees per year. Two ipsilateral hemivertebrae produce a more progressive scoliosis that is expected to increase by 3 to 4 degrees per year, exceed 50 degrees by the age of 10 years, and reach 70 degrees at skeletal maturity, with a greater risk for the development of a severe structural compensatory curvature across the adjacent levels. Two opposing hemivertebrae separated by one or more normal vertebral segments can occur either in the same region of the spine (often thoracic), referred to as a hemimetameric shift, or farther away from each other. A hemimetameric shift affecting the thoracolumbar or lumbosacral spine is more likely to create an unbalanced deformity and may require surgical treatment (▶ Fig. 6.3).

A semisegmented hemivertebra produces a slowly progressive scoliosis that does not usually exceed 40 degrees at the completion of growth. Treatment may not be required if the curve is small unless it is located in the lumbosacral junction. Lumbosacral fully segmented or semisegmented hemivertebrae cause an oblique take-off of the spine and require early surgical treatment in order to prevent the development of a rapidly progressive structural compensatory scoliosis in the lumbar region as the spine attempts to balance. An incarcerated hemivertebra has limited growth potential and produces minimal deformity that does not require treatment. An unsegmented hemivertebra commonly occurs in the thoracic spine and has no ability to grow because it is fused to the adjacent proximal and distal vertebrae, and it does not cause a deformity.

The extent of a unilateral unsegmented bar corresponding to the amount of tethering effect produced, as well as the presence of contralateral vertebral growth, will define the rate of progression of a congenital scoliosis. Longitudinal growth of the spine occurs from the superior and inferior end plates of every vertebra. Open disk spaces on the side opposite to the bar suggest retained growth potential and as a consequence a higher risk for curve progression. The mean rate of deterioration of a scoliosis due to a unilateral unsegmented bar is 5 degrees per year, with the majority of curves exceeding 50 degrees by age 10 years and requiring early surgical treatment. If the unilateral unsegmented bar is combined with a contralateral hemivertebra at the same level, the unbalanced vertebral growth has the worst prognosis, with a rate of scoliosis progression that increases to 6 degrees per year. Most curves deteriorate beyond 50 degrees by 2 years of age.

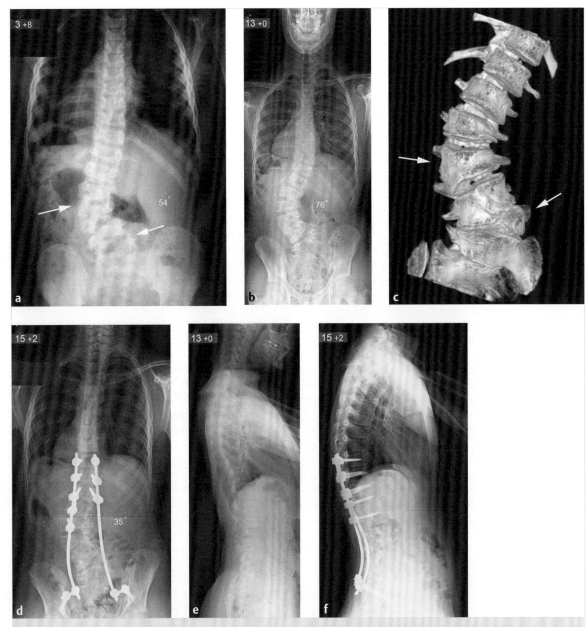

Fig. 6.3 Radiograph of a patient with congenital scoliosis due to the presence of two opposing hemivertebrae producing a hemimetameric shift at age 3 + 8 years (*arrow*, **a**). The scoliosis remained stable until puberty, when evidence of significant deterioration was noted (**b**). Computed tomography with three-dimensional reconstruction (**c**) demonstrated two contralateral hemivertebrae (*arrows*). The patient underwent a posterior spinal fusion, which achieved good balance of the spine in the coronal plane (**d**). The preoperative lumbar flat back deformity (**e**) was also well corrected, with restoration of normal lumbar lordosis and a good global sagittal balance of the spine (**f**).

6.5.2 Congenital Kyphosis and Kyphoscoliosis

Congenital kyphosis or kyphoscoliosis due to a failure of vertebral formation (posterior or posterolateral hemivertebra) or to mixed anomalies (anterolateral bar with contralateral quadrant vertebra) carries the greatest risk for progression. Congenital kyphosis or kyphoscoliosis often affects the thoracolumbar spine; if the curve is located in the thoracic region, the risk for neurologic complications is significantly increased. The severity of kyphosis is proportional to the degree of anterior failure of vertebral formation, and this is greater in the presence of two adjacent defects of formation. A posterolateral quadrant vertebra produces a kyphoscoliosis that progresses at a mean of 2.5 degrees per year before the age of 10 years and 5 degrees per year during puberty, exceeds 80 degrees by the age of 11 years, and carries the greatest risk for neurologic compromise. A kyphoscoliosis due to an asymmetric butterfly vertebra progresses at 1.5 degrees per year before age 10 years and 4 degrees per year during puberty. An anterior unsegmented bar creates a slowly progressive kyphosis at a mean rate of 1 degree per year before 10 years and less than 2 degrees per year during puberty, with no risk for spinal cord compression. An anterolateral unsegmented bar has a worse prognosis than an anterior bar because it produces a kyphoscoliosis that exceeds 90 degrees at skeletal maturity. A kyphoscoliosis due to an anterolateral bar with a contralateral quadrant vertebra carries the greatest risk for deterioration, progressing at a mean rate of 5 degrees per year before age 10 years and 8 degrees per year during puberty.

Spinal cord compression can occur in congenital kyphosis or kyphoscoliosis due to a posterior hemivertebra or posterolateral quadrant vertebra at a reported prevalence of 10 to 12%. The onset of symptoms is usually during adolescence with a variable degree of deformity, and if left untreated, the condition always results in paraplegia.

Further Reading

Bush CH, Kalen V. Three-dimensional computed tomography in the assessment of congenital scoliosis. Skeletal Radiol 1999; 28: 632–637

Christ B, Wilting J. From somites to vertebral column. Ann Anat 1992; 174: 23–32

Evans DJR. Contribution of somitic cells to the avian ribs. Dev Biol 2003; 256: 114–126

Huang R, Zhi Q, Neubüser A et al. Function of somite and somitocoele cells in the formation of the vertebral motion segment in avian embryos. Acta Anat (Basel) 1996; 155: 231–241

Huang R, Zhi Q, Schmidt C, Wilting J, Brand-Saberi B, Christ B. Sclerotomal origin of the ribs. Development 2000; 127: 527–532

Huang R, Zhi Q, Wilting J, Christ B. The fate of somitocoele cells in avian embryos. Anat Embryol (Berl) 1994; 190: 243–250

Kawakami N, Tsuji T, Imagama S, Lenke LG, Puno RM, Kuklo TR Spinal Deformity Study Group. Classification of congenital scoliosis and kyphosis: a new approach to the three-dimensional classification for progressive vertebral anomalies requiring operative treatment. Spine 2009; 34: 1756–1765

McMaster MJ, Ohtsuka K. The natural history of congenital scoliosis. A study of 251 patients. J Bone Joint Surg Am 1982; 64: 1128–1147

McMaster MJ, Singh H. Natural history of congenital kyphosis and kyphoscoliosis. A study of 112 patients. J Bone Joint Surg Am 1999; 81: 1367–1383

Morin B, Poitras B, Duhaime M, Rivard CH, Marton D. Congenital kyphosis by segmentation defect: etiologic and pathogenic studies. J Pediatr Orthop 1985; 5: 309–314

Nakajima A, Kawakami N, Imagama S, Tsuji T, Goto M, Ohara T. Three-dimensional analysis of formation failure in congenital scoliosis. Spine 2007; 32: 562–567

Newton PO, Hahn GW, Fricka KB, Wenger DR. Utility of three-dimensional and multiplanar reformatted computed tomography for evaluation of pediatric congenital spine abnormalities. Spine 2002; 27: 844–850

Roaf R. Vertebral growth and its mechanical control. J Bone Joint Surg Br 1960; 42-B: 40–59

Shahcheraghi GH, Hobbi MH. Patterns and progression in congenital scoliosis. J Pediatr Orthop 1999; 19: 766–775

Tsou PM. Embryology of congenital kyphosis. Clin Orthop Relat Res 1977: 18–25

Tsou PM, Yau A, Hodgson AR. Embryogenesis and prenatal development of congenital vertebral anomalies and their classification. Clin Orthop Relat Res 1980: 211–231

7 Surgical Treatment of Congenital Spine Deformity

Athanasios I. Tsirikos

Congenital vertebral anomalies can produce a severe deformity of the spine in the coronal and/or sagittal plane with often a rotational component, which requires accurate diagnosis and early treatment. If the problem is recognized when the patient is at a young age, prophylactic surgery can be performed, which can prevent the development of a significant deformity. Knowledge of the different types of vertebral abnormalities and their natural history alerts the clinician to the long-term prognosis, so that early surgical treatment can be undertaken whenever this is appropriate. A thorough initial assessment is required to exclude associated intraspinal and systemic anomalies. Surgical techniques range from in situ fusion and convex hemi-epiphysiodesis to vertebral column resection followed by spinal reconstruction and the placement of growth preservation devices.

7.1 Patient Evaluation

A detailed clinical assessment of every patient with a congenital deformity of the spine is of prime importance to identify associated abnormalities affecting multiple organ systems; these can have major implications not only on spinal care but also on the overall well-being of the patient. The assessment should include a thorough physical examination, including repeated measurements of height, weight, arm span, and body mass index (BMI) at every clinical visit; these will indicate the progress of skeletal growth, which can have a direct effect on the deterioration of a spinal deformity. A low BMI correlates strongly with reduced pulmonary function and restrictive lung disease, indicating thoracic insufficiency syndrome. Patients with congenital vertebral anomalies need to be assessed for concurrent abnormalities of the ribs and thoracic cage with regular pulmonary function tests, including measurements of inspiratory and expiratory chest capacity, as well as lung volumes. Thoracic insufficiency is a dreaded complication that often occurs in patients with complex congenital vertebral defects in conjunction with spondylocostal or spondylothoracic dysplasia and Jarcho–Levin syndrome, and it can result in a major constriction of respiratory function and a short life expectancy.

7.2 Associated Skeletal and Systemic Anomalies

The vertebrae, neural structures, and musculoskeletal, cardiovascular, and genitourinary systems develop during similar stages of embryogenesis. As a consequence, embryonic insults affecting one or more of these systems

simultaneously can be expected. The incidence of abnormalities affecting other organ systems in patients with congenital deformities of the spine, especially those due to mixed vertebral anomalies, can be greater than 61%. The patients in this group present with isolated defects involving one or more systems, or their clinical picture can be the expression of one of the following syndromic conditions: VATER (coexistence of vertebral, anorectal, tracheaesophageal, and renal anomalies); VACTERL (all of the above with the addition of cardiac and limb anomalies); Goldenhar (oculo-auriculo-vertebral) syndrome; Noonan syndrome (congenital cardiac disease, short stature, cervical fusions, Chiari I malformation, pectus carinatum or excavatum, low muscle tone); and Poland syndrome (ipsilateral hand and pectoralis major anomalies).

7.2.1 Musculoskeletal Anomalies

Spinal Column

The evaluation of a patient with a congenital deformity of the spine should include the entire length of the vertebral column because anomalies can concomitantly affect different areas and not necessarily produce a clinically obvious curvature. Klippel–Feil syndrome manifests with a short neck, low posterior hairline, and congenital fusion of two or more cervical vertebrae; this has to be excluded because it may result in limitation of neck movement and, over time, segmental instability at levels proximal or distal to the abnormality. Congenital cervical anomalies are particularly associated with a congenital scoliosis affecting the thoracic or lumbar spine. A common location for a unilateral unsegmented bar with or without a contralateral hemivertebra or mixed congenital vertebral defects is the area around the cervicothoracic junction, and these anomalies may be associated with Klippel–Feil syndrome. As a consequence, they can produce an elevation of the convex shoulder and head tilt toward the concavity of the scoliosis.

Other Skeletal Anomalies

Other skeletal abnormalities associated with a congenital deformity of the spine include craniofacial malformations, radial club hand, thumb hypoplasia, developmental hip dysplasia, club foot, cavus foot, vertical talus, and deficiencies or atrophies of the upper or lower limbs.

Congenital Elevated Scapula (Sprengel Shoulder)

Congenital elevated scapula occurs in patients with congenital spinal deformities at a prevalence of 7% and is mostly associated with a cervicothoracic or thoracic scoliosis due to a unilateral failure of vertebral segmentation. The combination of a congenital high scapula lying on the convexity of a congenital upper thoracic scoliosis creates a significant deformity due to elevation of the shoulder line and occasionally impairment of shoulder function. In such a situation, surgical treatment is often needed for both problems—to address the scoliosis and to reduce the scapula to its anatomically normal position in relation to the spine. However, when a Sprengel deformity is located on the concavity of a scoliosis, it often partly compensates for the cosmetic deformity produced by the elevation of the contralateral shoulder on the convexity of the curve. This minimizes shoulder asymmetry, and surgical treatment to restore the scapula to its normal location is usually not required.

Rib Anomalies

The ribs and chest wall form in close association with the vertebral column; abnormalities affecting thoracic cage development have been recorded in 19.2% of the patients with congenital deformities of the spine followed in our center. These developmental rib and chest wall anomalies may be simple (79%) or complex (21%) and are due to a failure of either segmentation or formation of the ribs (▶ Fig. 7.1). The most common simple anomaly of the ribs is a localized fusion of two to three consecutive ribs; the most common complex abnormality is a combination of fused ribs with an adjacent large thoracic wall defect.

Congenital rib anomalies usually occur on the concavity of a thoracic or thoracolumbar congenital scoliosis caused by a unilateral failure of vertebral segmentation. A likely explanation for the close association between rib abnormalities and this type of congenital scoliosis is a localized embryologic error occurring during the initial developmental stage that results in a failure of segmentation of both the primitive ribs and vertebrae on the same side. The rib abnormalities do not appear to have an adverse effect on the degree or rate of progression of the deformity; these are determined primarily by the vertebral segmentation defect, which produces a severe unilateral imbalance in the longitudinal growth of the spine. The main driving force for the development of scoliosis in this group of patients is the unilateral failure of vertebral segmentation, the effect of which greatly exceeds any adverse effect due to rib fusions.

A long congenital thoracic scoliosis associated with fused ribs may affect thoracic function and growth of the lungs in young children and lead to thoracic insufficiency syndrome. This condition is usually due to a congenital failure of vertebral segmentation, which inhibits longitudinal growth of the spine and in turn vertical development of the thoracic cage. The coexistence of rib fusions will further restrict chest development on the concave side of the scoliosis and result in underdevelopment of

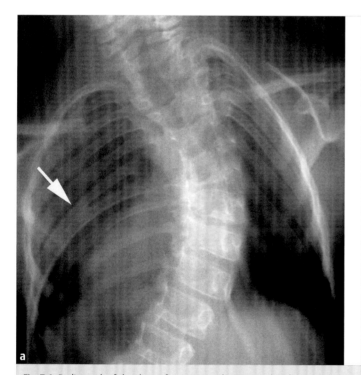
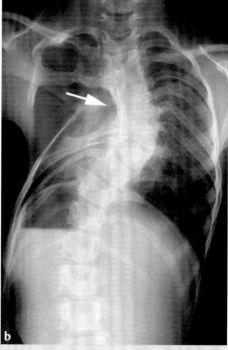

Fig. 7.1 Radiograph of the chest of a patient with congenital scoliosis (a) shows a congenital fusion (simple anomaly) of the seventh and eighth ribs (*white arrow*). Radiograph of the chest of a patient with a congenital scoliosis (b) demonstrates a chest wall defect and congenital rib fusions adjacent to a unilateral unsegmented bar (*white arrow*).

the lungs and restrictive pulmonary disease. An imbalance in the mechanical thrust of the ribs may adversely affect spinal growth as well as the function of trunk muscles and thus increase pressure within the thorax. Rib and chest wall abnormalities have been observed less frequently in patients with congenital lumbar or lumbosacral scoliosis, congenital kyphoscoliosis, or pure kyphosis.

7.2.2 Intraspinal Abnormalities

Intraspinal anomalies can be associated with a scoliosis that is not due to congenital vertebral defects (scoliosis associated with spinal dysraphism). More commonly, spinal dysraphism may occur in conjunction with congenital vertebral anomalies that include Chiari or Dandy–Walker malformations, syringomyelia, tethering of the cord, diastematomyelia, dural bands or cysts, intradural lipomas, and tight filum terminale (▶ Fig. 7.2). More than one dysraphic change can affect the same patient, and these are more prevalent in association with a congenital scoliosis due to mixed or vertebral segmentation abnormalities. The incidence of spinal dysraphism is 18 to 37%, with tethered cord most frequently encountered in patients with a congenital scoliosis.

Patients with congenital deformities of the spine and intraspinal anomalies may be completely asymptomatic; the absence of neurologic deficits or cutaneous lesions overlying the vertebral column does not rule out a dysraphic change. The presence of a cutaneous lesion such as a hairy patch, skin dimple or tag, vascular pigmentation, or hemangioma increases the possibility of an underlying dysraphic anomaly. Children with intraspinal pathology may present with neurologic signs and symptoms varying from subtly asymmetric leg tendon or abdominal reflexes to gait disturbance, severe motor and sensory deficits, bowel and bladder dysfunction, foot deformities, and lower limb muscle atrophy or contracture.

A detailed neurologic examination is mandatory to detect deficits. This should include an evaluation of motor and sensory function as well as the tendon reflexes in both upper and lower limbs; the examiner should assess for signs of nerve root tension and symmetry of the abdominal reflexes and should exclude the presence of clonus. Magnetic resonance (MR) imaging of the entire spine should be routinely performed when congenital vertebral anomalies are identified on plain radiographs, especially if surgical treatment is planned. MR imaging of the brain is indicated in a patient with a Chiari malformation, which can produce an increased fluid collection in the ventricles and raised intracranial pressure. Intraspinal abnormalities can occasionally affect the risk for and rate of deformity progression more than the associated congenital vertebral defects. The surgical correction of a spinal deformity can result in severe neurologic complications if it is undertaken before the dysraphic pathology is treated, particularly in the case of a fixed cord due to distal tethering, a diastematomyelia (typically a split cord due to a bony spur or fibrous band), or herniation of the cerebellar tonsils through the foramen magnum. The intraspinal anomaly is usually addressed first, with subsequent surgery to treat the progressive spinal deformity. Recent reports have indicated possible benefits of the simultaneous treatment of both types of pathology during the same procedure.

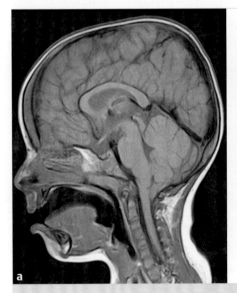 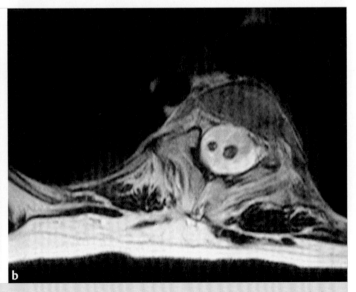

Fig. 7.2 (a) Lateral magnetic resonance image of the head and neck shows a Chiari malformation with cerebellar descent through the foramen magnum. (b) Axial magnetic resonance image across the thoracic spine demonstrates a split spinal cord due to diastematomyelia.

7.2.3 Cardiac Defects

Congenital cardiac defects occur in 26% of patients with congenital deformities of the spine; the incidence is highest in patients with mixed anomalies and failures of segmentation. Ventricular and atrial septal defects are the most common, but more complex abnormalities, including tetralogy of Fallot, patent ductus arteriosus, and transposition of the great vessels, may be encountered. A cardiac review with echocardiography and an ultrasound examination is recommended as part of the initial patient evaluation. Severe cardiac anomalies may necessitate multiple surgeries at different stages of growth and must be addressed before correction of a spinal deformity is considered.

7.2.4 Genitourinary Abnormalities

Abnormalities of the kidneys, ureters, bladder, or urethra can occur in 20 to 35% of patients with a congenital scoliosis. These can vary from unilateral absence of a kidney, which may be asymptomatic, to obstructive uropathy including duplicate or mega-ureters, horseshoe kidney, ectopic kidney, renal hypoplasia, and hypo- or epispadias. Renal ultrasound can be used as an initial routine screening test; up to one-third of patients with anomalies require urologic treatment. MR imaging of the spine that includes the abdomen can also demonstrate the abnormalities.

7.2.5 Gastrointestinal Anomalies

Anomalies of the gastrointestinal tract can occur in 5 to 15% of patients with congenital scoliosis and include esophageal atresia, trachea-esophageal fistula, congenital diaphragmatic hernia, and anorectal malformations.

7.3 Imaging

Plain radiographs of the spine can facilitate recognition of the anatomical pattern and the classification of congenital vertebral anomalies, as well as the detection of curve progression and the response to treatment. The radiographs are taken with the patient standing except in the case of infants before walking stage; radiographs can be obtained while they are supine or sitting. As the patient's development progresses from the supine to the sitting stage, apparent curve deterioration may be observed and does not necessarily signify true aggravation of the deformity. A lateral radiograph is necessary to exclude associated kyphosis, which carries the highest risk for neurologic complications.

Posteroanterior and lateral radiographs can be obtained to determine the type of vertebral abnormality, measure the size of the curvature, and assess growth potential around the area of the vertebral anomalies.

Curve progression can be documented by using consistent anatomical landmarks on serial radiographs; errors in the Cobb angle measurement can vary between 3 and 12 degrees. Defining the growth potential of the vertebral abnormality provides an indication of the risk for curve deterioration until skeletal maturity. A fully segmented hemivertebra with normal disk spaces and end plates both above and below can be considered an example of maximal asymmetric growth and increased risk for scoliosis progression compared with a semisegmented or incarcerated hemivertebra, and this can usually be recognized on plain radiographs. The prognosis of a patient with a unilateral unsegmented bar to a large degree depends on whether open, normal-appearing disk spaces are present on the opposite side, indicating active growth plates and an increased deforming force. Radiographs, including supine traction and side-bending views as well as views obtained with the patient lying against a bolster, can also be used during surgical planning to assess the flexibility of the deformity in the coronal and sagittal planes.

The advent of computed tomography (CT) has improved the ability to determine in detail the spatial anatomy of vertebral abnormalities, including posterior element defects. The three-dimensional reconstruction of CT scans has become an integral part of surgical planning, with a reported 100% accuracy in recognizing anomalies that were discovered during surgery but were undetected on plain films. MR imaging of the spine has replaced myelography as the procedure of choice to detect occult spinal dysraphism, and all patients with a progressive deformity that requires surgical treatment should undergo this procedure, as should patients with abnormal neurologic findings and symptoms or coexisting cutaneous lesions over the spine. Spinal MR imaging will also demonstrate canal stenosis and cord compression in patients with a posterior or posterolateral hemivertebra and a kyphotic or kyphoscoliotic deformity, as well as the response to surgical treatment.

7.4 Treatment

The cornerstone of treatment in children with congenital deformities of the spine is an accurate early diagnosis of those types of vertebral anomalies that carry a maximal risk for producing progressive curves and have the potential to cause neurologic compromise. This will allow adequate decision making and surgical planning to prevent the development of a severe deformity. The surgeon's skill in treating patients with congenital spinal deformities consists not only of the ability to conduct complex and technically very challenging procedures that involve significant risks for major medical and neurologic morbidity but also the experience to recognize at a young age aggressive deformities, anticipate a poor prognosis, and initiate early prophylactic surgery.

7.4.1 Observation

Close monitoring of all patients with congenital vertebral anomalies is required in order to detect the progression of congenital and structural compensatory curves at an early stage and apply appropriate treatment. The type of vertebral abnormality and spinal deformity will define the natural history and prognosis. Patients should be followed until skeletal maturity, usually at 6- to 12-month intervals, with serial radiographs; closer screening is needed during periods of rapid skeletal growth through the first 3 years of life and again through puberty. The clinical examination should include a neurologic assessment at every visit in order to diagnose subtle changes in neurologic function that may alert the clinician to the need for earlier spinal or neurosurgical treatment.

Certain failures of vertebral formation (unsegmented or incarcerated hemivertebra) and segmentation (block vertebra) can be predictably expected to remain fairly stable or change by only a few degrees at follow-up, and these are unlikely to require surgical treatment. In contrast, unilateral failures of segmentation (unilateral unsegmented bar with or without a contralateral hemivertebra at the same level) or fully segmented hemivertebrae have a significant deforming potential and usually require early surgery.

7.4.2 Bracing

Brace treatment is not effective to control congenital curves, which are structurally abnormal and rigid. In addition, the application of a brace and the exertion of corrective forces through the rib cage in young children can produce or exacerbate chest wall deformities. Bracing may be used to slow or prevent the deterioration of a structural compensatory curve developing across the levels cephalic to or caudal to a congenital scoliosis. An underarm brace can also be used following resection of a hemivertebra and segmental instrumented fusion of the proximal and distal vertebrae in order to control a scoliosis that spans more levels above and below. This preserves spinal growth and delays the need for a longer fusion at a later age.

7.4.3 Surgical Treatment

Surgical correction is indicated when curve progression is documented. It is also indicated as a prophylactic measure in the presence of vertebral anomalies that carry an unfavorable prognosis and are likely to produce severe deformities and/or neurologic complications. Good examples are the following: (1) scoliosis due to a unilateral unsegmented bar with or without a contralateral hemivertebra at the same level; (2) kyphosis due to a posterior hemivertebra; (3) kyphoscoliosis due to a posterolateral quadrant vertebra or an anterolateral unsegmented bar

with a contralateral quadrant vertebra. The patient's age is not necessarily a limiting factor when surgical correction is undertaken for curvatures that are expected to progress rapidly.

Global spinal imbalance and trunk decompensation in relation to the type and location of the deformity should also be taken into consideration during decision making regarding surgical treatment. Congenital scoliosis affecting transitional areas of the spine is likely to be more disfiguring. Cervicothoracic curves produce a significant deformity due to shoulder asymmetry and neck tilt and are likely to require stabilization. In addition, congenital scoliosis in the lumbosacral junction is very deforming because it produces an oblique take-off of the spine, often with marked pelvic obliquity and the consequent development of a structural compensatory lumbar curve that progresses rapidly. Surgical correction of a congenital lumbosacral curve is indicated at an early stage of growth, ideally before the development of a structural compensatory lumbar scoliosis. If the patient presents with an already established structural compensatory curve, this may need to be included within the fusion levels, resulting in larger compromise of spinal growth.

The goal of surgery is to produce a balanced spine with a stable thoracic cage, delay the need for fusion to preserve spinal growth and development of the chest, and limit the number of vertebral segments included within the fusion to maintain flexibility of the spine. Neurosurgical procedures to correct associated dysraphic lesions, such as tethered cord, diastematomyelia, and Chiari I malformation, reduce the neurologic risk during deformity correction. Intraoperative monitoring of the spinal cord during deformity surgery by recording somatosensory and motor evoked potentials is mandatory to reduce the risk for neurologic complications, which is particularly high when kyphotic curves are corrected. Changes in baseline monitoring potentials should be addressed immediately through a joint approach by the surgeons, anesthesiologists, and neurophysiologists. The blood supply to the spinal cord in patients with extensive congenital vertebral and intraspinal anomalies is abnormal, and therefore every effort must be made to minimize intraoperative blood loss and limit hypotension. Equally, distraction techniques should be avoided in the presence of vertebral and neuroaxial abnormalities. Before surgery or after anterior spinal releases, halo-gravity, halo-femoral, or halo-pelvic traction for a few weeks can be effective to achieve a gradual increase in curve flexibility and a greater correction during the later stage of the procedure.

Surgical options include the following: in situ fusion, convex hemi-epiphysiodesis (growth arrest procedure); deformity correction through posterior spinal fusion by means of instrumentation associated with releases and facetectomies; deformity correction through spinal osteotomies followed by fusion; deformity correction through vertebral column resection and fusion; and growth preservation techniques (growing rod, vertebral expandable prosthetic titanium rib [VEPTR]). Often, more than one technique is required for the same patient to address complex deformities affecting different levels of the spine.

In Situ Fusion

In situ fusion is best indicated in young patients who have a small congenital curve due to a unilateral unsegmented bar with or without a contralateral hemivertebra at the same level or a mixed anomaly. The aim is to stabilize the deformity because correction of the deformity with a bone graft cannot be expected. The procedure should be performed as prophylactic treatment when progression has been documented and the curvature is still minimal. In the presence of a failure of vertebral segmentation or a mixed anomaly that limits longitudinal growth of the spine, an early fusion does not have adverse effects on the patient's predicted height and development. Complete facetectomies and posterior decortications should be followed by bone grafting to achieve a solid fusion. Iliac crest autograft remains the gold standard but can be safely obtained only in older children; in younger patients, quantities are insufficient and the risk for associated donor site morbidity is greater. Autologous rib graft can be harvested through the posterior spinal approach and a subperiosteal exposure; this can be supplemented by allograft bone. The arthrodesis should include one level above and below the levels of the vertebral anomalies followed by the application of a plaster jacket for 3 to 4 months. A spinal cast cannot be used for cervicothoracic or upper thoracic curves, but in the presence of segmentation or mixed abnormalities, the risk for nonunion is smaller.

If the patient is small, pediatric instrumentation can be used in conjunction with the in situ fusion to provide a more stable fixation, reduce the risk for nonunion and bending of the fusion mass, which can occur in 14% of patients, and allow some degree of correction across the levels above and below the segmentation anomaly. The risk for the crankshaft effect, which can result from continuous anterior vertebral growth when a solid posterior fusion has been attained, can be eliminated by the addition of an anterior fusion performed through an open or thoracoscopic approach.

Congenital thoracic scoliosis due to a unilateral unsegmented bar with or without a contralateral hemivertebra can be treated effectively with an isolated anterior convex fusion (no need for an additional posterior in situ fusion) and the placement of an autologous rib strut extending one level above and below the vertebral abnormality. This eliminates the concave tethering effect and convex deforming force by converting the affected level to a block segment with no residual growth potential. Increased blood loss should be expected in young children with a small body weight during preparation of the vertebral bodies to position the rib strut graft.

A localized posterior in situ fusion with bone graft is also indicated for patients who have a congenital kyphosis of up to 50 degrees and who are younger than 5 years of age in order to produce a posterior bony tether; the fusion should extend at least one level above and below the most sagittally tilted vertebra. Preserving residual anterior vertebral growth in the presence of a solid posterior fusion will allow some degree of spontaneous kyphosis correction during the remaining stages of growth, but this is difficult to predict. The risk for nonunion following initial surgery is high because of the mechanical disadvantage of the bone graft, which is under tension. Placement of a spinal jacket is indicated for a period of 3 to 4 months. There should be a low threshold for exploration of the fusion mass to repair a pseudarthrosis or augment a weak fusion if progression of the deformity by more than 5 degrees is observed within the first months after cast removal. In congenital lordosis, an anterior in situ fusion alone can be sufficient to control the deformity.

Convex Growth Arrest (Hemi-epiphysiodesis)

This procedure can be performed through a combined anterior and posterior approach to the spine at the convex side of the curve, preferably in young children with a short, modest congenital scoliosis due to a thoracic hemivertebra. The convex half of the disk and adjacent end plates are removed at the level of the hemivertebra, as well as across one segment proximal and one segment distal. The posterior hemi-epiphysiodesis extends along the same levels, and the concave side is not exposed. The procedure eliminates the deforming force across the convexity and can allow a gradual spontaneous reduction of the scoliosis over time as a consequence of contralateral vertebral growth; however, the final outcome is variable, with long-term results demonstrating 0 to 20 degrees of total correction. A hemi-epiphysiodesis performed in the presence of a unilateral unsegmented bar, which prevents concave growth, acts like an in situ fusion and is not expected to reduce the size of the curve.

An isolated anterior convex growth arrest with an autologous rib strut graft obtained during thoracotomy is as successful as the combined procedure in controlling congenital thoracic scoliosis due to a hemivertebra. This has a localized kyphogenic effect resulting from the presence of normal remaining posterior growth and therefore preserves the normal sagittal contour of the spine. In contrast, an isolated anterior hemi-epiphysiodesis in the lumbar spine can produce a hypolordotic or kyphotic deformity. In this case, the convex growth arrest can be best performed through a combined anterior and posterior approach to the spine. In general, the development of hemivertebra resection techniques, especially through posterior approaches to the spine, can produce predictably superior results and have limited the role of hemi-epiphysiodesis.

Hemivertebra Excision

Hemivertebra excision is indicated for patients with progressive congenital scoliosis, kyphoscoliosis, or kyphosis due to a lateral, posterolateral, or posterior fully segmented or semisegmented hemivertebra. The advantage of the procedure is that it removes the abnormal vertebral segment and eliminates the deforming force, providing a better ability to balance the spine. It can be used even for severe curves in which a localized in situ fusion or a convex hemi-epiphysiodesis would be unable to produce adequate global spinal alignment. The procedure is technically challenging and should be performed by surgeons with a high level of expertise because of the increased risk for neurologic complications.

Hemivertebra resection should ideally be performed in children around the age of 2 years, when the anatomy is easier to identify because the vertebrae are more ossified, a fusion can be achieved more predictably, and pedicle screw instrumentation can be used. The procedure is safer when the hemivertebra is located below the level of the spinal cord, where the neural elements are more amenable to manipulation. The ideal indication for a hemivertebra excision is a lumbosacral hemivertebra, which is associated with an increased risk for an oblique take-off of the spine and severe deformity. Caution must be exercised because the sacrum is often posteriorly deficient in a patient with a wide spina bifida, which makes the application of instrumentation challenging. Hemivertebra resection can also be performed safely in the thoracic spine. More than one ipsilateral hemivertebra can be excised during the same or separate procedures, depending on the patient's reaction during surgery.

A lateral or posterolateral hemivertebra can be excised through either a combined sequential anteroposterior or an isolated posterior approach to the spine. Simultaneous anterior and posterior exposure of the spine can also be achieved with the patient in the lateral decubitus position, which allows resection of the hemivertebra and adjacent disks, followed by the placement of posterior compressive instrumentation to correct the deformity. Compared with the posterior-only procedure, a combined anteroposterior hemivertebra resection can significantly increase the amount of intraoperative blood loss as a result of vertebral body bleeding in an open space during the anterior stage.

The isolated posterior procedure is less invasive and includes initial removal of the abnormal posterior elements followed by hemivertebra excision in a piecemeal manner through the pedicle. The lateral wall of the hemivertebra is removed through a subperiosteal exposure to protect the segmental and major vessels anteriorly. The disks above and below the hemivertebra are excised, and the disk on the side opposite to the hemivertebra is released to allow compression of the remaining convex gap through the instrumentation. Spinal instrumentation is superior to casting for achieving and maintaining deformity correction. Despite the ability to stabilize the spine with small modern instrumentation, postoperative support through a plaster jacket is advised for 3 to 4 months after hemivertebra excision. Wedge resection of a posterior hemivertebra causing a pure congenital kyphosis is best done through a posterior approach to the spine, which provides better access to the anomalous vertebra than does the anterior approach, followed by segmental stabilization and fusion.

Congenital scoliosis or kyphoscoliosis due to a hemivertebra may occasionally extend across a longer segment of the spine. In that case, after hemivertebra excision, the instrumented fusion may have to span more levels and so will have a greater impact on vertebral growth (▶ Fig. 7.3). Alternatively, the patient can be fitted with an underarm brace as an additional measure to control adjacent level deformity, preserve growth, and delay the need for extension of the fusion until a later age.

Instrumented Correction and Fusion

This is indicated for older patients with stiff congenital curves, in whom global balancing of the spine with partial deformity correction can be achieved across the adjacent mobile segments cephalic and caudal to the anomalous vertebra (▶ Fig. 7.4). The use of pedicle screw and hook or all pedicle screw instrumentation allows some degree of deformity correction and solid spinal fixation, which will enhance fusion. Because of the presence of posterior element fusions or defects, the vertebral anatomy may be difficult to recognize, and the application of instrumentation can be challenging. The application of distraction forces on the concavity of a congenital scoliosis and in the presence of a kyphosis should be avoided as much as preoperative skeletal traction because of the increased neurologic risk.

The addition of an anterior spinal release can address the risk for the crankshaft phenomenon in young children; it can also increase curve flexibility, mainly across the normal vertebral segments included in the deformity above and below the abnormalities, and it provides the cosmetic benefit of the anterior thoracoplasty. Staging an anterior spinal release and posterior instrumented fusion allows the application of traction for a few weeks between the two procedures, with the aim of achieving a greater correction of severe deformities. This requires continuous monitoring of neurologic function, which can be affected by the exertion of distraction forces on the spinal column and cord.

In a patient with a sharply angular congenital kyphosis, a posterior implant may become prominent under the

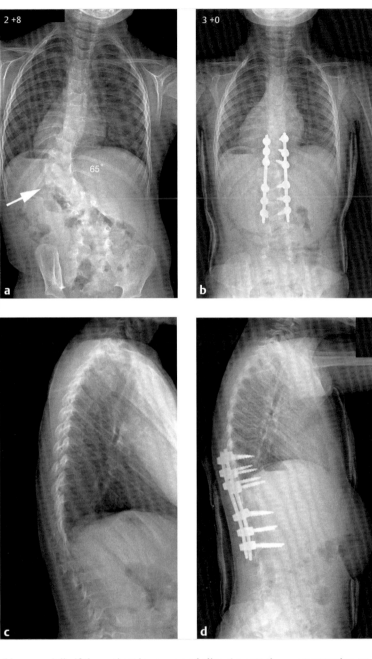

Fig. 7.3 Posteroanterior (**a**) and lateral (**c**) radiographs of a patient with a severe congenital kyphoscoliosis and marked spinal imbalance due to the presence of a fully segmented posterolateral hemivertebra. Surgical resection of the hemivertebra followed by instrumented fusion restored spinal balance in the coronal and sagittal planes at age 2 + 8 years (**b, d**). A spinal jacket was applied after surgery for 3 months to provide additional stability.

skin, especially if the patient is young and slim. An anterior arthrodesis with a vascularized or free rib strut autograft can provide support to the spine and achieve fusion if posterior instrumentation cannot be used. This should be followed by postoperative casting for 3 to 4 months to increase stability until fusion of the rib graft has occurred.

Spinal Reconstruction with Osteotomies and Vertebral Column Resection

Complex spinal reconstruction can be performed through multisegment closing wedge and pedicle subtraction osteotomies or vertebral column resection followed by instrumented fusion. This is reserved for patients who have very severe, rigid, and neglected deformities that produce a highly unbalanced spine with marked decompensation of the trunk, fixed pelvic obliquity, or associated neurologic compromise. Such extreme deformities may require resection of part of the vertebral column, and this can be done through either a posterior-only or an anteroposterior approach to the spine, depending on the type and location of the congenital vertebral anomalies.

A posterior approach is particularly indicated in patients who have significant congenital kyphosis or kyphoscoliosis with or without neurologic complications

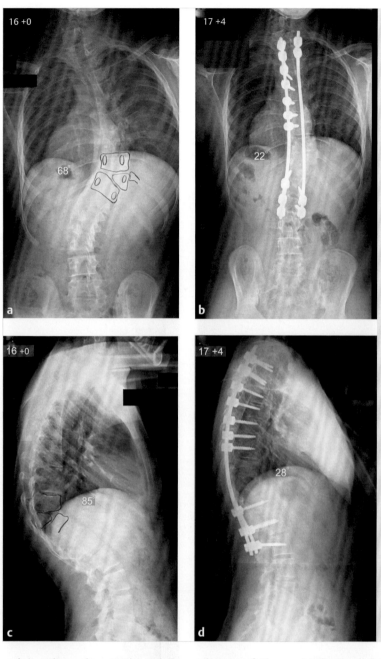

Fig. 7.4 Posteroanterior (**a**) and lateral (**c**) radiographs of an adolescent patient with a severe congenital kyphoscoliosis due to a posterolateral quadrant vertebra in the thoracolumbar junction. The patient underwent a posterior spinal fusion, which achieved good correction of the deformity in the coronal and sagittal planes (**b, d**).

and in whom the anterior column and apex of the deformity are positioned posteriorly. The posterior-only subperiosteal resection also has the advantage of preserving the segmental vessels, which may be abnormal, especially around the levels of the vertebral anomalies; thus, the neurologic risk is less in comparison with that of an anteroposterior resection, in which the convex vessels have to be sacrificed.

Posterior-only procedures allow severe deformities to be corrected through a single approach but are technically demanding. In addition, they are medically and neurologically risky because dural and spinal cord manipulation is required, significant blood loss limits

visualization of the anterior column and can be life-threatening in small patients with a small total volume of blood, and spinal column instability may develop that can displace the osteotomy intra- or postoperatively. The anterior vertebral column can also be accessed in a costo-transversectomy via a posterior approach, particularly in patients who have severe congenital scoliosis or kyphoscoliosis with an extreme degree of rotation requiring circumferential deformity correction.

Spinal osteotomies through previous fusion masses may be needed during revision surgery to address residual or recurrent congenital curves. Osteotomy of a unilateral unsegmented bar can be performed at the apex of the curve, often in association with a contralateral hemi-vertebra resection through a posterior approach to the spine in order to achieve acute correction of a severe deformity followed by instrumented fusion.

Growth Preservation Techniques

Trunk height and often thoracic cage development are reduced in children who have complex congenital deformities in comparison with those who have normal spines, and the reduction is directly proportional to the number and extent of vertebral anomalies. The growth of the spinal column is greatest during the first 5 years of life, by which time the sitting height reaches two-thirds of its adult level. Children younger than 5 years with severe congenital or structural compensatory curves present a treatment challenge because every effort should be made to avoid early fusion, which will cause further stunting of spinal growth.

Instrumentation without fusion in the form of *growing rods* has been extensively used in patients with early onset scoliosis of idiopathic or syndromic etiology.

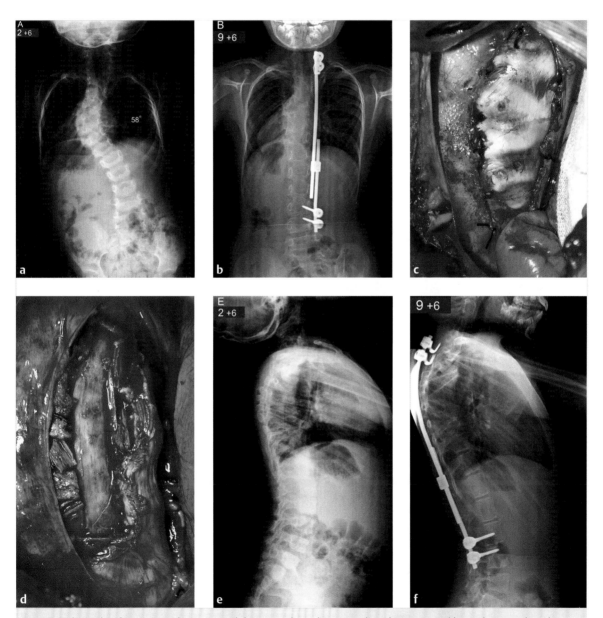

Fig. 7.5 Radiographs of a patient with a congenital thoracic scoliosis due to a unilateral unsegmented bar with a contralateral hemivertebra (**a, e**). At age 2 + 6 years, the patient underwent an anterior convex hemi-epiphysiodesis with the use of a rib strut (**c, d**) and simultaneous placement of a concave growing rod construct. Consecutive lengthening procedures gradually achieved full correction of the scoliosis, maintained good sagittal balance, and preserved spinal growth (**b, f**).

Growing rods can also be applied in patients with congenital scoliosis, in whom the experience is more limited, to prevent deformity progression, maximize growth of the spine, and delay definitive fusion until a later age. A growing rod would be indicated in a child with scoliosis due to a unilateral failure of segmentation, in combination with a limited anterior convex fusion, to control the adjacent level deformities above and below the levels of the fusion (▶ Fig. 7.5). Equally, it would be indicated in a child with a long congenital thoracic scoliosis due to a hemivertebra treated by a convex growth arrest as an adjunct to prevent deterioration of the curve across the segments cephalic and caudal to the hemivertebra. A prerequisite is the presence of adequate anatomical landmarks to allow the placement of foundation anchors in the upper thoracic and lumbar regions.

The placement of growing rods involves limited subperiosteal exposure of the spine at the proximal and distal ends for the insertion of hooks and/or screws, along with segmental bone grafting to reinforce the construct foundations. The rods are placed under the fascia and linked either through end-to-end or lateral domino connectors. Unilateral or bilateral constructs can be used. Complications of growing rods include rod breakage, hook dislodgment, and screw pullout, which occur most commonly with unilateral constructs. In addition, gradual stiffening of the spine and spontaneous fusions result in a limited ability of the spine to lengthen over time, which happens earlier if a bilateral construct has been used. All lengthening procedures, which typically are done at 6-month intervals, have a kyphogenic effect, and the development of proximal junctional kyphosis is one of the most severe and difficult to correct complications of growing rods. Supportive bracing may reduce the risk for implant failure while the growing rods are in place.

Rib fusions produce a tethering effect and a constricted thorax, with reduced development of the lung parenchyma. A progressive congenital deformity can further compromise the height of the chest and respiratory function. Early thoracic fusions to address aggressive congenital deformities, especially before the age of 8 years, when most lung growth and alveolar development occurs, will impair growth of the spine and rib cage and cause a restrictive lung disease predisposing to thoracic insufficiency syndrome. The *vertical expandable prosthetic titanium rib* (VEPTR) has been developed to address severe congenital rib and chest wall deformities that lead to thoracic insufficiency syndrome. Thoracic wall anomalies can occur in isolation, together with vertebral segmentation abnormalities, or as part of a syndromic condition, such as spondylocostal dysostosis or spondylothoracic dysplasia.

Campbell et al suggested that extensive rib fusions affecting the hemithorax on the concavity of a congenital scoliosis in growing children can act as a powerful lateral tether to further unbalance the development of the spine, and they described the "windswept" thorax. To overcome the problem of congenital scoliosis associated with chest wall anomalies producing thoracic insufficiency, Campbell et al. developed the surgical technique of expansion thoracoplasty, in which the concave segments of fused ribs are osteotomized and the hemithorax is lengthened and stabilized by serial rib distractions with the VEPTR. This includes a rib-to-rib and a rib-to-spine device secured at the anchor points with the use of hooks. The rods are lengthened every 4 to 6 months through interconnectors in a way similar to that used for growing rods. The VEPTR complication rate is comparable with that of growing rod techniques. Complications include rod breakage, hook dislodgment, implant migration, wound infections, brachial plexus injury, and rib fractures. The adverse effects of expansion thoracotomy and subsequent scarring on an already compromised chest have not been clarified. Recent studies have indicated that the increased volume of the constricted hemithorax and the total lung volumes obtained during initial chest expansion are maintained at follow-up. Consensus has not been reached on the role of the VEPTR and any possible advantages over traditional growing rods in the treatment of congenital scoliosis with no associated rib fusions or thoracic insufficiency.

Further Reading

Andrew T, Piggott H. Growth arrest for progressive scoliosis. Combined anterior and posterior fusion of the convexity. J Bone Joint Surg Br 1985; 67: 193–197

Basu PS, Elsebaie H, Noordeen MH. Congenital spinal deformity: a comprehensive assessment at presentation. Spine 2002; 27: 2255–2259

Beals RK, Robbins JR, Rolfe B. Anomalies associated with vertebral malformations. Spine 1993; 18: 1329–1332

Campbell RM Jr Hell-Vocke AK. Growth of the thoracic spine in congenital scoliosis after expansion thoracoplasty. J Bone Joint Surg Am 2003; 85-A: 409–420

Campbell RM Jr Smith MD, Mayes TC et al. The characteristics of thoracic insufficiency syndrome associated with fused ribs and congenital scoliosis. J Bone Joint Surg Am 2003; 85-A: 399–408

Deviren V, Berven S, Smith JA, Emami A, Hu SS, Bradford DS. Excision of hemivertebrae in the management of congenital scoliosis involving the thoracic and thoracolumbar spine. J Bone Joint Surg Br 2001; 83: 496–500

Holte DC, Winter RB, Lonstein JE, Denis F. Excision of hemivertebrae and wedge resection in the treatment of congenital scoliosis. J Bone Joint Surg Am 1995; 77: 159–171

Klemme WR, Denis F, Winter RB, Lonstein JW, Koop SE. Spinal instrumentation without fusion for progressive scoliosis in young children. J Pediatr Orthop 1997; 17: 734–742

Klemme WR, Polly DW Jr Orchowski JR. Hemivertebral excision for congenital scoliosis in very young children. J Pediatr Orthop 2001; 21: 761–764

McMaster MJ. Occult intraspinal anomalies and congenital scoliosis. J Bone Joint Surg Am 1984; 66: 588–601

Ruf M, Harms J. Hemivertebra resection by a posterior approach: innovative operative technique and first results. Spine 2002; 27: 1116–1123

Ruf M, Jensen R, Letko L, Harms J. Hemivertebra resection and osteotomies in congenital spine deformity. Spine 2009; 34: 1791–1799

Thompson AG, Marks DS, Sayampanathan SR, Piggott H. Long-term results of combined anterior and posterior convex epiphysiodesis for congenital scoliosis due to hemivertebrae. Spine 1995; 20: 1380–1385

Tsirikos AI, McMaster MJ. Congenital anomalies of the ribs and chest wall associated with congenital deformities of the spine. J Bone Joint Surg Am 2005; 87: 2523–2536

Winter RB, Moe JH, Eilers VE. Congenital scoliosis. A study of 234 patients treated and untreated. Part 2. Treatment. J Bone Joint Surg Am 1968; 50: 15–47

Winter RB, Moe JH, Lonstein JE. Posterior spinal arthrodesis for congenital scoliosis. An analysis of the cases of two hundred and ninety patients, five to nineteen years old. J Bone Joint Surg Am 1984; 66: 1188–1197

Winter RB, Moe JH, Wang JK. Congenital kyphosis. Its natural history and treatment as observed in a study of 130 patients. J Bone Joint Surg Am 1973; 55: 223–256

8 Surgical Treatment: The Nottingham Experience

John K. Webb and Nasir A. Quraishi

Early onset scoliosis is a heterogeneous condition. The prognosis and natural history vary widely, depending on whether the cause is congenital, idiopathic, syndromic, or neuromuscular. The majority of cases of early onset idiopathic scoliosis resolve spontaneously. Fewer than 10% of cases progress, but unless they are treated early, progression may be rapid and lead to severe deformity. Therefore, the early recognition and stabilization of potentially progressive curves are key to the successful treatment of this complex problem. An ideal method of stabilizing early onset idiopathic scoliosis in a growing child should (1) correct and stabilize the curve, (2) allow normal growth of the spine, and (3) prevent the crankshaft phenomenon, which is due to disproportionate anterior vertebral growth. Unfortunately, there is no known surgical or nonsurgical treatment method that addresses all of these factors adequately.

The growth rate of the spinal column varies bimodally with age, with the most rapid growth taking place from birth to the age of 2 years and further rapid growth occurring at adolescence. Although the spine has a major effect on the development of the lungs and thoracic cavity, cross-sectional volume also depends on the growth of the ribs, both in length and degree of rib obliquity. The thoracic volume increases to 30% of its adult size by 5 years of age and to 50% of its adult size by 10 years of age. Curve progression or early fusion can limit the thoracic volume, which in turn can lead to respiratory failure and early mortality.

Because of the dismal natural history of early onset scoliosis and the unfavorable effects of early fusion, a variety of surgical techniques have been used in an attempt to avoid, delay, or limit spinal fusion. These "growth-friendly" techniques and implants provide curve control and limit early spinal fusion.[1] Casting techniques were commonly used for the treatment of scoliosis before the introduction of spinal instrumentation.[2] Skin complications have been reported, and attention to meticulous technique is essential. Growth-friendly implants to control thoracic spinal deformity and minimize its adverse impact on the growth and development of the spine and thorax can be based on distraction techniques; these include growth rods and the vertical expandable prosthetic titanium rib (VEPTR; Synthes, West Chester, Pennsylvania). Implants can also be based on guided growth (e.g., Luque trolley, Shilla procedure) or compression techniques (e.g., tethers, staples). In larger curves, preoperative halo traction is sometimes used before instrumentation in an effort to decrease neurologic risk, obtain better correction, and improve pulmonary function before surgery. The use of traction in early onset scoliosis with curves larger than 80 degrees and curves associated with kyphosis before the placement of growth-friendly instrumentation has been described.[3]

In 1990, the senior author [JKW] first reported the use of segmental spinal instrumentation in which Luque rods were used without fusion for early onset idiopathic scoliosis. The principle was to leave a part of the Luque rods straight at either end, beyond the overlapped section, to allow the spine to grow along the rods. The Luque rods acted like a trolley to guide spinal growth while maintaining correction until the adolescent growth spurt, when the construct might fail because of growth of the spine beyond the limit that the construct could hold. The Luque trolley (LT) could then be replaced with definitive instrumentation for final curve correction and fusion.

Over the years, the configuration of the LT has evolved to some extent, but the basic principle has remained the same. In 1999, a short-term result (up to 5 years) was published.[4] This showed that LT instrumentation alone did not prevent curve progression (Cobb angle corrected from 56 degrees [range, 46–67 degrees] to 43 degrees [range, 24–55 degrees]). Additional convex epiphysiodesis resulted in curve resolution in some patients; the mean preoperative Cobb angle was 65 degrees (range, 40–95 degrees), the mean Cobb angle was 26 degrees (range, 8–66 degrees) after the combined surgery, and it was 32 degrees (range, 0–86 degrees) at the 5-year follow-up. The 5-year growth was 2.9 cm (49% of that expected for age- and gender-matched normal subjects; range, 31–71%) for LT only and 2 cm (32% of expected for age-and gender-matched normal subjects; range, 11–53%) for convex hemi-epiphysiodesis (CE) and LT. These results emphasized that the LT construct alone was ineffective to prevent curve progression, but when used in conjunction with CE, it supported spinal growth while either the curve resolved or correction was maintained. During further follow-up, deterioration of the curve at around the time of the adolescent growth spurt was noted in some of the patients, as expected, and they were treated with definitive instrumentation and fusion. Surprisingly, the curves of many patients did not deteriorate, and they not require any further surgery despite having significant spinal growth. In this chapter, we describe our technique of CE and LT for patients with early onset idiopathic scoliosis and their long-term follow-up at a minimum age of 16 years.

8.1 Surgical Technique

8.1.1 Convex Epiphysiodesis

A convex thoracotomy was performed through the rib two levels above the apex. The apex was exposed, and

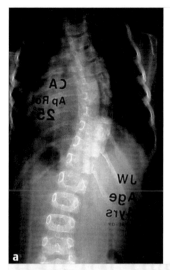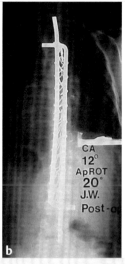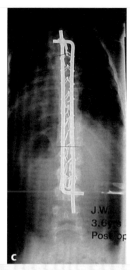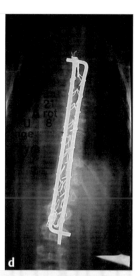

Fig. 8.1 (**a**) A 4-year-old boy with a 44-degree right thoracic curve. (**b**) Radiograph obtained immediately after initial surgery with a convex hemi-epiphysiodesis and Luque trolley growing rod and an I construct with projected straight ends to accommodate growth. (**c**) At 3.6-year postoperative follow-up, the curve is well maintained (12 degrees) with the instrumentation while growing along the rods. (**d**) At 5-year follow-up (patient 9 years of age), the spine continues to grow beyond the limits of the projected straight ends of the rod at the superior end, and the curve tends to deteriorate (21 degrees).

the apical disks and adjacent growth plates that did not correct on side-bending films were excised on the convex side back to the posterior longitudinal ligament (three to five levels around the apical vertebra). The excised rib furnished graft for that side. The combination of LT and epiphysiodesis was staged; the epiphysiodesis was done first, with a mean interval of 5 weeks between the procedures.

8.1.2 Segmental Spinal Instrumentation without Fusion

We employed a posterior extraperiosteal approach with diathermy to prevent new bone formation. The facet joint capsules were preserved. Sublaminar wires were passed at each level and the end vertebrae double-wired. Before 1988 (14 patients), Luque rods were used in an overlapped *I* configuration (▶ Fig. 8.1). The straight ends of the rods were kept 3 to 5 cm longer beyond the curved end of the other rod at either end, which allowed the spine to grow along its length. After 1989, because the proximal straight end tended to project prominently under the skin, the configuration was changed to an overlapped *u* shape (▶ Fig. 8.2, ▶ Fig. 8.3, ▶ Fig. 8.4). Postoperative bracing was not used in any case. Spinal cord monitoring with sensory evoked potentials and motor evoked potentials was done in all cases.

8.1.3 Our Results

From 1984 to 1992, we operated with CE and LT on 31 patients who had progressive deformity due to early

onset idiopathic scoliosis. The mean age of the patients at surgery was 4 years and 4 months (range, 1.5–9 years). The mean time between the diagnosis of scoliosis and surgical correction was 2 years and 7 months (range, 4 months–6 years). All the patients were Risser grade 0 at the time of initial surgery. The indication for surgery was documented curve progression and an apical rib–vertebral angle difference (RVAD) exceeding 20 degrees with or without overlap of the rib head on the apical vertebra on the convex side. Six patients had failed brace treatment, which had been tried in selected cases before 1989 but was not used thereafter. Of the 31 patients treated, 23 (14 boys and 9 girls), who had reached a minimum 16 years of age at final follow-up, were reviewed. The mean preoperative Cobb angle of the main thoracic curves was 62 degrees (range, 30–90 degrees). Definitive fusion and removal of the LT was required at a mean age of 14.5 years (range, 9–23 years) because of progression of scoliosis in nine of the 23 patients (mean Cobb angle, 61 degrees) and because of the development of junctional kyphosis in four of the 23 patients. In 10 patients, correction was maintained until skeletal maturity without definitive fusion (mean Cobb angle at final follow-up, 29 degrees), with curve regression actually noted in three of the 23 patients.

Instrumented segmental growth was calculated as the difference between the length of the instrumented segment, measured between the midpoints of the upper and lower instrumented end plates, after initial surgery and the length at the time of definitive surgery or final follow-up. The length was corrected for magnification. Mean instrumented segmental growth was

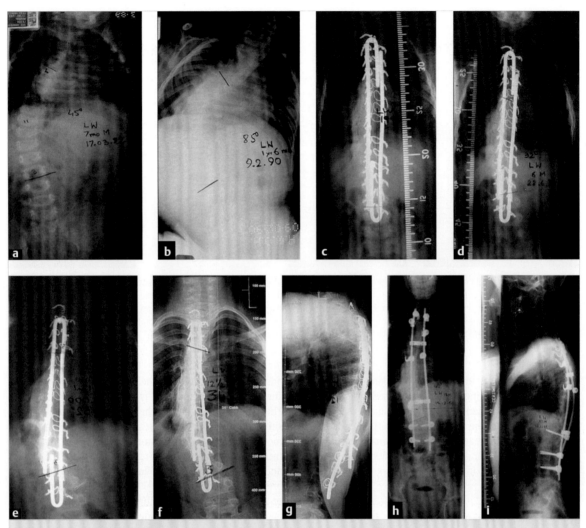

Fig. 8.2 (**a, b**) A 7-month-old boy presented with a 45-degree right thoracic curve. (**b**) When the patient was 18 months of age, the curve rapidly deteriorated to 85 degrees. He was treated at this time with convex hemi-epiphysiodesis and the Luque trolley growing rod technique (overlapped u construct). (**c–e**) The curve was maintained at 32 degrees, permitting significant spinal growth along the rods until the boy was 11½ years old. (**f, g**) During his adolescent growth spurt (at 12½ years of age), the curve started to deteriorate, with decompensation of the coronal and sagittal balance. (**h, i**) The Luque trolley was removed, and a definitive fusion was performed at 12½ years of age. The final curve magnitude was 45 degrees.

3.17 cm ± 1.44 SD (range, 1–5 cm). This was 32% of the expected growth. Scoliosis progression was predicted by the preoperative apical convex RVAD ($p = 0.03$, logistic regression). Excessive instrumented segmental growth was predictive of junctional kyphosis but not of scoliosis progression. Age at operation and initial curve size were not found to be significantly predictive of the need for definitive surgery. Finally, 72% (10 of 14) of the patients with overlapped *l* rod constructs and 33% (three of nine) of the patients with overlapped *u* rod constructs had curve progression and required definitive fusion.

8.1.4 Complications

The most common complication was broken wires (11 cases), noted particularly toward the ends of the LT instrumentation; these appeared with increasing growth of the instrumented segment. Often, they were asymptomatic. The other common complication was prominence of the rods[5] toward the end of the instrumented segment, and this was more frequently noted with the *l* rod construct. Trimming of the prominent rod at the proximal end was required in one patient. Deep infection was noted in three patients, and two of them required either

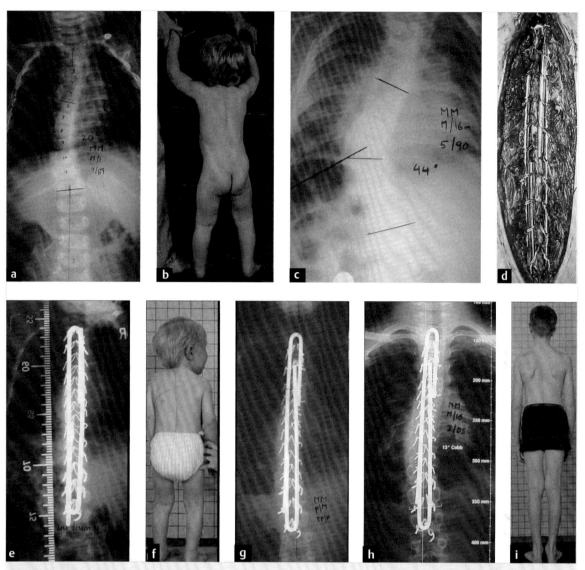

Fig. 8.3 (**a, b**) A 12-month-old boy presented with a 20-degree left thoracic curve and dextrocardia. (**c**) When he was 16 months of age, the curve rapidly deteriorated to 44 degrees. (**d–f**) At 2 years of age, he was treated with convex hemi-epiphysiodesis and the Luque trolley growing rod technique (overlapped u construct). (**g**) The curve was maintained at 32 degrees, permitting significant spinal growth along the rods until the boy was 11½ years old. (**g–i**) During his adolescent growth spurt, the curve remained stable at 25 degrees until he reached skeletal maturity at 16 years of age, without the need for any definitive surgery.

removal or trimming of the rod. Junctional kyphosis was noted in four patients. Postoperative chest infection developed in one patient. Horner syndrome developed after the primary surgery in one patient, which resolved spontaneously.

8.2 Predictive Factors for Definitive Surgery

Definitive surgery with removal of the LT and fusion with (12 patients) or without[1] instrumentation was needed in

13 patients at a mean age of 14.5 years (range, 9–23 years). Posterior instrumentation consisted of the Universal Spinal System (USS; Synthes, Oberdorf, Switzerland) in nine patients and Cotrel–Dubousset instrumentation in three patients. The indications for definitive surgery were progression of scoliosis during the adolescent growth spurt in nine patients and the development of kyphosis with prominence of the LT rods under the skin in four patients. The nine patients with deteriorating scoliosis developed a mean Cobb angle of 61 degrees (range, 55–75 degrees), which was corrected to 47 degrees (range, 24–55 degrees) following definitive surgery. This is

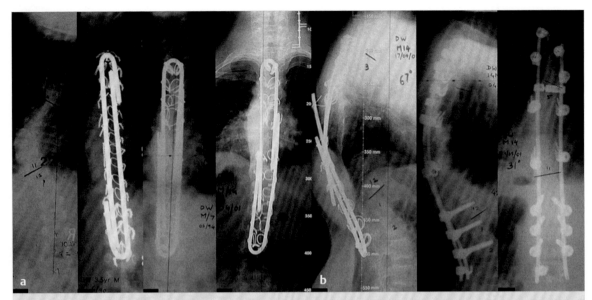

Fig. 8.4 (a) A 60-degree progressive left thoracic scoliosis in a 1½-year-old child was treated with a Luque trolley growing rod (overlapped u construct), and the Cobb angle was corrected to 28 degrees. (b) At 7 years of age, the patient had outgrown the Luque trolley growing rod construct, and the Luque trolley rods were exchanged, with a longer overlap of the u construct. At 14 years of age, when he entered the adolescent growth spurt, he had further growth of the spine (5 cm total growth). The scoliosis was maintained at 28 degrees, but progressive kyphosis developed at the apex of the curve, at the junction of the overlapped proximal and distal rods. He underwent a definitive surgery with posterior instrumented fusion (Universal Spinal System; Synthes, Oberdorf, Switzerland).

indicative of the decreased flexibility of the spine caused by the LT growing rod instrumentation despite a careful extraperiosteal dissection to prevent fusion. Large, stiff curves developed in two patients. One of them required an anterior release followed by posterior instrumentation in the same stage. The other patient required an anterior osteotomy, followed by halo traction and posterior instrumentation as a staged procedure. Solid fusion was noted around the apex of the curve at the time of removal of the LT rods in three patients; one of them had had previous infection. These patients were treated with posterior instrumentation and costoplasty. One patient had only costoplasty at 23 years of age without instrumentation. The other four patients had a moderate deterioration of scoliosis (mean Cobb angle, 48.5 degrees; range, 40–55 degrees) but developed a more severe kyphosis deformity. Junctional kyphosis was noted either at the proximal[1] or distal[1] end of the instrumented segment, or near the apex of the curve[2] at the junction of the proximal and distal Luque rods. All these patients were treated with removal of the LT rods and posterior instrumentation and fusion. Correction was maintained in 10 patients until skeletal maturity without the need for any further surgery. The mean Cobb angle in this group at final follow-up was 27 degrees (range, 13–45 degrees). Regression of the curve, compared with the curve immediately after the initial surgery, was noted in three patients.

The factors that could possibly influence progression of the scoliosis curve following initial surgery were age at initial surgery, Cobb angle at initial surgery, growth of the instrumented segment, type (l or u) of the LT construct, and preoperative RVAD. It was expected that excessive growth of the instrumented segment (mean, 3.17 cm; range, 1–5 cm) beyond the limit permitted by the overlap of the LT growing rod construct would lead to deterioration of the curve and the need for definitive surgery. Contrary to this expectation, growth of the instrumented segment was actually smaller in the definitive surgery group (mean, 2.96 cm ± 1.51 SD) than in the no-surgery group (mean, 3.45 cm ± 1.36 SD), although the difference was not significant ($p = 0.45$). When growth was compared based on the indications for definitive surgery, the four patients with progressive kyphosis[4] had significantly greater growth in the instrumented segment (mean, 4.25 ± 0.96 SD) than did the nine patients with progressive scoliosis (mean, 2.39 ± 1.36 SD; $p = 0.032$).

The l construct, in which straight ends extended beyond the overlapped section to accommodate spinal growth, was used in 14 patients earlier in this series. Only a limited section could be used as extended straight ends because the ends projected prominently under the skin. The overlapped u construct caused no such problem and was used in nine patients later in this series. Of the 14 patients with an l rod construct, 10 (72%) required definitive surgery because of progressive scoliosis[6] or because of progressive kyphosis at the proximal (one patient) or distal ends (one patient) of the instrumentation. On the other hand, only three (33%) of the nine patients with an overlapped u rod construct needed definitive surgery at a later date; surgery was required for progressive scoliosis in one and for progressive kyphosis in the other two at the junction of the proximal and distal halves of the *u* rods near the apex of the curve.

The preoperative apical convex RVAD differed significantly between the two groups ($p = 0.001$). In the definitive surgery group, the mean RVAD was 58.54 degrees ± 14.03 SD, whereas it was 31.90 degrees ± 7.99 SD in the no-surgery group. A logistic regression analysis was done to identify the factors predictive of the need for definitive surgery in adolescence, comparing ages at initial operation. Only the RVAD was found to be significantly predictive ($p = 0.03$) of the need for definitive surgery in adolescence.

8.3 Comparisons with Other Techniques

In 1972, Mehta described a radiologic method for predicting curve progression in early onset idiopathic scoliosis on the basis of the apical RVAD and overlap of the rib head on the apical vertebra on the convex side.[2] This is a well-established method of identifying early onset idiopathic scoliosis with the potential for rapid curve progression, and these patients may be selected for early intervention and stabilization. Ideally, the surgical treatment of early onset idiopathic scoliosis should be able to correct the deformity and maintain the correction and growth, without the need for bracing. The common denominator of these techniques is accommodating growth while correcting scoliosis, but most studies have included patients with scoliosis having other causes (e.g., congenital scoliosis, neuromuscular scoliosis) as well as patients with early onset idiopathic scoliosis.

8.3.1 Distraction-Based Growing Rods

Distraction-based implants correct spinal deformity and maintain the correction via spinal distraction, in a manner not unlike that in which the original Harrington rods functioned. These distraction-based implants can be attached to the spine, ribs, or pelvis depending on the patient's age, the characteristics of the curve, and the available bone stock.

Traditional growth rods and the vertical expandable prosthetic titanium rib (VEPTR) provide similar options for the management of young children with scoliosis. Although Bess et al[7] and Akbarnia et al[5] demonstrated increased curve correction and overall T1-S1 growth with frequent lengthening, more recent studies have shown an increased risk for complications with each procedure and less length gained with each subsequent lengthening. Controversy exists regarding the optimal timing for the implantation of a growth rod as well as for the optimal lengthening intervals. Typical results include those of Akbarnia et al,[8] who reported 23 children with progressive early onset scoliosis who underwent treatment with dual growing rods. The Cobb angle improved from 82 degrees preoperatively to 36 degrees at the time of fusion. T1-S1 length increased from an average of 23 cm preoperatively to 32.6 cm at the time of fusion. Complications occurred in 11 (48%) of 23 patients. Innovations such as low profile designs, growing connectors, dual rod application, and the use of rib fixation and/or pedicle screws have enabled surgeons to control deformity better.

8.3.2 Vertical Expandable Prosthetic Titanium Rib

VEPTR placement was originally indicated for patients with rib fusions, but currently the VEPTR functions very much like the traditional growing rod. Compared with the growing rod, the VEPTR features circumferential rib anchors, telescopic lengthening that allows twice the amount of lengthening, and a lengthening mechanism that allows expansion in the kyphotic segment of the thoracic spine; in contrast, axial connectors generally need to be placed at the thoracolumbar junction. Several studies have demonstrated the efficacy of the VEPTR in controlling curve magnitude and promoting spine growth. Campbell and Hell-Vocke[6] reviewed 27 children with congenital scoliosis and fused ribs who underwent expansion thoracostomy and VEPTR insertion. At a mean follow-up of 5.7 years, scoliosis had decreased from a mean of 74 degrees preoperatively to 49 degrees. Mean thoracic spine growth per year was 0.80 cm. The presence of an unsegmented bar seemingly did not prevent spine growth; expansion thoracoplasty led to an average 7.3% increase in the length of the bar at a 4.2-year follow-up. Complications are similar to those of traditional growing rods, including wound problems, rib fracture, and creeping fusion. Iliac *s*-hook migration has also been reported, and debate continues regarding the appropriate means of anchoring to the pelvis in patients with growing constructs.

8.3.3 Vertebral Body Stapling

Vertebral body stapling is a new technique used for adolescent and juvenile idiopathic scoliosis. As predicted by the Hueter-Volkmann principle, increased pressure across a growth plate in the vertebral body slows growth. Although this phenomenon has been observed in experimental animal spine models, experience in the 1950s with the stapling of large congenital curves was disappointing. More recently, flexible tethers attached to vertebral anchors have been used to modulate spinal growth. Using tethers in animal models, Newton et al[9] demonstrated vertebral wedging, which might correct scoliosis.

Modern vertebral body staples consist of a shape-memory alloy (i.e., nitinol) that allows the staple to clamp down into a *c* shape when it is warmed to body temperature. Literature reviewing the effect of stapling in scoliosis is limited. Betz et al[10] followed 28 children who had adolescent idiopathic scoliosis treated with vertebral body stapling for 2 years. A procedure was considered successful when a curve corrected more than 10 degrees or corrected to within 10 degrees of the preoperative measurement. With use of the stapling technique, 86% of lumbar curves and 80% of thoracic curves of less than 35 degrees were successfully corrected. There were no major neurovascular injuries or staple migration. Curves of more than 35 degrees did not do well with stapling, and the authors recommended alternative treatments. Compression-based implants require continued innovation, and close follow-up is needed to assess the optimal indications and potential complications. Also needed is a commitment to foster these novel implants through the regulatory process. Still, early work has documented proof of concept.

In our long-term follow-up, beyond the adolescent growth spurt, of patients treated with CE and LT, nearly 43% (10 of 23) of them maintained curve correction and spinal growth and did not even require a definitive surgical intervention. This was thought to be a tremendous achievement for a difficult clinical problem, with a single surgical intervention in childhood achieving the ultimate goals of treatment. Naturally, the authors tried to look for the factors that could predict such success. Age at initial operation and curve size did not predict the need for definitive surgery. The RVAD, however, was a strong predicting factor, and our findings emphasize the importance of this radiologic parameter in predicting the malignant growth potential of these idiopathic curves in infants.

It was expected that when the spine grew beyond the ability of the instrumentation to contain the curve, curve progression would ensue and definitive surgery would be needed. Contrary to this expectation, instrumented segmental growth was larger in the group that did not need definitive surgery. When the instrumented segment failed to contain the curve because of excessive growth of the spine, it failed more often in kyphosis, but the magnitude of the scoliosis remained the same. The group that required definitive surgery had relatively smaller instrumented segmental growth. When the instrumented segment of the spine failed to grow linearly along the Luque rods, either because of stiffness of the instrumentation or inadvertent fusion, it tended to grow laterally, contributing to the progression of scoliosis. When reoperation was required, the curves were often stiff, with an abundance of soft tissue, and sometimes even fusion around the apex of the curve. The mean angle of scoliosis correction at definitive surgery was only 23% (from 61 to 47 degrees).

The evolution of the instrumentation construct had a large effect on outcome. Curve progression and the requirement for definitive fusion were noted in 72% (10 of 14) of the patients with an overlapped *l* rod construct but in only 33% (three of nine) of the patients with an overlapped *u* rod construct. It appears that the *u* rod construct directed spinal growth linearly and therefore prevented lateral growth from contributing to curve progression. This led to further evolution of the instrumentation technique. The initial *u* construct was incomplete, with one arm half length and the other arm full length, and when the proximal and distal rods were put together, the cross section at any level showed only three rods. This configuration directed liner growth of the spine but led to kyphosis in the midzone when spinal growth exceeded the limit. The technique was therefore further revised to have a complete *u* configuration, with a full length of both arms of the *u*, in both rods. Therefore, after placement of the construct in the spine, a cross section showed four rods at any level. This arrangement apparently prevents the development of kyphosis during excessive spinal growth at the junction of the proximal and distal rods in the middle of the curve.

A more recent modification is a combination of four individual rods. The proximal pair is designed with a claw construct at the cranial end (now pedicle screws), and the distal pair is fixed to the spine with pedicle screws at the caudal end and sublaminar wires in the midsection, permitting the rods directing linear spinal growth to slide. The claw construct and the pedicle screws prevent rotation of the spine around the rods, which cannot be controlled by sublaminar wiring alone. A long-term outcome of these newer configurations will be presented in the future.

8.4 Conclusion

The LT growing rod construct appeared to achieve the goals of the surgical treatment of early onset idiopathic scoliosis. It permitted spinal growth; it also corrected and maintained correction of the scoliosis, without the need for bracing. A definitive surgery can be anticipated at the adolescent growth spurt, particularly in patients with malignant growth potential, as predicted by a large RVAD. The use of an overlapped *u* construct of the LT growing rod was more successful in containing the curve without the need for any further intervention, even when the operation was performed at an early age. The RVAD was able to predict malignant growth potential of the curve.

References

[1] Gomez JA, Lee JK, Kim PD, Roye DP, Vitale MG. "Growth friendly" spine surgery: management options for the young child with scoliosis. J Am Acad Orthop Surg 2011; 19: 722–727

[2] Mehta MH. The rib-vertebra angle in the early diagnosis between resolving and progressive infantile scoliosis. J Bone Joint Surg Br 1972; 54: 230–243

[3] D'Astous JL, Sanders JO. Casting and traction treatment methods for scoliosis. Orthop Clin North Am 2007; 38: 477–484, v

[4] Pratt RK, Webb JK, Burwell RG, Cummings SL. Luque trolley and convex epiphysiodesis in the management of infantile and juvenile idiopathic scoliosis. Spine 1999; 24: 1538–1547

[5] Akbarnia BA, Breakwell LM, Marks DS et al. Growing Spine Study Group. Dual growing rod technique followed for three to eleven years until final fusion: the effect of frequency of lengthening. Spine 2008; 33: 984–990

[6] Campbell RM Jr Hell-Vocke AK. Growth of the thoracic spine in congenital scoliosis after expansion thoracoplasty. J Bone Joint Surg Am 2003; 85-A: 409–420

[7] Bess S, Akbarnia BA, Thompson GH et al. Complications of growing-rod treatment for early-onset scoliosis: analysis of one hundred and forty patients. J Bone Joint Surg Am 2010; 92: 2533–2543

[8] Akbarnia BA, Marks DS, Boachie-Adjei O, Thompson AG, Asher MA. Dual growing rod technique for the treatment of progressive early-onset scoliosis: a multicenter study. Spine 2005; 30 Suppl: S46–S57

[9] Newton PO, Farnsworth CL, Faro FD et al. Spinal growth modulation with an anterolateral flexible tether in an immature bovine model: disc health and motion preservation. Spine 2008; 33: 724–733

[10] Betz RR, Ranade A, Samdani AF et al. Vertebral body stapling: a fusionless treatment option for a growing child with moderate idiopathic scoliosis. Spine 2010; 35: 169–176

Part 3

Infantile Idiopathic Scoliosis

3

9 Surgical Intervention

Adrian Gardner and David Marks

Surgical intervention in the management of noncongenital early onset scoliosis and infantile idiopathic scoliosis is indicated if there is a failure of conservative management (either casting or bracing) or if the deformity is considered too severe at presentation for conservative treatment to have any real prospect of success. The aims of the surgical treatment of early onset scoliosis and infantile idiopathic scoliosis are to control the spinal deformity while maximizing both cardiac and respiratory development and allowing the spine to grow and gain the most "normal" length possible. Surgical intervention takes many different forms, but essentially these consist of distraction-based posterior instrumentation systems, growth guidance instrumentation, or anterior spine–based tethers. All of these methods of managing early onset scoliosis have their indications, contraindications, and specific complications. In reality, however, there can be no one "right" answer for the management of all forms of spinal deformity, which continues to be a difficult and taxing problem. The aim of this chapter is to introduce these concepts and indicate where the different types of operative intervention may be employed, to consider the specific pathologies that may be addressed, and to discuss the contraindications and complications of each particular type of operative intervention.

9.1 Classification of the Operative Treatments of Early Onset Scoliosis

Skaggs et al have described a classification of growth preservation techniques in early onset scoliosis:[1]

- Nonoperative
  - Observation
  - Bracing
  - Casting
- Operative
  - Posterior distraction systems
    - Growing rods (single or dual, manual or remote lengthening)
    - Vertical expandable prosthetic titanium rib
    - Hybrid spine-to-rib construct
  - Growth guidance
    - Luque trolley
    - Shilla / Shilla-like
  - Anterior tether-based
    - Screw cable / ligament
  - Osteotomy

These are subdivided into nonoperative and operative groups. The nonoperative group includes serial observation,

casting (with or without traction), and bracing. All of these techniques are indicated in certain circumstances and have been used worldwide with great success. They are covered elsewhere in this book and are not the subject of this chapter.

The operative group is subdivided into three groups:

1. Distraction-based techniques include "growing rods" (either single or dual), the vertical expanding prosthetic titanium rib (VEPTR), and "hybrid" spine-to-rib constructs. What is common to all these systems is the requirement for intermittent lengthening of the construct (through either serial reoperation or some form of external (usually magnetic drive) distraction.

2. Growth guidance instrumentation is aimed at allowing the spine to "grow" along a predetermined "path"; the instrumentation is used to guide growth in the appropriate direction. This does not depend on serial lengthening procedures. This was the original segmental instrumentation concept of Luque, developed initially in the Luque trolley (and modern pedicle screw–based derivations) and subsequently refined in the Shilla technique.

3. Anterior tether based systems function by placing nonfusion instrumentation across the growth plates of the vertebral bodies—a cable, a ligament, or multiple staples—in an attempt to retard growth on the convex side of the spine in the hope that the concave side will "catch up" with the induced asymmetric growth.[2]

The effort to preserve growth is based on the understanding that we currently have about how early fusion inhibits spinal growth and growth of the thorax. This inhibition then interferes with the development of both the heart and lungs and leads to morbidity and early mortality through respiratory failure, as demonstrated by Pehrrson et al.[3] Subsequent work by Karol et al has shown that failure to attain a minimum vertebral height of the thoracic spine of 18 cm at maturity is strongly correlated with respiratory morbidity in early adult life. Consequently, all growth preservation systems are aimed at attaining at least 18 cm of thoracic spinal height, if not more, to maximize thoracic growth and development of the underlying organs.[4]

Surgical growth preservation attempts to match as closely as possible the normal growth of the spine and thorax, as documented previously by Dimeglio et al, with the overall aim of reaching as closely as possible a spine of normal length and normal three-dimensional development of the thoracic cage and underlying organs.[5]

9.2 Distraction-Based Instrumentation

9.2.1 Growing Rods

This posterior distraction-based instrumentation system was Harrington's original concept in the 1960s for the management of scoliosis following polio. A strut was placed on the concave side of the apex of a deformity to prevent the deformity from increasing in size. The strut was then lengthened periodically in an attempt to maintain any correction obtained at the index surgery. Any growth obtained was of secondary concern and is considered only briefly in Harrington's papers. However, no rotational control was associated with this instrumentation because the hooks did not lock to the rods. Consequently, significant crankshaft developed, and unchecked anterior growth in the presence of a posterior tether sometimes resulted in an even worse deformity than had been present initially. The other complication was a fracture rate of more than 66% during the lifetime of the construct.[6]

Second-generation posterior distraction based mechanisms were brought to the fore with implant systems such as the pediatric ISOLA Spine System (DePuy Synthes Spine, Raynham, Massachusetts), which has been the basis of the growing rod program in Birmingham. The construct employs either single or dual rods placed posteriorly to the spine with combination hook or screw foundations at both the proximal and distal ends of the curve. The Birmingham approach is always to use a dual rod construct, with the foundations typically placed in the upper thoracic spine and midlumbar spine. The approach is through a long posterior skin incision followed by subperiosteal exposure only of the vertebra required for the foundations. The procedure, analogous to a Wiltse-type approach, can be performed through four small incisions lateral to the midline over the foundations, with the rods then tunneled between the skin bridges. The rods are placed in a submuscular plane (or subcutaneous plane) to minimize skin problems and maximize soft tissue cover. Tandem growing connectors are placed over the relatively straight sagittal thoracolumbar junction outside the lumbar lordosis or thoracic kyphosis (▶ Fig. 9.1). This approach allows the greatest part of the curve, including the apex, to remain undisturbed during implantation because no periosteal stripping of the posterior musculature from the back of the spine is required.

At regular intervals (dictated by pathology, but usually every 6 months), the construct is lengthened. This is a day case procedure in which a small incision is made over the tandem connectors without disturbing the midline. The upper rod is then distracted away from the lower construct to lengthen the spine. This process is repeated until maturity is reached or the spine autofuses and becomes stiff, such that further lengthening procedures

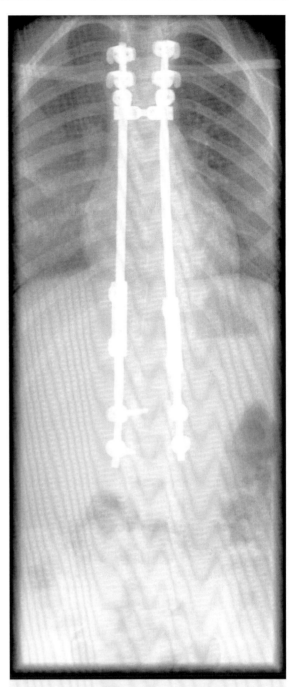

Fig. 9.1 Posteroanterior radiograph of a posterior growing rod construct.

are not possible. Studies have shown that approximately seven lengthening procedures are possible before the spine stiffens and lengthening achieves little and becomes increasingly difficult.[7] The timing of starting the growing rod program must take this limitation into account in conjunction with matching the growth velocity of the child. Thus, the average age for the implantation of growing rods is approximately 6 years. However, each case must be reviewed on an individual basis, and failure to control the curve may force operative intervention at an earlier age.

Once maturity has been reached, if there is still evidence of an articulation with patent facet joints or well-preserved disk spaces across the apex of the vertebral body, then a final fusion procedure is often recommended. The posterior implants are exposed and the rods exchanged. Further correction can be obtained through osteotomies of the posterior spinal elements. The posterior elements of the spine are then decorticated. Fusion is stimulated by adding either allograft or artificial bone to the autograft harvested from the posterior elements of the spine. This can be supplemented with iliac crest autograft from the posterior superior iliac spine as required.

Studies of the original cohort of pediatric ISOLA growing rod instrumentation patients through to graduation and beyond as studied and documented by the Growing Spine Study Group (which included the Birmingham cohort) has shown that a dual growing rod technique resulted in 5.7 ± 2.9 cm of spinal growth during a treatment period of 4.37 ± 2.4 years, with a greater growth rate for those lengthened at intervals of 6 months or less than for those lengthened at intervals longer than 6 months.[8]

Growing rods are suitable for a curve requiring instrumentation when fixation is possible at both the proximal and distal aspects of the curve, and in recent times these have evolved to become a screw-based construct distally and a screw or screw-and-hook construct proximally. Growing rods are contraindicated if it is not possible to obtain sound fixation to the spine or if the child is not suitable or will become unsuitable for multiple reoperations, even if these are of a lesser magnitude than the initial insertion of instrumentation. Newer materials have meant that growing rods, pedicle screws, and hooks can now be manufactured in titanium, so that the imaging difficulties that arose with steel implants in magnetic resonance (MR) imaging scanners have now been minimized. The infection rates also seem to have been reduced.[9]

Although posterior growing rods are initially inserted with the assistance of spinal cord monitoring, monitoring is not always employed for lengthening procedures. Neurologic complications following a lengthening of growing rods have been reported anecdotally. These have ranged through the entire spectrum, from a temporary loss of motor and sensory function that returned fully on removal of the distraction to permanent incomplete neurologic loss. Good practice dictates that a wake-up test always be performed in the operating theater following any lengthening procedure, with the instruments kept sterile until the child has passed the wake-up test satisfactorily and is seen to move both arms and legs purposefully with normal power *to command*. This is done even if multimodal monitoring has been used throughout the lengthening procedure.

The complications of growing rods are threefold. First, there is a risk for infection in the construct. This is because the spine and implant are exposed on multiple occasions through the same incision over a period of many years. The soft tissue in this area will become stiff and scarred, with a poor vascular supply, which adds to the overall risk. The infection rate has decreased with the use of titanium implants rather than steel because of the surface oxidation properties of titanium. Infection is managed similarly to any orthopedic infection, with débridement and often VAC (vacuum-assisted closure; Kinetic Concepts, Inc., San Antonio, Texas) therapy. A persistent deep infection can make it necessary to remove all instrumentation, including hooks, screws, and rods, to eradicate the infection. On removal of the implants, control of the scoliosis is lost, and the deformity can recur rapidly. An alternative method of curve control must then be employed, such as a brace or plaster, while the infection is cleared. Once this occurs, then re-instrumenting the spine to continue the growth program or converting to another form of construct can be considered.

The quoted infection rate for a growing spine construct over the *life span of the construct*, including the multiple reoperations for lengthening, rod revision, etc., is 10.4%.[9] Infection rates are increased in a growing spine construct by poor care in the surgical approach to lengthening, but also through a subcutaneous placement of the rods and poor skin over the prominent implant (especially in smaller children). Certain conditions, namely Prader–Willi syndrome, mucopolysaccharidosis, and graft-versus-host disease, predispose to infection.

The second complication of growing rods is rod fracture. This is thought to be due to cyclical loading of the construct over the unfused apex of the spine through many years of spinal movement during normal day-to-day life. This issue is well-known in orthopedic implant surgery. Ultimately, if a fusion does not consolidate, the implant will loosen or break. Breakage was originally observed in the original series of Harrington growing rods and has subsequently been observed in all growing rod systems. The Growing Spine Study Group has investigated this problem and has published its findings: a rod fracture rate of 15% with a re-fracture rate of 33%. The rod fracture rate is less if a dual rod over a single rod construct (11% vs. 36%) is used, presumably because the force is shared between the two rods.[10]

In the case of a rod fracture, there is currently controversy as to whether fracture of one rod mandates that all of the other rods in the construct be replaced. The reasoning here is that all of the rods have undergone the cyclical loading that has led to the rod fracture and are therefore at increased risk for fracture. A recent review of the Birmingham growing rod series has revealed that 80% of second rod fractures occur in the rod that originally failed, regardless of which rods were revised and replaced after the first rod fracture. It does seem that this finding indicates unequal loading of the construct leading to repeated fractures of just one rod. Our practice now is to revise only the fractured rod when a first rod fracture occurs and to replace all rods after a second rod fracture to minimize the operative insult to the patient.[11]

The final major complication related to growing rods is sagittal malalignment. It is a misunderstanding that "growing rods grow" the spine. What actually occurs is the inherent relative overgrowth of the anterior spine, which seems to be the final common pathway of early onset scoliosis / infantile idiopathic scoliosis. This overgrowth causes a crankshaft phenomenon to occur in the presence of the fixed posterior tether of the rods. Extending the growing rods then "takes *up* the slack" of the anterior crankshafting, increasing the vertical height of the spine *and* reducing the size of the curve. Children will often appear to "know" when they are due for a lengthening because they will describe the onset of pain around the spine and chest, usually in the month before surgery. This pain may be related to the relative anterior spinal overgrowth, and it is often observed that the pain is relieved by surgery. If premature spontaneous posterior fusion has occurred and anterior growth has been observed to continue, then these lead to anterior spine rotation and worsening of the deformity through a true crankshaft phenomenon. In this situation, thoracoplasty may be indicated for cosmesis in the presence of an ugly chest wall deformity.

Junctional kyphosis remains a difficult problem with the use of any posterior distraction system. Time will tell whether the systems of the new generation are any less likely than the older ones to cause junctional kyphosis. Posterior distraction can lead to significant junctional issues at both the proximal and distal ends of the construct. By the very nature of the mechanism of action of growing rods, posterior distraction is kyphogenic, especially at the proximal end of the construct. Proximal junctional kyphosis can be a significant problem above the growing spine construct, leading to hardware failure and pullout of the proximal anchors. There have been anecdotal reports of unsupported screw-only constructs pulling out backward and causing catastrophic neurologic injury through screw transection of the spinal cord.[12] Thus, there is a role for proximal hooks to protect the construct from screw pullout at the proximal foundation, either as a claw or in combination with screws.

At the end of the growing process, following the final fusion procedure and discharge of the child, there is a return to theater rates for other spinal surgery, related either to the growing rods or to other areas of the spine. If fusion does not occur soundly following definitive fusion, pseudarthrosis will be seen. This will lead to rod fracture, with the subsequent sudden onset of pain and/or the development of a palpable mass in the skin. Progression of the residual deformity may also occur, requiring revision fusion and rod exchange.

After a definitive fusion, pain distal to the instrumented and fused segments resulting from degenerative changes in the disk and facet joints can also be a reason for further operative intervention at a later date—decompressive and/or fusion surgery in adulthood. The problem of distal junctional kyphosis in posterior distraction systems is currently poorly understood, but as more children with growing rods age, it will undoubtedly come to more surgeons' attention.

In an effort to avoid multiple surgeries to lengthen posterior growing rods, with their attendant complications, new technologies have developed to automate the distraction process with magnetic actuators. Automation has been achieved with both the Phenix (Soubeiran, France) and MAGEC (Ellipse Technologies, Irvine, California) devices. These are magnetic field–activated devices that allow interval lengthening to be accomplished as a nonoperative outpatient procedure, eliminating the need for small, repeated interval surgeries. Early experience with the MAGEC implant, as reported by Akbarnia et al,[13] has been positive and represents a significant breakthrough in the treatment of these children. However, long-term follow-up (in excess of 10 years) will be required for an accurate assessment of this and other innovative techniques in early onset scoliosis surgery and their place in the management of early onset scoliosis. Unfortunately, it currently is not possible for a child with a MAGEC implant in situ to undergo MR imaging because the device becomes heated while in the magnetic field of the scanning machine. This issue is being addressed by the manufacturers (▶ Fig. 9.2).

9.2.2 Vertical Expansile Prosthetic Titanium Rib

The VEPTR (vertical expanding prosthetic titanium rib) was originally designed to deal with Jeune syndrome, and its use was rapidly expanded to include congenital and exotic scoliosis (scoliosis with associated rib fusion and thoracic cage volume depletion; ▶ Fig. 9.3). The VEPTR allows distraction of the fused chest wall element to increase the space available for development of the underlying lung. The VEPTR acts through a proximal rib anchor; the distal foundation is a rib anchor to the lower ribs, a spine anchor through pedicle screws or hooks, or a pelvic anchor through a Dunn–McCarthy hook that sits over the iliac crest. The choice of anchors depends on the pathology being treated, the length of curve, and the aim of the intervention. As with the growing rod, manual distraction is required to allow the total length of the construct to be increased on an interval basis, typically every 6 months. General anesthesia must be administered on an inpatient basis for a short time, but the procedure is a day case. The VEPTR, and specifically the VEPTR II (Synthes, West Chester, Pennsylvania), can be employed in

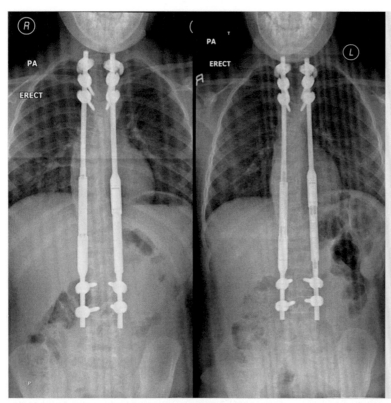

Fig. 9.2 Posteroanterior radiographs of a MAGEC rod construct before and after lengthening.

early onset scoliosis because it offers proximal rib attachment in a kyphotic situation through contouring of the proximal rod. This is very helpful, especially when it would be difficult to place proximal spine anchors with a growing rod system because of either anatomy or position. Using proximal rib anchors leaves the proximal spine undisturbed, which may be beneficial in reducing proximal junctional kyphosis or in allowing new fixation points if these are required for future surgery. The specific complication unique to the VEPTR in comparison with a standard growing rod is proximal migration of the rib anchor through the ribs, irritating the brachial plexus and causing brachial plexopathy. This can be seen acutely during a lengthening procedure or over time between lengthening procedures. Some centers report the use of nerve monitoring of the brachial plexus during lengthening specifically to avoid this complication. When attached distally to the pelvis, the Dunn–McCarthy hook can migrate distally through the iliac wing, so that revision surgery and repositioning of the implant are required.

The VEPTR implant is by its very nature situated away from the spine and over the posterior chest wall. There is less muscular tissue here in the young child, so the implants can be more prominent. It is therefore important to place the initial incision and muscle dissection to allow a full-thickness musculocutaneous flap to cover the implant. Secondary chest wall stiffness and decreased lung compliance are beginning to be reported as late sequelae of VEPTR, analogous to the spine stiffness seen with growing rods.[14]

The Birmingham experience with the VEPTR device has included patients with exotic scoliosis and thoracic insufficiency syndrome. Along with expansion thoracoplasty the device has been used as a growing system for patients with early onset scoliosis. Its use in early onset scoliosis has been particularly helpful because proximal rib cradle placement is easier than proximal spine fixation in small children with aggressive curves. Rib cradles can also be placed around more than one rib, providing better fixation in small and relatively fragile bones. The implant has been placed on the concavity of the curve, and the position away from the midline allows a better soft tissue cover.

In a recent attempt to overcome the specific problems inherent to individual implants, surgeons have combined systems and principles in hybrid constructs. Typical among these is the combination of multiple rib anchors and spinal hooks connected to a growing rod implant fixed distally to the spine. Early reports of this hybrid technique suggest that implant-related complications are fewer than with either a traditional growing rod construct or a VEPTR construct, but long-term results are awaited (▶ Fig. 9.4).[10]

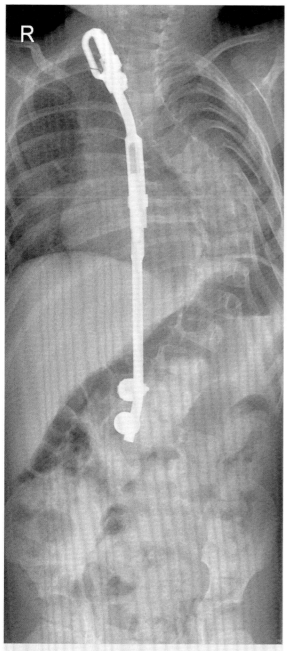

Fig. 9.3 Posteroanterior radiograph of a vertical expandable prosthetic titanium rib construct used in early onset sclerosis.

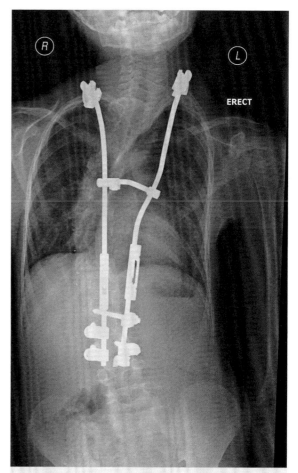

Fig. 9.4 Posteroanterior radiograph of a posterior growing rod construct with proximal rib anchors.

9.2.3 Anterior Nonfusion Anterior Release

As an adjuvant therapy to posterior distraction-based technologies in patients with very large or stiff infantile curves, there remains a role for anterior surgery analogous to the anterior release used in adolescent idiopathic scoliosis surgery. This technique of nonfusion anterior release combines anulotomy and nuclectomy and involves

a 270-degree incision to the anulus to expose the nucleus, which is then removed with very fine rongeurs without traumatizing the growth plate (▶ Fig. 9.5). The technique attempts to prevent anterior fusion and preserve end plate growth, whereas the total diskectomy of the adolescent idiopathic anterior release leads to fusion. In addition, the approach does allow access to the concave tether in the scoliosis, thus improving flexibility, especially across the apex, and certainly improving the initial correction and possibly the long-term results in terms of longitudinal growth and maintenance of deformity correction. The procedure can be performed without transecting and ligating the segmental vessels, and therefore it is suitable for use in those children whose scoliosis is associated with intradural anomalies. Traditionally, it has been carried out through a small thoracotomy, although it can also be done thoracoscopically if appropriate equipment and training are available. This procedure is used for curves of approximately 60 degrees or larger and for curves that do not correct on suspension or on bending radiographs. A

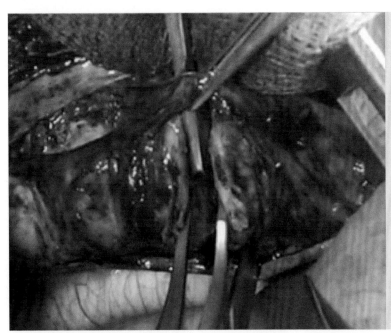

Fig. 9.5 Clinical photograph of anulotomy and nuclectomy, a nonfusion anterior release.

review of a series of this procedure from the scoliosis unit in Birmingham has shown that initial curve correction is much better than it would be without the release. Fusion did not occur over the segments treated with the nonfusion anterior release, and spinal growth occurred both anteriorly and posteriorly afterward.[15] This technique has been applied in Birmingham combined with both posterior distraction systems (spine-to-spine and spine-to-rib hybrids) and with the VEPTR device, with good results.

9.2.4 Growth Guidance

The principle of growth guidance is to "persuade" the spinal deformity to correct by directing growth of the spine along a predetermined path (the rods) with minimal surgical interference. Guidance promotes growth in an appropriate direction to control the scoliosis and prevent compression of the intrathoracic organs. This is done through the posterior implantation of a rod and bone anchors that are fixed to the vertebra but are not locked to the rods and so can "slide" along the rods without growth inhibition or posterior tethering. The original system based on this idea was the Luque trolley, popularized by Eduardo Luque. This consisted of a series of multilevel segmental sublaminar wires placed around *l* rods. The Luque trolley was a very low-profile construct and allowed growth without interval surgery. The downside of the Luque trolley is that the placement of multiple sublaminar wires requires periosteal stripping of the entire posterior elements over the instrumented levels. This can and did lead to autofusion posteriorly, creating a posterior tether and causing the crankshaft phenomenon, with associated failure of

longitudinal growth. Reports of the success of the Luque trolley in the literature are mixed.[16]

The concept of a Luque trolley idea was revisited recently by Mehdian et al of Nottingham, in the United Kingdom, and Ouellet et al of Montreal, Canada,[17,18] in an attempt to counter the problem of autofusion by using pedicle screw foundations and fewer or no wires. These investigators describe proximal and distal fixation with overlapping rods between held together by wires (Mehdian et al) or a sliding screw with a new design (Ouellet et al). As growth progresses, the proximal and distal foundations move away from each other while the sliding rods maintain control of the curve without inhibiting growth. Although the control of deformity has undoubtedly been enhanced, long-term follow-up will be required to identify whether the issue of premature fusion has been resolved.

Recently popular as an alternative to the Luque trolley is the Shilla procedure. It addresses the concerns about a large exposure of the back of the immature spine by using a short-segment anterior and posterior apical fusion, typically over three or four levels, for maximal correction. Pedicle screws are then placed transmuscularly under image guidance into the upper and lower ends of the spine (the upper thoracic spine and midlumbar spine) to be instrumented without exposure of the spine in the midline. A sliding mechanism is created with Shilla caps, which are end caps that screw to the tulip head of the pedicle screw and torque to the screw but not to the rod, allowing the screw to slide on the rod.

McCarthy and McCullough reported their 5-year follow-up with the technique at the Scoliosis Research Society meeting in 2012. They reported that growth occurred across the length of the construct, although not to the same degree as a posterior distracting technology such as growing rods or the VEPTR. The complication rate was comparable with that of an equivalent group of growing rods, and it was lower in terms of infection. Each patient underwent on average 2.7 procedures, whereas the projected number of surgeries with a posterior distraction technique is on average 9.9 per patient. The rate of implant revision due to broken rods was 32.5% (13 of 40 patients), which is greater than that for a growing rod technique.[19] Unfortunately, again because of the nature of the implant, which is a stainless steel construct, it is not possible to obtain good MR images once the Shilla implant has been placed, and therefore it may not be suitable for those children who have had surgery because of scoliosis secondary to an intradural lesion or syringomyelia or a malformation such as an Arnold–Chiari malformation. The classic Shilla technique is also contraindicated if a child is not fit to undergo a thoracotomy for creating an anterior fusion over the apex of deformity, although some surgeons perform the Shilla technique with only a posterior apical fusion, avoiding the thoracotomy completely. The results of this modification are currently awaited (▶ Fig. 9.6).

9.3 Anterior Tether-Based Technologies

Vertical growth of the spine occurs at the growth plates of the vertebral bodies rather than at the posterior elements of the spine. Additionally, the rotation in scoliosis is driven anteriorly, and this does seem to be the seat of the primary pathology. Anterior tether–based procedures in early onset scoliosis are experimental; their use in juvenile scoliosis is currently limited to small case study series. The tether concept is aimed at altering the primary pathology directly rather than, like posterior technologies, aimed at steering growth in an appropriate direction. The other difference in comparison with posterior systems for the operative treatment of immature scoliosis is that anterior systems appear to be truly "fusionless" and do not end with a fusion and instrumentation of the scoliosis curve. As with the other concepts, final confirmation of the anterior tether will come only with follow-up well into skeletal maturity. Nevertheless, the potential for future continued progress is exciting.

Anterior techniques originally started with vertebral body stapling in congenital scoliosis. The results were disappointing, mainly because of technical issues with the implants. The technique was reintroduced by Betz et al with the use of the nitinol staple.[20] The staples are inserted across the disk spaces at multiple levels over the convex side of the apex of the curve. Nitinol is an alloy that changes shape in response to changes in temperature and has been designed in such a way that body temperature causes the spikes of the staple to come close together, providing compression over the disk space. The staples can be inserted thoracoscopically, eliminating the need for a thoracotomy, or via a minimally invasive approach to the subdiaphragmatic spine. Because there is no other instrumentation to the vertebral body, ligation of the segmental vessels around the waist of the vertebral bodies is not required. The published results of this technique in patients with juvenile scoliosis who have smaller curves have been promising, although it appears that curves over a certain size are resistant to stapling and progress despite this procedure. The current guidance is to consider other, supplemental posterior spine-to-rib hybrid constructs or abandon stapling altogether and use anterior vertebral body tethers if a thoracic curve measures 35 to 45 degrees and does decrease on bending radiographs to 20 degrees or less. Patients for whom bracing is suitable are those for whom anterior vertebral body stapling is suitable, and the difficulties of noncompliance with bracing can be avoided.[20] It is important to note that this technique has not been described for curve control in early onset scoliosis, although the principle would be very similar. Another variant of the staple has been developed by Wall.[21] This device attempts tethering of the vertebral growth plate along with some compression of the convex side of the disk. The technique is still experimental in clinical trials and is not currently licensed for use in early onset scoliosis.

A recent, exciting development in the fusionless treatment of deformity is anterior vertebral body tethering through the placement of a flexible ligament over

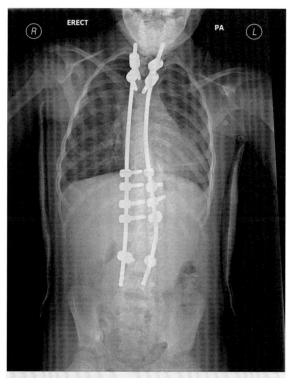

Fig. 9.6 Posteroanterior radiograph of a Shilla procedure.

multiple vertebral bodies across the apex of the curve. Fixation to the spine is with screws placed through the vertebral body in a coronal plane, similar to any anterior spinal instrumentation. This technique has been used in vivo in juvenile scoliosis by Crawford and Lenke with success,[22] although currently it is not widely available for routine use and is contraindicated if the child is not fit for a thoracotomy or thoracoscopic approach to the spine. The suggested indications are idiopathic (or idiopathic-like) scoliosis in a patient older than 8 years of age with growth remaining, Risser stage 0–2, and a thoracic curve between 35 and 60 degrees that is flexible to below 30 degrees. Careful follow-up is required for these patients because it is possible with growth to reverse the curve and cause scoliosis to develop in the opposite direction.

9.4 Conclusion

The aim of surgical intervention in early onset scoliosis is to obtain and maintain correction of the spine. However, this intervention must also allow the spine and thorax to develop to their maximum potential and facilitate the development of the underlying cardiorespiratory system. Surgical treatment is fraught with difficulties related to what is inevitably a prolonged path of growth taking many years. Three different surgical philosophies exist:

- Posterior distraction, either manually or magnetically, by using growth rods with proximal spine anchors, the VEPTR with proximal rib anchors, or a hybrid of the two;
- Growth guidance with either the Luque trolley or a Shilla procedure;
- Anterior stapling and ligament tethers.

There are advantages and disadvantages to each, yet each has its place in managing these various and challenging deformities. During the period of treatment, it may well be suitable to change from one philosophy to another or to recruit another method, depending on the growth and individual requirements of the child in question.

Finally, the surgeon must always remember to approach these challenging patients with respect. Respect for the curve but above all respect and compassion for the child and family who have to bear these treatments for what is often a very long time.

References

[1] Skaggs DL, Akbarnia BA, Flynn JM, Myung KS, Sponseller PD, Vitale MG Chest Wall and Spine Deformity Study Group. Pediatric Orthopaedic Society of North America. Scoliosis Research Society Growing Spine Study Committee. A classification of growth friendly spine implants. J Pediatric Orthop 2014; 34: 260–274

[2] Aronsson DD, Stokes IA, McBride C. The role of remodeling and asymmetric growth in vertebral wedging. Stud Health Technol Inform 2010; 158: 11–15

[3] Pehrsson K, Bake B, Larsson S, Nachemson A. Lung function in adult idiopathic scoliosis: a 20 year follow up. Thorax 1991; 46: 474–478

[4] Karol LA, Johnston C, Mladenov K, Schochet P, Walters P, Browne RH. Pulmonary function following early thoracic fusion in non-neuro-muscular scoliosis. J Bone Joint Surg Am 2008; 90: 1272–1281

[5] Dimeglio A, Canavase F. The growing spine: How spinal deformities influence normal spine and thoracic cage growth. Eur Spine J 2012; 21: 64–70

[6] Klemme WR, Denis F, Winter RB, Lonstein JW, Koop SE. Spinal instrumentation without fusion for progressive scoliosis in young children. J Pediatr Orthop 1997; 17: 734–742

[7] Sankar WN, Skaggs DL, Yazici M et al. Lengthening of dual growing rods and the law of diminishing returns. Spine 2011; 36: 806–809

[8] Akbarnia BA, Breakwell LM, Marks DS et al. Growing Spine Study Group. Dual growing rod technique followed for three to eleven years until final fusion: the effect of frequency of lengthening. Spine 2008; 33: 984–990

[9] Kabirian N, Akbarnia BA, Pawelek JB, Alam M, Mundis GM Jr, Acacio R, Thompson GH, Marks DS, Gardner A, Pawelek JB, Sponseller PD, Skaggs DL. Deep surgical site infection following 2344 growing-rod procedures for early onset scoliosis. J Bone Joint Surg Am 2014; 96: e128

[10] Yang JS, Sponseller PD, Thompson GH et al. Growing Spine Study Group. Growing rod fractures: risk factors and opportunities for prevention. Spine 2011; 36: 1639–1644

[11] David M, Gardner A, Jennison T, Spilsbury J, Marks D. The impact of revision of one or more rods on refracture rate and implant survival following rod fracture in instrumentation without fusion constructs in the management of early-onset scoliosis. J Pediatr Orthop B 2014; 23: 288–290

[12] Skaggs KF, Brasher AE, Johnston CE, Purvis JM, Smith JT, Myung KS, Skaggs DL. Upper thoracic pedicle screw loss of fixation causing spinal cord injury: A review of the literature and multicenter case series. J Pediatr Orthop 2013; 33: 75–79

[13] Akbarnia BA, Cheung K, Noordeen H et al. Next generation of growth-sparing techniques: preliminary clinical results of a magnetically controlled growing rod in 14 patients with early-onset scoliosis. Spine 2013; 38: 665–670

[14] Akbarnia BA, Emans JB. Complications of growth-sparing surgery in early onset scoliosis. Spine 2010; 35: 2193–2204

[15] Choudhury M, Siddique I, Gardner A, Spilsbury J, Marks D. Nonfusion anterior release with growing rod instrumentation in early onset scoliosis—does it work? Presented at: Britspine; April 30, 2010; Liverpool, UK

[16] Mardjetko SM, Hammerberg KW, Lubicky JP, Fister JS. The Luque trolley revisited. Review of nine cases requiring revision. Spine 1992; 17: 582–589

[17] Mehdian H, Boreham B, Hammett T, Clamp J, Quraishi N. Segmental self-growing rod constructs in the management of early onset neuro-muscular scoliosis. Presented at: Scoliosis Research Society 47th Annual Meeting and Course; September 5–8, 2012; Chicago, IL

[18] Ouellet J, Klein K, Steffen T, Von Rechenburg B. A new gliding anchor for self-growing rods: trolley screw. Presented at: Scoliosis Research Society Annual Meeting and Course; September 5–8, 2012; Chicago, IL

[19] McCarthy R, McCullough F. Five-year follow-up of 40 patients with the original Shilla procedure. Presented at: Scoliosis Research Society Annual Meeting and Course; September 5–8, 2012; Chicago, IL

[20] Betz R, Ashgar J, Samdani A. Non-fusion anterior stapling. In: Akbarnia B, Yazici M, Thompson G, eds. The Growing Spine. New York, NY: Springer-Verlag; 2011:569–577

[21] Wall E. Update on hemibridge. Presented at: 6th International Congress on Early Onset Scoliosis and Growing Spine (ICEOS); November 15–16, 2012; Dublin, Ireland

[22] Crawford CH III Lenke LG. Growth modulation by means of anterior tethering resulting in progressive correction of juvenile idiopathic scoliosis: a case report. J Bone Joint Surg Am 2010; 92: 202–209

10 Growth as a Corrective Force

Min Mehta (transcribed by Colin Nnadi)

10.1 Introduction

One of the world's leading proponents of the treatment of early onset scoliosis, Min H. Mehta, FRCS, made a rare public appearance on September 8, 2011, in Christ Church, Oxford, United Kingdom. Miss Mehta had not given a public talk in the United Kingdom for more than a decade, so it was an honor to have her in our company. She is best known for establishing the importance of the rib–vertebra angle difference as a prognostic index in the evaluation of early onset scoliosis, and she also popularized the casting technique as a treatment option for patients with early onset scoliosis.

What follows is the lecture she presented on that day, edited for print and ease of reading. A summary of the casting technique popularized by Miss Mehta for the treatment of early onset scoliosis is also provided toward the end of this chapter.
– Colin Nnadi

I have not progressed very far since my 2005 paper in *The Bone & Joint Journal* was published because there are many things I still do not know. However, I am quite sure that we must pay attention to the smaller curves when they are small because that is the time when the health care professional can be optimally effective in correction. This is not true for all cases, but it does hold true for many patients.

Scoliosis is a spectrum disorder resulting in varying degrees of deformity (▶ Fig. 10.1). At one end of the scale, curves spontaneously resolve; for a long time, this is where treatment was focused. It is important to understand why the curves resolve. Some progress in a benign, gentlemanly manner, whereas other curves are malignant, rapidly destroying scoliosis. They are a mystery. At the other end of the scale is the dysmorphic group with various associated anomalies. This is the spectrum of curves that we must look at and appropriately treat—that is how I saw it at the time. There are also two distinct phenotypes of scoliosis—namely, the sturdy phenotype (patients will get better) and the slim / slender phenotype (patients will not get better).

Examining the child is the first step in the treatment plan. With a very young child, the diaper must be removed. This is absolutely fundamental. As seen in ▶ Fig. 10.2a, although the child is being supported, a convex curve is present to the right; the diaper is just about slipping off and is obscuring half of the child's body. Let the parents handle the child because children trust their parents. A health care professional is a stranger to them. In ▶ Fig. 10.2b, the head is rotated away from the side of curve convexity; also note contralateral pelvic tilt.

Early on, it is important to adopt these very basic patterns in an examination of early scoliosis. The child's head should be examined because oftentimes asymmetry of the skull is associated with scoliosis (▶ Fig. 10.3). Anteriorly, a slight prominence on the left side and a slight flattening on the right side can be seen and may develop into a severe deformity.

Scoliosis can also affect a child's face (▶ Fig. 10.4). Although facial asymmetry is commonly seen among the general population, if a child presents to you with a curvature of the spine, pay great attention to the facial asymmetry because this feature indicates that scoliosis is likely to progress, sometimes very rapidly. A short

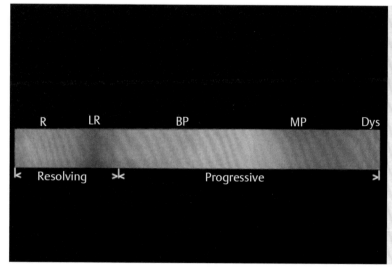

Fig. 10.1 Scoliosis is a spectrum disorder that results in varying degrees of deformity. R, Resolving; LR, Late Resolving; BP, Benign Progressive; MP, Malignant Progressive.

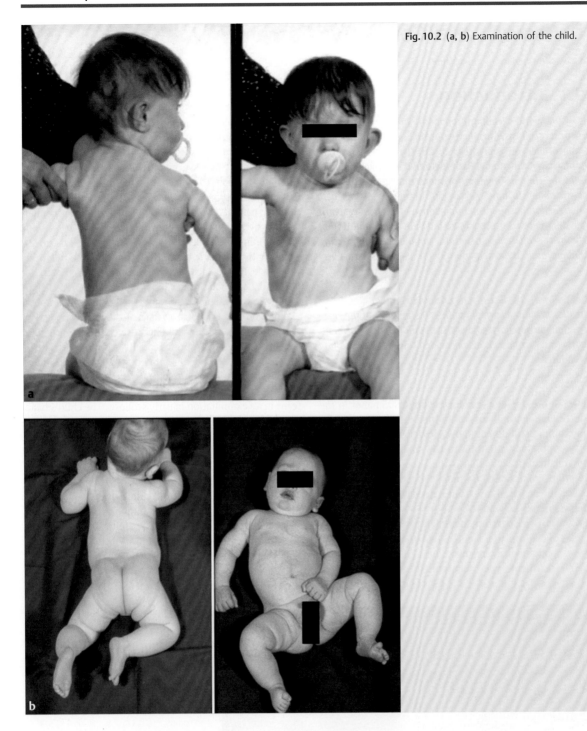

Fig. 10.2 (a, b) Examination of the child.

period between appointments is the rule for babies in such a scenario, but not for adolescent patients with scoliosis.

Take note of the femur during the examination. As suggested previously, allow the parent to handle the child. By touching the child only occasionally and talking to the parents, it is likely that the child will become inquisitive and gradually trust you to examine him or her, thus enabling the health care professional to make an early diagnosis.

▶ Fig. 10.5 a shows the image of a broad-backed youngster who is slender; he is already beginning to show a curve on his left side, indicating early scoliosis. ▶ Fig. 10.5 b is the image of a child without scoliosis, but the child is slightly lordotic; therefore, it would be prudent to follow-up with him to ensure that a curvature does not develop.

Assess the flexibility and rigidity of the curve. Floppiness and hypotonia are well-known features. When you are observing and palpating these features, let the parent do the work for you—an approach that is simple and offers a greater picture of what is happening with the child's spine.

There are many different features of scoliosis. There are hypotonic floppy children, and there are some children with spasticity—a gibbus or joint laxity is quite often seen in these children. Resisting head rotation to the curve convexity (i.e., the child does not like going to the right side because the entire spine is being moved) is a relatively regular feature. Furthermore, and perhaps most importantly, there are other idiopathic anomalies—at least in the sense that nothing is obvious.

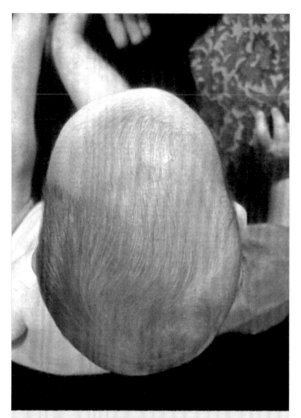

Fig. 10.3 Asymmetry of the skull.

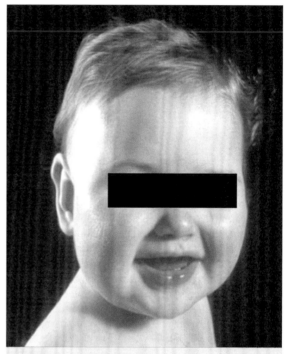

Fig. 10.4 Facial asymmetry.

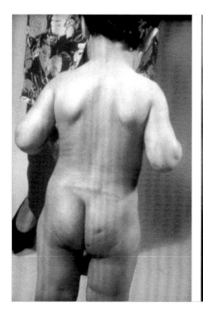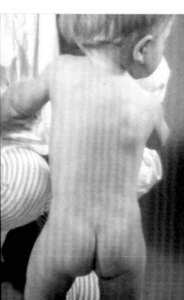

Fig. 10.5 Different phenotypes.

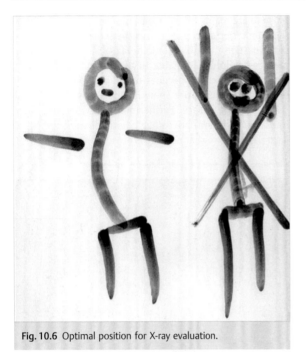

Fig. 10.6 Optimal position for X-ray evaluation.

Ensure that the baby is lying down and being handled by the parent. Note the degree of asymmetry; the head will tilt to one side, while the pelvis will tilt to the other. There may also be a hint of scoliosis on the left side, with the head rotated in the contralateral direction. (These are features seen regularly but not always recorded.)

During a radiographic evaluation, there are rather obvious things that health care professionals must do. Do not stretch the patient's arms when obtaining radiographs because doing so reduces the curve (▶ Fig. 10.6). As mentioned previously, the best way to perform this task is to let the parents gently hold the child with his or her arms outstretched.

▶ Fig. 10.7 presents radiographs of two children whom I met years ago in the maternity ward. There is a rotatory element. One child is 2 months of age, and the other is aged 6 months. In the 1970s, the medical community was not quite sure what to do with them. My training seemed to suggest that the 2-month-old child must have a very severe curve. The curve in the 6-month-old child was 14 degrees. After reviewing their records and assessing the patterns, I found that the 14-degree curve was likely to progress, while the other one was likely to resolve. I also performed a small series to understand what was happening to the growing spine, taking the series right through the stages so that some of the people were older (ranging from 12 to 51 years of age).

And in those days, health care professionals paid no attention to the rotation of the curve; by contrast, it was the degree of the Cobb angle that was important. However, curves sometimes looked innocuous, but quite a lot

of rotation was present. Two curves can be seen; the first one is the little curve, there is a small blob, which is the transverse process, and the second one above it is the body (see ▶ Fig. 10.7). Rotating them at 15-degree intervals changes the picture, and quite often, it is the rotation that leads to severe problems in the future.

As the picture moves from 30 to 45 degrees of rotation, a straight back can be seen at 60 degrees, and the curvature is then absent because of rotation. Therefore, it is crucial that health care professionals pay a great deal of attention to the rotatory element when they examine children with scoliosis.

The spine of the 2-month-old infant shows a 6-degree difference in the rib–vertebra angle compared with the spine of the 6-month-old child (see ▶ Fig. 10.7). Although the curve was larger, it was definitely hidden. The curve of the 6-month-old child is worse because it had a large rib–vertebra angle difference (RVAD). The age of 6 months is the point in time when treatment should begin.

The 14-degree curve following treatment is revealed in ▶ Fig. 10.8a, and the other child's spine, which grew straight, is shown in ▶ Fig. 10.8b. Therefore, the Cobb angles are not the only indicators to look for.

Curves as severe as this can—and do—occur. Refer to the degree of rotation. The spine is badly rotated, and once rotation is present, no amount of surgery or novel techniques will normalize the alignment of the spine.

At what stage can health care professionals discern what is going to happen? The rib–vertebra angle is important in the early differentiation of resolving and progressive curves because this angle may help determine which curve will do what. Once the rib–vertebra angle is known, the health care professional can establish which curve may resolve and which may progress, and therefore which curve will require early treatment. For example, a curvature with a large difference between the rib and spine is not likely to resolve. The angle of the rib to the spine also gives the health care professional a rather clear prognosis of what will happen. If the rib–vertebra angle is less than 20 degrees, then the curve may be likely to resolve, provided that the child is treated early.

Radiography is also important and should be obtained at 3 months, then repeated no more than 2 months after the initial radiograph.

In progressive scoliosis, the RVAD is usually more than 20 degrees, and it may remain the same or increase within 2 months. Conversely, in resolving scoliosis, the RVAD is less than 20 degrees and gets better after 2 months; therefore, the RVAD is very important. Treatment is appropriate when it is apparent that the RVAD has been increasing after 2 months. Waiting any longer than this means that it is too late for treatment.

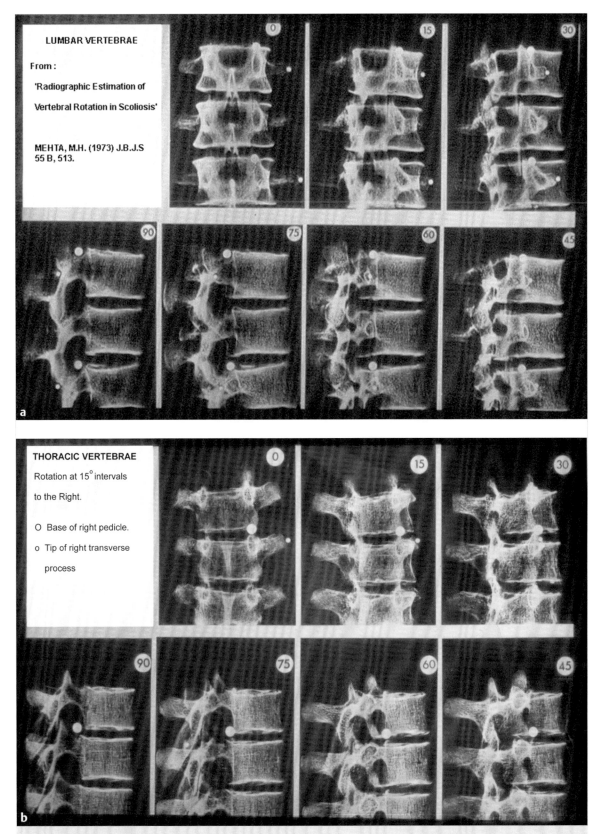

LUMBAR VERTEBRAE

From :

'Radiographic Estimation of

Vertebral Rotation in Scoliosis'

MEHTA, M.H. (1973) J.B.J.S
55 B, 513.

THORACIC VERTEBRAE

Rotation at 15° intervals

to the Right.

O   Base of right pedicle.

o   Tip of right transverse

    process

Fig. 10.7 (a, b) Radiographs of a 2-month-old and 6-month-old.

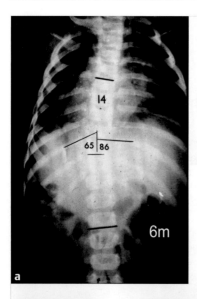

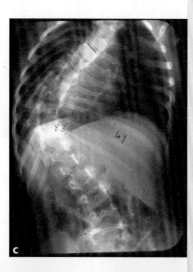

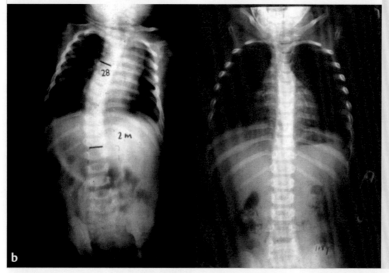

Fig. 10.8 (a) Fourteen degree curve in a 6-month-old. (b) Resolving curve in 2 month old (RVAD is less than 20). (c) Eighty-three degree curve in a 4-year-old.

Case Study

In the case of one child who was 3 months of age, the rib–vertebra angle was measured, and there was symmetry of the rib cage. However, when the child was 5 months of age, a curve that looked relatively benign could be seen, but the parents were fearful because the rib–vertebra angles were asymmetric. At 7 months and 8 months, the curve looked worse, and by 1 year it was much worse. At this point, palliative treatment was likely to be the only option. This case serves as a warning—that is, the more appropriate action to take is to begin watching these children much earlier than the medical profession does now, and to do so more frequently, because children grow fast. At the first sign of deterioration, health care professionals should take action. After that point, it is often too late. Every clinician is different, and so is every child; children do not conform to a specific rule, so treatment must be individualized to prevent the development of scoliosis.

Phases 1 and 2 were devised to help health care professionals decide when to take action. If there is any doubt, look at the head of the rib in relation to the vertebra; if it is phase 2, immediate action should be taken. If there is any doubt in phase 1, watch very carefully because it can soon become phase 2. The spine can be normalized up to a point during the phase 2 stage; beyond that stage, however, very little can be done.

A familiar pattern of growth should now be visible to the reader, peaking in the first few years, then becoming slower and slower as a child grows until there is a peak at adolescence. Generally, the child will increase in height (20 cm) during the first year of life, but the child may grow only 12 cm during the second year. Therefore, that first year is a phenomenal period of growth. Once the child reaches adolescence, the rate of growth only matches that of the second year of life. So, if scoliosis is to be prevented, health care professionals should avoid telling parents to "come back in 6 months"; even 3-month periods are likely to be unacceptable. Instead, the health care professional should examine the child, and if there is a slight increase in the RVAD, treat the child to ensure that the spine will grow completely straight.

It is unfortunate that there are children with 20-degree curves who have never received early treatment. Spinal fusion is avoidable, provided action is taken very early on, but it is still a condition seen in many cases. In order to take action early, health care professionals must change their mindsets. Children grow at a phenomenal speed, so supplying a plaster jacket after the child has grown past that point on the graph is useless. Current treatment options are better than those in the past, but the principle of treatment still remains the same: to get rid of scoliosis forever, treat patients early (▶ Fig. 10.9).

In one particular case, an individual presented with a small curve but was never treated. Later, that same patient presented with a disastrous increase to a 63-degree deformity with an overlap of the ribs and rotation of the vertebrae. There was no cure; the placement of rods was

the only option. Another case was that of a 4-year-old child with underlying genetic factors whose condition resembled syndromic scoliosis. The child should have been quickly treated to prevent the condition from becoming worse. It is the same with the curves in the lower back. Yet another child presented with small curves that very rapidly progressed to big curves (▶ Fig. 10.10).

Another patient, approximately 6 to 9 months of age, presented to my clinic. The child was not walking at that time. A plaster jacket was applied and moulded to align the ribs. The ribs on the prominent side were being pushed, allowing the body to grow symmetrically by getting a nice large rib window in the concavity. There was also a large window to allow the child's chest to expand.

Growth can be used as a corrective force in early treatment. While a patient is still growing, early treatment will result in the absence of scoliosis in a large number of patients. Of course, there are some whose scoliosis is

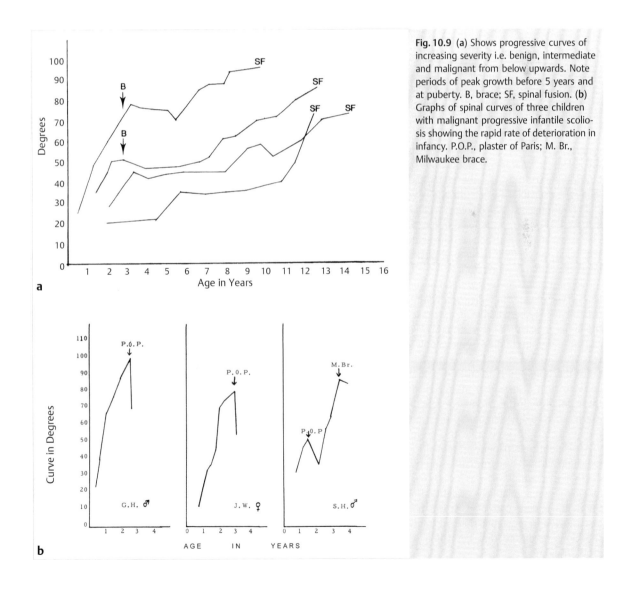

Fig. 10.9 (a) Shows progressive curves of increasing severity i.e. benign, intermediate and malignant from below upwards. Note periods of peak growth before 5 years and at puberty. B, brace; SF, spinal fusion. **(b)** Graphs of spinal curves of three children with malignant progressive infantile scoliosis showing the rapid rate of deterioration in infancy. P.O.P., plaster of Paris; M. Br., Milwaukee brace.

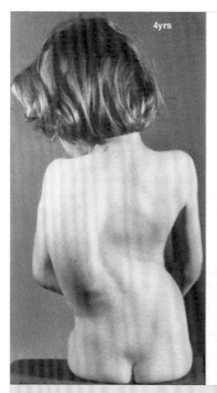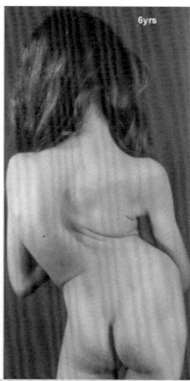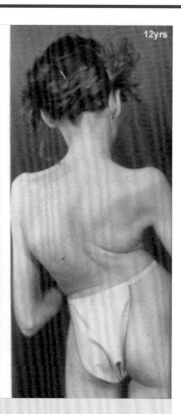

Fig. 10.10 Untreated curve with rapid progression.

syndromic; in these cases, the prognosis is not the same. If you look at what is commonly called the general population with scoliosis (i.e., the idiopathic group), you can apply the principle of using growth as a corrective force.

If treatment is started early, good results can be achieved. However, is there a difference with bad curves? The cases mentioned above represented small curves; one such curve that became disastrous was only 12 degrees when it was first noticed.

Even if patients present with large curves, if you persevere in the manner in which you want the child to grow, treatment may be possible. It may take a long time, but the spine is likely to grow straight. When scoliosis was caught "early" in children, some people used to say that it was cruel to put a child into a plaster jacket, but I feel quite the opposite. It is cruel to allow these curves to grow to such a stage that plaster is the only option for these children. If the curves are caught early, then they can be corrected within a very short period of time, and then that child can grow up with a normal spine.

A 14-month-old patient presented for the first time to my clinic with a 43-degree curve and rotation of about 15 degrees. By the time she was 3 years of age, her spine was already growing relatively straight, although the derotation had not quite corrected. At this point, the child was just allowed to grow, but she had frequent hospital consultations to ensure that her spine was continuing to grow straight.

Another patient, aged 9 months, presented to my clinic with a double curve and rotation of 50 degrees. It was a massive distortion for such a young child and should never have been allowed to progress that far.

Many little curves become big curves and never spontaneously resolve. In such cases—and they do frequently occur—immediate action should be taken, and these patients should be treated right away. It may be "only" a small curve, but that small curve can grow very large in a short amount of time. Health care professionals must begin to anticipate these situations and move into a different mindset.

However, what if you suspect that there is a syndrome? Perhaps a syndromic element can be seen. If a syndromic scoliosis is suspected, then it must be treated early because the condition always progresses. Regardless of the size of the Cobb angle or the RVAD, if you suspect that there is an underlying problem, treat the scoliosis first; investigations into the underlying problem can occur at a later time.

In one such case, a small, 8-day-old infant was intubated because there was obviously something wrong with his spine, but no treatment was provided at the time for the scoliosis. At 6 months of age, the patient developed severe scoliosis. He presented to my clinic with this severe deformity. There was a high degree of rotation and crowding of the ribs, and a curve above and one below. An operation would have been futile, so he was put into a plaster jacket. At 5 years of age, a curve was still present, but the child was living a relatively normal life. And although the child was involved in an unfortunate road accident when he was 10 years of age, he had had a quality life, which is important.

Late referrals are not appropriate. Yes, it can take time to obtain a referral, but if you suspect that a child has scoliosis, inform the parents that it is important that their child be seen the next day if the clinic is full. Parents will do anything for their children, and it may be easier to talk to the parents and tell them what is being done and why. We must teach parents about huge delays of 12 to 19 months for treatment. Once parents begin talking to each other, they will become better detectives early on in the diagnosis of scoliosis.

10.2 Commentary

Miss Mehta stresses in this lecture the importance of early treatment once a curve has been detected. However, how early is "early," and what is a reasonable time scale? Treatment involves the serial application of plaster jackets while the child is under general anesthesia. Is this option acceptable, given that emerging evidence suggests that there are risks of neurotoxicity from repeated anesthesia in children? Can orthotic skills be refined enough to provide adequate bracing at such a young age?

The importance of early treatment cannot be overstated, but the clinical prognostic indicators guiding the decision-making process should not be forgotten. Physical characteristics such as facial asymmetry, floppiness, spasticity, and joint laxity can be observed during a meticulous examination of the child. The radiologic markers by way of the relationship between the rib heads and the upper corners of the vertebral bodies are—and should remain—an important part of the armamentarium in the battle against progressive curves. The presence of rotation also heralds the likelihood of progression and cannot be overlooked.

The outlook for children with poorly treated curves is at best a lifetime of ill health and at worst early mortality; therefore, it is imperative that health care professionals avail themselves of the optimal knowledge and acquire the skills to manage this debilitating and complex condition.

Further Reading

Mehta MH. Growth as a corrective force in the early treatment of progressive infantile scoliosis. J Bone Joint Surg Br 2005; 87: 1237–1247

11 The Mehta Casting Technique

Min Mehta (transcribed by Colin Nnadi)

Min Mehta popularized the casting technique for the treatment of early onset scoliosis. The Mehta casting technique is based on the Cotrel elongation, derotation, *and* flexion technique. Its principal concept is that forces are applied in longitudinal, transverse, and rotatory directions. Early treatment is key.

Factors to consider when the child is being examined include the following:

- Curve pattern (single, double, or triple)
- Lumbar or thoracic curve
- Structural or compensatory curve
- Location of the apex
  - Above T8: over the shoulder
  - Below T8: under the arm
- Ideally, upper thoracic curves require neck inclusion (but may cause compliance issues)
- Risk for truncal imbalance with a structural upper thoracic curve
- Rib prominence / lumbar prominence
- Shoulder asymmetry
- Pelvic obliquity
- Limb length discrepancy

Key essentials of the technique include the following:

- Radiographic equipment in the operating theater
- Surgeon and surgeon assistant
- Casting frame
- Plaster technicians
- Plaster of paris
- Body stockinettes (two)
- Wool
- Felt pads
- Adequate time
- General anesthesia

The casting frame (▶ Fig. 11.1) consists of a Risser trolley and an overhead frame. Pulleys with a ratcheting mechanism attached to the ends and sides of the frame allow the application of traction. The head, shoulder (shoulder bar at the level of the axilla), sacrum (sacral bar just below the buttocks at the level of the greater trochanter), and legs (slings) are supported. For patients with a lumbar curve, flexion of the hips helps to derotate the curve.

11.1 Summary of the Procedure

The child is under general anesthesia. A body stockinette is placed over the trunk. Halter traction is applied through a windlass at the head and foot ends of the casting frame. The patient's head is put into a halter strap and attached to the windlass at the head of the frame (▶ Fig. 11.2). Two pelvic straps are wrapped around the waist overlying the body stockinette; they pass above the iliac crests and are tied at the level of the greater trochanter. Each strap runs under the ipsilateral leg to attach to the windlass at the foot end of the casting frame; the legs are supported by slings attached to the overhead crossbar of the casting frame.

A second body stockinette is applied so that the pelvic straps are situated between two layers of stockinette. They can be easily pulled out at the end of casting. A layer of 4-inch Bandage Ortho Wool is then applied over the stockinettes and snugly wrapped around the trunk (▶ Fig. 11.3). The layers should not be bulky so that the clinician's ability to achieve a good mold to the plaster is not compromised. A Velband roll is placed over the symphysis pubis to help mold the

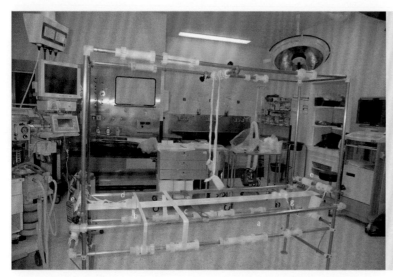

Fig. 11.1 Casting frame.

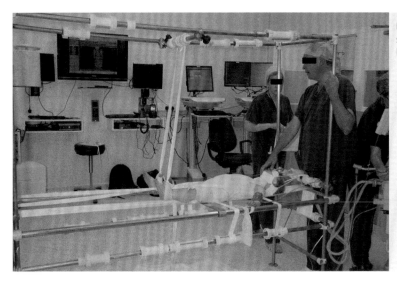

Fig. 11.2 Patient's head is put into a halter strap and attached to the windlass at the head of the frame.

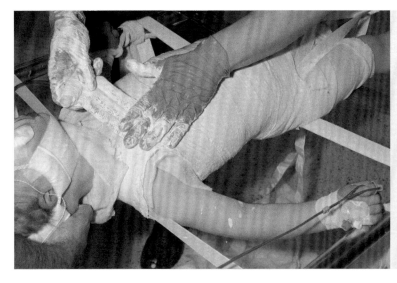

Fig. 11.3 Ortho Wool is applied over the stockinettes and snugly wrapped around the trunk.

plaster cast over the iliac crests and abdomen and to prevent too tight a fit around the child's abdomen. The Velband padding should be applied in such a way that there is adequate moulding with a good grip. Felt pads should be placed over all bony prominences to protect them and prevent pressure sores.

Hip flexion allows the derotation and correction of lumbar curves. Awareness of any shoulder asymmetry (arm positioning) and pelvic asymmetry / limb length discrepancy should be maintained, and with the ratchets, the traction of the straps should be adjusted as necessary.

The spine should be palpated during traction to determine the amount of curve correction needed. Once the surgeon is satisfied with the patient's positioning, plaster of paris is applied. A few minutes should be allowed to pass before the clinician begins to mold the plaster as follows:

- The rib / lumbar prominence is derotated by displacing the apex of the prominence anteriorly with posterolateral pressure for a thoracic curve and lateral pressure for a lumbar curve.
- The frontal portion of the cast extends distally to the symphysis pubis to allow hip flexion to 100 degrees.
- The cast extends distally at the back to the mid buttocks to allow gluteal hygiene.

A fiberglass layer is applied, and an epigastric window is cut with an oscillating saw to allow abdominal expansion and ease of breathing (▶ Fig. 11.4). A window is also cut over the concavity of the curve on the side opposite the apex to allow passive correction. Another contralateral window may be applied for lumbar curves. The cast should be changed, on average, every 2 to 4 months and in response to curve changes. More frequent changes may be necessary in younger children.

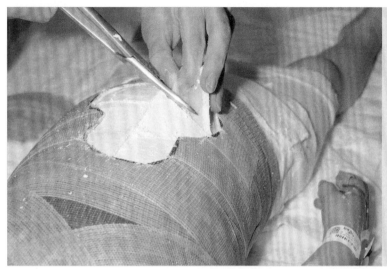

Fig. 11.4 A fiberglass layer is applied, and an epigastric window is cut with an oscillating saw.

It is worth noting that historically, derotation was applied through a strap that was attached to the side bar on the concavity of the curve, then passed under the patient and attached to a pulley on an overhead bar on the convexity of the curve. Presently, the surgeon applies derotation manually with anteriorly directed, posterolateral pressure over the apex of the curve while moulding the plaster.

Further Reading

Cotrel Y, Morel G. La technique de l'EDF dans la correction des scolioses. Rev Chir Orthop 1964; 50: 59–75

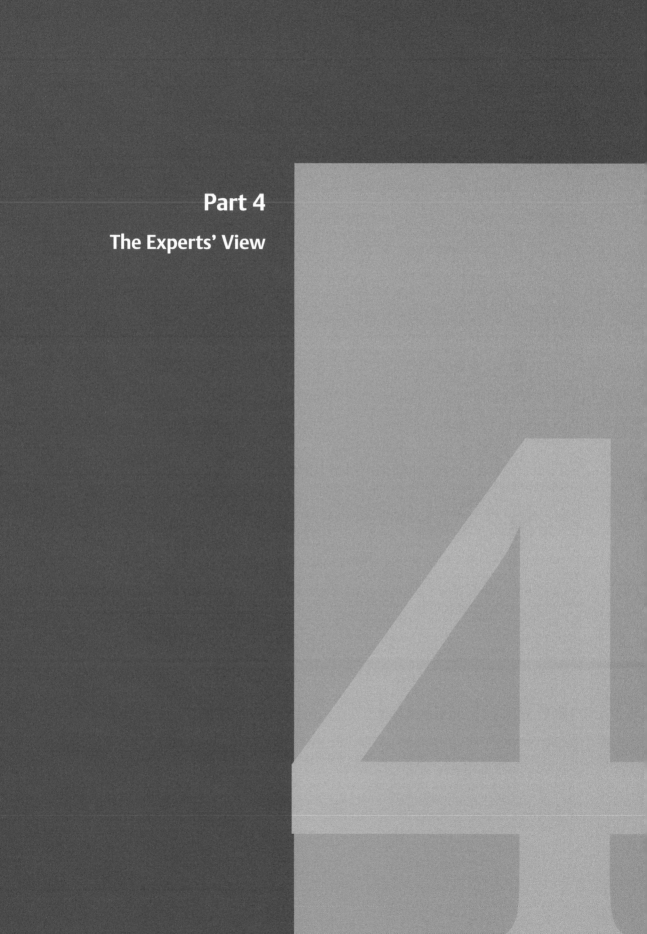

Part 4
The Experts' View

12 Dual Growing Rod Treatment

Matthew J. Goldstein and Behrooz A. Akbarnia

The preservation of spinal growth and prevention of pulmonary compromise in early onset scoliosis pose particularly challenging problems for clinician and patient alike. Maintaining spinal growth and achieving the necessary thoracic height are critical for expansion of the thoracic cavity and the prevention of thoracic insufficiency syndrome.

Alveolar multiplication is thought to continue up until 9 years of age, and the attainment of a vertical thoracic height of 22 cm may afford 80% of the normal forced vital capacity.[1] With these values in mind, it is essential for the clinician to understand spinal and thoracic cavity growth patterns. The first peak in spinal growth occurs during the first 5 years of life, when the T1-S1 height increases at a rate of approximately 2 cm per year. At this time, the thoracic and lumbar spine reaches approximately two-thirds of its adult height. Approximately 6 cm is gained between the ages of 6 and 10 years, and 10 cm between 10 and 18 years.[2] Dimeglio and Bonnel[3] showed that normal T1-T12 thoracic height in newborn children without scoliosis is 11 cm; it reaches 18 cm at 5 years, 22 cm at 10 years, and 26.5 cm in female adults and 28 cm in male adults. The average adult spine measures 42 to 45 cm at skeletal maturity.

Operative treatment in this patient population should be reserved for those with progressive curves in whom nonoperative measures, including casting and bracing, have failed. The correction of surgical deformity ideally aims to restore, maintain, and promote cardiopulmonary and visceral growth. Research in the treatment of this difficult problem strives for more definitive, less invasive or noninvasive options. As our knowledge and understanding of the pathophysiology and biomechanics of scoliosis increase and as more reliable, less invasive options become available, outcomes are expected to improve.

In the absence of rib anomalies or resectable congenital deformities, growth-friendly, distraction-based techniques, such as dual growing rods, currently remain the preferred and most commonly used surgical treatment for children with early onset scoliosis.

12.1 Historical Context

Fusionless instrumented techniques for early onset scoliosis have evolved to be more reliable since Harrington's account in 1962.[4] He described a concavity-placed single rod anchored with two hooks. Hook dislocation and rod breakage ultimately obliged technique modification. Moe et al[5] later depicted a modification of Harrington's technique through the serial lengthening of subcutaneous rods placed with a limited subperiosteal exposure at the anchor sites. They also modified the rod geometry to reduce scar formation and allow sagittal contouring. Despite improvements, similar instrumentation problems were encountered. To address anchor and rod failure, Marchetti and Faldini[6] introduced the technique of end-of-construct (foundation) fusion in 1978. Serial lengthening procedures were then performed on the mobile spine after the initial fusion procedure. Other, later notable modifications included the use of sublaminar wires, segmental fixation without arthrodesis, and Luque rod instrumentation.

Modern day growing rods as we know them were introduced in the last decade. Despite advances in technique and instrumentation, the reported outcomes and complications with the use of modern growing rods, especially single rods, have been variable and have resulted in premature fusion in some patients.

In 2000, Akbarnia and Marks[7] introduced the use of dual growing rods with posterior segmental instrumentation and limited arthrodesis of the foundations. In 2005, Akbarnia et al described the technique that most surgeons use today.[8] It has become the most commonly applied technique for dual growing rod surgery and is discussed in detail in this chapter.

12.2 Patient Evaluation

12.2.1 Physical Examination, Clinical and Radiographic Assessment

Patients with early onset scoliosis are often referred by their primary care physicians because of concern about spinal deformity. A thorough and systematic history and physical examination are critical and should be performed on all patients. The prenatal and birth history, as well as the record of achieving age-appropriate developmental milestones, should be included. Questions should be asked about factors predisposing a child to scoliosis, such as family history. The physical examination should include measurement of the height, weight, and arm span as well as an evaluation of the skin, head, neck, chest, pelvis, and extremities. A thorough neurologic examination is paramount, and abdominal reflex testing should be done; its absence may signal an underlying neuroaxial anomaly. The evaluation of the spine should include forward bending and an assessment of spinal flexibility. This may have to be done over the clinician's knee. Scoliometry is valuable in the clinical evaluation of trunk rotation. Limb lengths should be measured, and pelvic obliquity should be assessed. Gait should be observed in the ambulatory child when possible.

A clinical assessment for early onset scoliosis should always include plain roentgenograms (anteroposterior, lateral, and full-length views) of the spine, including the neck, pelvis, and hips, to evaluate the degree of coronal and sagittal malalignment as well as scoliosis. Bending roentgenograms provide valuable information regarding curve flexibility. Traction or bolster films should also be considered. In idiopathic early onset scoliosis, measurement of the rib–vertebral angle difference (RVAD) and overlap (phase 1 or phase 2) should be evaluated to predict progression. Magnetic resonance (MR) imaging should be considered to rule out concomitant pathology involving the neuraxis and visceral structures. Computed tomography (CT) with three-dimensional reconstructions is useful for further evaluating the deformity, better visualizing any congenital anomalies, and planning surgery (e.g., pedicle screw length). To reduce cumulative exposure of the patient to radiation, an attempt should be made to schedule imaging with other specialties should more than one organ system need to be evaluated.

A multidisciplinary team approach to pre- and postoperative care is employed because many of these patients pose challenges to medical management. Pulmonary function testing should be considered before surgical intervention when possible. A preoperative laboratory and nutritional evaluation should include a complete blood cell count with total lymphocyte count, a comprehensive metabolic panel with albumin and prealbumin levels, and a bleeding profile. Appropriate medical clearances should be obtained before surgery, with a thorough anesthesia and, if necessary, pulmonary evaluation.

12.3 Treatment

12.3.1 Nonoperative Treatment

Nonoperative treatment options for early onset scoliosis include observation, bracing, and casting (▶ Fig. 12.1). Some authors have reported utility with halo traction, but this is less desirable in our view and is reserved for selected patients with severe and rigid curves as a preoperative adjunct to correction. The flexibility of the immature rib cage may limit the transmission of force on the spine and as a whole may render nonoperative treatment ineffective. Nonetheless, nonoperative treatment modalities should be exhausted before surgical intervention is undertaken. Serial casting, such as the technique of Mehta and Morel,[9] has recently gained popularity as a surgery-delaying tactic; it includes repeated cast changes, with the patient under general anesthesia, every 4 to 6 weeks until a brace may be used. A cervicothoracic lumbosacral orthosis (CTLSO), such as the Milwaukee-type brace, is preferred to control a thoracic curve. An underarm brace, or thoracolumbosacral orthosis (TLSO), is less effective at controlling a thoracic deformity. The over-the-shoulder TLSO Kalibus brace has been historically

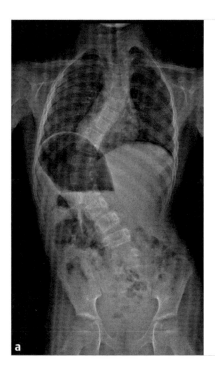
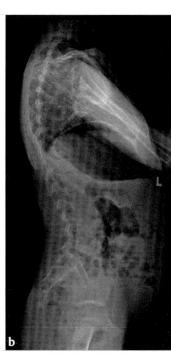

Fig. 12.1 Preoperative posteroanterior (a) and lateral (b) radiographs of an 8-year-old girl with idiopathic early onset scoliosis. The T7-L3 left thoracolumbar scoliosis measured 66 degrees. The patient underwent bracing with a thoracic lumbosacral orthosis for 18 months.

recommended for patients as young as less than 1 year of age who have early onset scoliosis. Bracing failure, noted as curve progression or brace intolerance secondary to skin or pressure issues, should prompt consideration for surgery. Earlier correction may be considered for patients with more significant thoracic curves to prevent potential pulmonary complications.

12.3.2 Operative Indications and Timing

The optimal timing and indications to pursue operative intervention remain in question. In a level 4 survey of international surgeons treating early onset scoliosis,[10] the surgeons reported that their primary indication for growing rod treatment included curves greater than 60 degrees in patients younger than 8 to 10 years of age, with 6 months as the preferred time between lengthening procedures. Other reported indications included rigid curves, brace intolerance, and syndromic diagnoses. Despite this consensus, in actual practice, the mean curve at rod insertion was at 73 degrees at a patient age of 6 years. Lengthening procedures occurred at 8.6 months. Skeletal maturity and Risser 3 (or greater) measurements were reported as markers of the time to perform final fusion.

As is detailed in another chapter, the earlier that operative intervention is undertaken, the greater is the likelihood that complications will be encountered.[11] For this reason, prolonging observation or nonoperative treatment as long as possible may be ideal. However, most authors agree that nonfusion treatment for early onset scoliosis, such as dual growing rods, should be initiated between the ages of 4 and 7 years.

12.3.3 Authors' Preferred Technique[12]

Index Procedure

The goal of the index procedure is partial correction, with the remaining correction accomplished through repeated lengthening and growth. The most significant gains in the coronal plane can be expected in the index surgery. The initial surgery is performed on an inpatient basis, with the patient under general anesthesia. After antibiotics have been administered and general endotracheal anesthesia has been induced, multimodality neuromonitoring with transcranial motor evoked potentials (Tc-MEPs), electromyography, somatosensory evoked potentials (SSEPs), and Hoffmann reflexes, as well as arterial blood pressure monitoring, is begun. A Cell Saver (Haemonetics, Braintree, Massachusetts) is used. After placement of the Foley catheter, smaller children are positioned on chest rolls on a flat-top Jackson table (Mizuh OSI, Union City, CA) and older patients on a Relton-Hall frame (Surgmed,

Dorval, Quebec, Canada). Fluoroscopic imaging is used to identify proximal and distal anchoring levels. A limited incision is made at the proximal and distal anchor sites. Unnecessary exposure of noninstrumented levels may lead to spontaneous fusion and should be avoided. The anchor sites chosen proximally are generally at the T2–T4 level, and distally at two to three levels below the lower-end vertebra of the major curve and usually at the stable vertebra or below; pelvic fixation is added in patients who require correction of pelvic obliquity. The number and levels of the fixation points should be determined by the underlying diagnosis and the amount of correction necessary at the index surgery. Four to six bilateral pedicle screws or hooks in a "claw" formation should be used for each foundation. When a hook construct is used, a cross-link is added to increase biomechanical strength. Cross-links are not usually used when an all-pedicle-screw construct is employed.[13]

A 4.5-mm stainless steel or titanium rod is often chosen in primary cases. Larger rods are reserved for large patients or revision situations. The rod is contoured for deformity correction, with care taken not to contour too much because excessive stress on the anchor sites may lead to failure. The region between T10 and L2 should be fairly straight to fit the connector; however, if more contouring is needed, a side-to-side connector can be used, and in that case, the rods can be contoured as needed. In addition, the rod segment ultimately placed within the tandem connector should not be contoured to fit into the connector and facilitate future distractions.

The rods are cut at the junction where future lengthening will be performed (most often at the thoracolumbar junction) and contoured. The rod is cut slightly longer to build in lengthening to the index procedure.

The rods are passed subfascially in a distal to proximal direction, with care taken not to penetrate the chest or spinal canal. The rods are then secured to their proximal anchors. The upper foundation is secured, and if hooks are used, a connector is added between the two rods for added stability. Tandem connectors are added from the distal onto the proximal rods. The longest tandem connector that can be accommodated is selected, and the set-screws are positioned medially to allow easy access in future lengthening procedures. Once the distal rods and foundation are secured, the tandem connectors are slid onto the distal rods and tightened. An initial lengthening is performed at this time outside the tandem connector against the distal anchors.

Fusion is then performed at the anchor sites by preparing the facet joints and the interlaminar and interspinous spaces with a high-speed cutting bur. These areas are packed with autograft or allograft / bone extenders as necessary.

Meticulous skin and subcutaneous closure is critical, given the expectation for multiple future surgeries. The surgeon should be prepared for complex wound closures

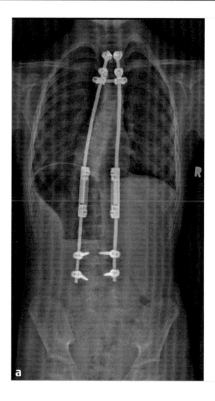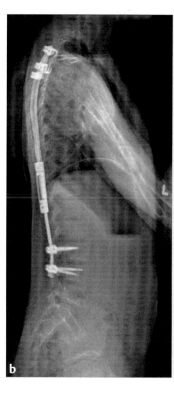

Fig. 12.2 Posteroanterior (a) and lateral (b) radiographs following index growing rod surgery. The Cobb angle corrected to 25 degrees, and the T1-T12 and T1-S1 heights initially improved from 183 to 198 mm and from 289 to 327 mm, respectively.

if necessary. A sterile dressing is applied. Final intraoperative radiographs are taken (▶ Fig. 12.2).

Postoperative Care

We employ a TLSO for the first 4 to 6 months postoperatively after the index procedure for anchor site protection. Once solid fusion is evident, the brace may be discontinued. A brace is generally not used after lengthening procedures.

Lengthening

Lengthening procedures are performed at approximately 6-month intervals on an inpatient or outpatient basis, depending on the individual patient. Positioning and neurophysiologic monitoring are similar to those used for the index procedure. The proximal setscrews within the tandem connector are identified by palpation or by fluoroscopy and marked. A single incision is used, often at the site of the previous incision. Bilateral exposure is obtained, with careful handling of the tissues to expose the rods, setscrews, and proximal ends of the tandem connectors and ensure that good soft tissue coverage is available for closure. We generally choose to lengthen the concavity of the curve first. The setscrew on the concave side is loosened first, but the setscrew on the convex side should also be loosened before lengthening is accomplished. A rod holder is placed proximal to the tandem connector on the concave side, and the distractor tool is

placed between the rod holder and connector to accomplish lengthening outside the tandem connector. While length is maintained, the setscrew on the concave side is released, and 5 to 10 mm of distraction is obtained. The setscrew is tightened, and the steps are repeated on the opposite side.

Lengthening may also be performed within the tandem connector. In this instance, the distractor is placed within the connector slot, the setscrew is loosened, a gentle distraction is performed, and the setscrew is retightened. The skin is closed in a manner similar to that used for the index surgery. Final intraoperative radiographs are taken (▶ Fig. 12.3, ▶ Fig. 12.4, ▶ Fig. 12.5).

Final Fusion

When the patient is of sufficient age (usually 11 to 13 years), additional lengthening no longer yields considerable benefit,[2] or instrumentation failure is encountered, the final fusion procedure is performed. The mean duration of growing rod treatment is 5 years. Additional correction is often possible after removal of the growing rod instrumentation at this time, with the majority of patients experiencing 21 to 50% curve correction.[14] Previously placed pedicle screws sites may be used with anchor exchange. It may be necessary to consider including additional levels (most often one or two levels) to the final fusion construct, but most often the proximal and distal foundations will be the same as those spanned by the growing rods.[14]

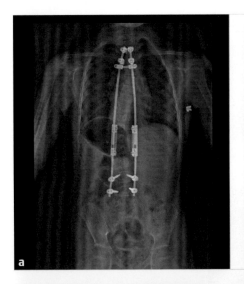
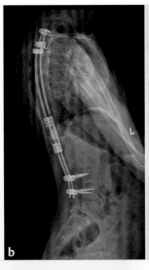

Fig. 12.3 Posteroanterior (**a**) and lateral (**b**) radiographs following the first lengthening procedure.

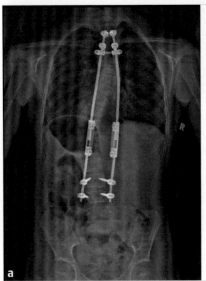
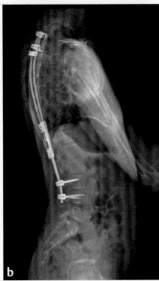

Fig. 12.4 Posteroanterior (**a**) and lateral (**b**) radiographs following the second lengthening procedure.

12.4 Outcomes

12.4.1 Operative Treatment: Single vs. Dual Rods, Device Types

Greater annual growth has been shown in patients undergoing more frequent lengthening procedures. In 2008, Akbarnia et al[15] did a retrospective case review of 13 patients (average age, 6.6 ± 2.9 years; average follow-up, 5.7 years) within the Growing Spine Study Group database who underwent subcutaneous dual growing rod treatment from 1990 to 2003. The patients had had no previous surgery and had noncongenital curves. Final fusion occurred at an average age of 11 years. The Cobb angle improved from 81 to 36 degrees after index surgery and to 27 degrees after final fusion. On average, the patients underwent a total of 5.2 lengthening procedures at 9.4-month intervals (range, 5.5–20 months). The T1-S1

length increased from 24.4 to 29.3 cm after initial surgery and to 35.0 cm after final fusion. Average growth was 1.46 cm per year. Those who underwent lengthening at intervals shorter than or equal to 6 months had better annual growth (1.8 cm) than did those who underwent lengthening less frequently (1.0 cm), and they also had significantly better scoliosis correction (79% vs. 48%). The upper foundation anchors were thoracic hooks in all patients. The lower foundation anchors were hooks alone in five patients, screws alone in five, a combination of hooks and screws in two, and hook/Galveston fixation to the pelvis in one patient.

Dual growing rod fixation constructs have been shown to be superior to single growing rod constructs with respect to correction and amount of growth. In 2005, Thompson et al[16] reported a level 3 retrospective comparison of 28 patients who were treated from 1992 to 2004 with a single growing rod or dual growing rods and

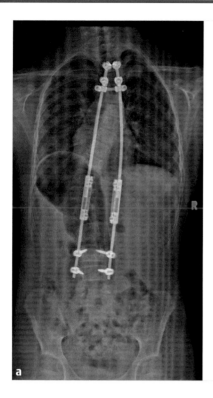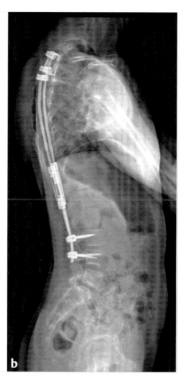

Fig. 12.5 Latest posteroanterior (**a**) and lateral (**b**) follow-up radiographs after the third lengthening. The Cobb angle measured 22 degrees, and the T1-T12 and T1-S1 heights measured 231 and 368 mm, respectively. No complications were encountered during the course of treatment.

who underwent a minimum of 2 years of follow-up. Of the 28 patients, five had a single submuscular growing rod with short apical fusion, 16 had a single growing rod alone, and seven had dual growing rods. Age at initial surgery and the interval between rod insertion and final fusion were similar across groups. Patients in the dual growing rod group underwent lengthening routinely at 6-month intervals. Of the three groups, the patients with dual growing rods had the best initial correction (48% vs. 39% vs. 57%), maintenance of correction (23% vs. 36% vs. 71%), amount of growth per year (0.3 vs. 1.04 vs. 1.7 cm), and percentage growth of T1-S1 (25% vs. 80% vs. 130%). However, frontal balance and sagittal balance were better in the single growing rod group, although sagittal alignment was not determined to be problematic in any group.

Consideration should be given to dual growing rod fixation with bilateral iliac fixation in selected patients. In a retrospective review of the Growing Spine Study Group database from 1990 to 2007 that analyzed the outcomes of patients who had growing rods fixed to the pelvis, Sponseller et al[17] reported improved correction in the coronal and sagittal planes with pelvic fixation. Furthermore, dual growing rods corrected pelvic obliquity better than a single growing rod, with iliac anchors more effective than sacral anchors. In their paper, they suggested bilateral iliac fixation with maximal anchor length and a rigid distal cross-link.

Eventually, lengthening procedures become less reliable and lead to "diminishing returns." Sankar et al[2] reported a retrospective multicenter study of 38 patients treated for early onset scoliosis whose mean follow-up

was 3.3 years; the patients underwent at least three lengthening procedures at 6.8-month intervals. The Cobb angle improved from 74 to 36 degrees after initial surgery and did not change with subsequent lengthening procedures. After the index surgery, the average gain in T1-S1 length for lengthening procedures was 1.76 ± 0.71 cm per year. However, the authors noted a significant decrease in this value with repeated lengthening procedures and with time. They refer to this phenomenon as the "law of diminishing returns" and suggest autofusion of the spine with prolonged internal immobilization to be the cause. The authors offer a word of caution that surgeons should not expect substantial distraction after repeated (six to eight) lengthening procedures.

12.4.2 Complications

Because these patients undergo frequent operations in the setting of multiple medical comorbidities, complications may be encountered. The patients should be followed with frequent clinical and radiographic evaluation. Complications include infection, wound dehiscence, curve progression, junctional kyphosis, instrumentation prominence or failure, and the crankshaft phenomenon. These are discussed in detail in the next chapter.

12.5 Future Directions and Emerging Techniques

In the future, distraction-based, growth-friendly surgery will focus on improving outcomes through the use of less invasive or noninvasive techniques. Minimally invasive techniques may reduce tissue damage and potentially reduce the number of operations and complications while optimizing outcomes. Additionally, the idea of lengthening procedures without the repeated need for anesthesia or open surgery is appealing. Exciting data published in 2012 by Akbarnia et al[18] showed promise for magnetically controlled growing rods. In a porcine model, the authors were able to achieve 80% of predicted spinal height through noninvasive means with the MAGEC system (Ellipse Technologies, Irvine, California). Since then, Cheung et al[19] have reported encouraging results in five patients, two with 24 months of follow-up, who underwent magnetically controlled, remote distractions on a monthly basis in the first human clinical series in which this device was used. In their series, the mean improvement in scoliosis was from 67 to 29 degrees. In addition, the length of the instrumented segment increased 1.9 mm. No complications were noted with this treatment, and patients reported no pain with lengthening procedures as measured by the Visual Analog Scale and stable Scoliosis Research Society questionnaire (SRS-30) scores. Similarly, Akbarnia et al[20] reported on 14 patients who underwent 68 distractions with a mean follow-up of 10 months. T1-T12 height gain through single rod distraction yielded 7.6 mm of total distraction, or 1.09 mm per month, whereas dual rod distraction yielded 12.12 mm of total distraction, or 1.97 mm per month. T1-S1 height gain through single rod distraction yielded 9.1 mm, or 1.27 mm per month, and dual rod distraction yielded 20.3 mm, or 3.09 mm per month. No major complications were observed, but one patient with superficial infection and one patient with a prominent implant were seen. Through innovations such as this, early onset scoliosis can be managed remotely with fewer operations, fewer anesthetic events, and, it is hoped, less morbidity for our patients.

12.6 Conclusion

Long-term outcome studies and advances in techniques have equipped us to manage patients with early onset scoliosis more effectively. Nonetheless, early onset scoliosis remains a considerable challenge. Progress is ongoing, with the focus on less invasive, more definitive options for confronting this problem. A novel, consensus-based classification of early onset scoliosis has been introduced to improve research efforts through standardization and ultimately improve care. This system is based on the etiology of the scoliosis (congenital / structural, neuromuscular, syndromic, or idiopathic), Cobb angle, degree of kyphosis (hypo-, normo-, or hyperkyphosis), and documented progression for a minimum of 6 months.[21] Future research should focus on acquiring a better understanding of the pathophysiology and natural history of early onset scoliosis, and the outcomes of our current treatment methods.

References

[1] Karol LA, Johnston C, Mladenov K, Schochet P, Walters P, Browne RH. Pulmonary function following early thoracic fusion in non-neuromuscular scoliosis. J Bone Joint Surg Am 2008; 90: 1272–1281

[2] Sankar WN, Skaggs DL, Yazici M et al. Lengthening of dual growing rods and the law of diminishing returns. Spine 2011; 36: 806–809

[3] Dimeglio A, Bonnel F. Le Rachis en Croissance. Paris, France: Springer; 1990:392–394

[4] Harrington PR. Treatment of scoliosis. Correction and internal fixation by spine instrumentation. J Bone Joint Surg Am 1962; 44-A: 591–610

[5] Moe JH, Kharrat K, Winter RB, Cummine JL. Harrington instrumentation without fusion plus external orthotic support for the treatment of difficult curvature problems in young children. Clin Orthop Relat Res 1984: 35–45

[6] Marchetti PG, Faldini A. End fusions in the treatment of some progressing or severe scoliosis in childhood or early adolescence. Presented to the Scoliosis Research Society, 1977 Orthop Trans 1978; 2: 271

[7] Akbarnia BA, Marks DS. Instrumentation with limited arthrodesis for the treatment of progressive early-onset scoliosis. Spine: State of the Art Reviews 2000; 14: 181–189

[8] Akbarnia BA, Marks DS, Boachie-Adjei O, Thompson AG, Asher MA. Dual growing rod technique for the treatment of progressive early-onset scoliosis: a multicenter study. Spine 2005; 30 Suppl: S46–S57

[9] Mehta M, Morel G. The non-operative treatment of infantile idiopathic scoliosis. In: Zorab P, Siezler D, eds. Scoliosis 1979. London, UK: Academic Press; 1979:71–84

[10] Yang JS, McElroy MJ, Akbarnia BA et al. Growing rods for spinal deformity: characterizing consensus and variation in current use. J Pediatr Orthop 2010; 30: 264–270

[11] Bess S, Akbarnia BA, Thompson GH et al. Complications of growing-rod treatment for early-onset scoliosis: analysis of one hundred and forty patients. J Bone Joint Surg Am 2010; 92: 2533–2543

[12] Mundis GM, Kabirian N, Akbarnia BA. Dual growing rods for the treatment of early-onset scoliosis. JBJS Essential Surg Tech 2013; 3: e6

[13] Mahar AT, Bagheri R, Oka R, Kostial P, Akbarnia BA. Biomechanical comparison of different anchors (foundations) for the pediatric dual growing rod technique. Spine J 2008; 8: 933–939

[14] Flynn JM, Tomlinson LA, Pawelek J, Thompson GH, McCarthy R, Akbarnia BA Growing Spine Study Group. Growing-rod graduates: lessons learned from ninety-nine patients who completed lengthening. J Bone Joint Surg Am 2013; 95: 1745–1750

[15] Akbarnia BA, Breakwell LM, Marks DS et al. Growing Spine Study Group. Dual growing rod technique followed for three to eleven years until final fusion: the effect of frequency of lengthening. Spine 2008; 33: 984–990

[16] Thompson GH, Akbarnia BA, Kostial P et al. Comparison of single and dual growing rod techniques followed through definitive surgery: a preliminary study. Spine 2005; 30: 2039–2044

[17] Sponseller PD, Yang JS, Thompson GH et al. Pelvic fixation of growing rods: comparison of constructs. Spine 2009; 34: 1706–1710

[18] Akbarnia BA, Mundis GM Jr Salari P, Yaszay B, Pawelek JB. Innovation in growing rod technique: a study of safety and efficacy of a magnetically controlled growing rod in a porcine model. Spine 2012; 37: 1109–1114

[19] Cheung KM, Cheung JP, Samartzis D et al. Magnetically controlled growing rods for severe spinal curvature in young children: a prospective case series. Lancet 2012; 379: 1967–1974

[20] Akbarnia BA, Cheung K, Noordeen H et al. Next generation of growth sparing techniques: preliminary clincial results of a magnetically controlled growing rod (MCGR) in 14 patients. Spine 201 3; 38: 66: 5–670

[21] Williams BA, Matsumoto H, McCalla DJ et al. Development and initial validation of a novel classification system in early onset scoliosis. J Bone Joint Surg Am 2014; 96: 1359–1367

13 Surgical Options: The Shilla Procedure

Richard E. McCarthy

The various etiologic diagnoses in early onset scoliosis all lead to a common pathway—namely, that of thoracic insufficiency syndrome. The diagnoses generally are classified as having idiopathic, syndromic, neuromuscular, or congenital causes. The long-term outcome of untreated early onset scoliosis is severe compromise of respiratory function, evidenced by pulmonary function study values that are less than 20% of predicted values; furthermore, respiratory compromise is correlated with early death according to the studies of Pehrsson et al,[1] who compared death rates in patients with infantile scoliosis with expected death rates in unaffected adults. Death due to respiratory compromise in children who have early onset scoliosis has been observed even in those younger than 10 years of age.

The previously accepted dictum of treatment with early fusion to produce a straight spine has resulted, in many cases, with short thoracic height, compromised pulmonary function, and early death.[2,3,4] The fallacy of this treatment method has been shown by many and has encouraged the development of expandable prostheses that promote an increase in thoracic height and an expansion of pulmonary capacity. However, what are the costs of this approach? Distraction techniques, commonly used in many centers, not only require repeated trips to the operating room for lengthening but also foster the development of proximal junctional kyphosis. This can be a source of an unsightly kyphotic deformity, with prominence of the spinal implants and potential skin breakdown over the implants. There is also a loss of growth centers around the anchor points, whether they are screws or hooks, where localized fusion is used to stabilize the anchor points and create platforms to be pushed apart through distraction.

Ankylosis and autofusion of the facet joints has been noted in patients followed to maturity as a consequence of the partial immobilization caused by the rods and results in the law of diminishing return with subsequent lengthening procedures and, in essence, a loss of potential growth.[5,6] Chest wall stiffness results from vertical expandable prosthetic titanium rib (VEPTR) treatment, and its ultimate effect on respiratory function is unknown. There is also evidence that repeated trips to the operating room cause cognitive delays and adversely affect early childhood development.[7] Skin problems, with an increased risk for infection and scarring, are commonplace in patients who undergo repeated lengthening procedures.

These issues raise questions as we plan the future treatment of early onset scoliosis. For instance, why not direct the corrective forces toward the most curved section of the spine, the apex? And why not place the anchor points where there is maximal deformity? If one is going to use the apex as the anchor point, why not correct the deformity in all planes, fixing rotation as well as coronal and sagittal misalignment? Furthermore, the normal growth rate of a child's spine is the rate at which the spine grows normally; growth does not occur as a sudden burst of distraction every 6 months with artificial lengthening.

Part of the answer to this dilemma has been addressed through a treatment modality known as growth guidance, which is analogous to directing the growth of a young tree. A stake is placed alongside the spine that allows the spine to proceed with its normal rate of growth, and the stake is held to an anchor that encourages straightening. Eduardo Luque used this technique in the 1970s and 1980s in what was characterized as the Luque trolley, in which wires were lashed to the posterior elements of the spine and around a smooth rod, allowing gradual elongation through growth. The problem with the anchor points was that dissection of the periosteum to place the wires resulted in premature fusion and inconsistent elongation, so that this technique fell into disfavor in most surgeons' hands.

A newer modification of the idea was developed in which pedicle screws were used as anchors, but the technique was inspired by the techniques for the manipulation and correction of spinal deformities demonstrated by Se Suk of Seoul, Korea.[8] The Shilla was born of a desire to harness spinal growth and guide correction more naturally. The apex of the curvature is corrected in all planes—coronal, sagittal, and axial—and is fused and firmly anchored to the rod while growing screws are placed through the muscle levels above and below the apex. The periosteum is not disrupted for growing screw placement, allowing normal patterns of growth and minimizing return trips to the operating room. This concept was tested in the laboratory in goats; studies showed that at the 6-month interval, all of the animals manifested growth across the expanse of their instrumentation and at both the upper and lower aspects of the construct.[9] The surgical technique is unique in that there is subperiosteal exposure only at the three or four levels at the apex of the curvature; the levels are identified with the use of small needles on the spinous processes and the C-arm. The apex is treated with Ponte osteotomies, bilateral pedicle screws at each level, and a derotation maneuver.[10] The fascia is released superiorly and inferiorly from this point 1 cm off the midline, allowing introduction of the Shilla growing screws through the muscle layer under fluoroscopic guidance. The cannulated screws are best placed with Jamshidi needles. Cannulated screws can be placed in a freehand manner as well. Either the screws

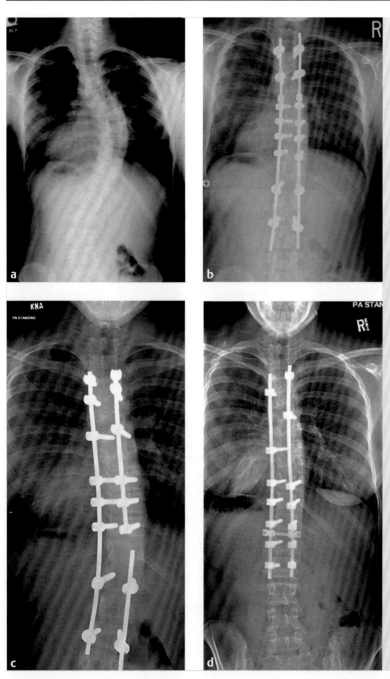

Fig. 13.1 (a) Preoperative radiograph of a 10-year-old who had juvenile idiopathic scoliosis with a 60-degree curve. (b) Postoperative radiograph with the Shilla in place. (c) Preoperative radiograph just before definitive fusion. (d) Postoperative radiograph after definitive fusion.

have a cap that fits to the top of the polyaxial portion or a closed head screw can be used, allowing the rod to slide through the center of the screw head. The rod is therefore captured but not bound by the screw head. The growing screws are placed at intervals above and below the apex and are sufficient to control the alignment and keep the curve as neutral as possible in the coronal and sagittal planes.

During the last 8 years, the Shilla technique has been used for many diagnoses, including idiopathic scoliosis, spina bifida, cerebral palsy, and multiple different syndromes, as well as for certain congenital curves. The data regarding these patients was first presented to the Scoliosis Research Society in 2008, when a cohort of 48 patients from two centers was reported; at that time, only 10 patients had had 2 years of follow-up. The average curve treated was 70 degrees, and the results reflected curve correction that was maintained over time, an increase in the space available for lung, and an increase in truncal height, both immediately after surgery and over time with further growth. In 2009, the number of procedures was analyzed, and among 22 patients with more than 2 years of follow-up, an additional 26 procedures after the initial index procedure had been recorded. It was calculated that if these patients had undergone lengthening procedures on a 6-month basis, an additional 115 surgical procedures would have been necessary, along with any unplanned procedures. In a report on a cohort of 40 patients in 2011, it was emphasized that any return to the operating room constituted a complication and that this group of patients, with 52 additional trips to the operating room, had been spared the anticipated 250 procedures they would have undergone if treated with a surgical distraction technique.

Several things were learned from this surgical experience. One of these was a recognition of the need for the preoperative release of stiff curves, or at least a period of preoperative traction, to acquire the mobility necessary for correction to be achieved at one sitting. It was also noted that direct vertebral derotation was an important part of the surgical treatment. For stiffer curves, it was found that a temporary rod on the convexity is helpful to gain provisional correction, and with the use of coronal benders, the apex can be pushed toward a concave rod, the permanent rod required to maintain correction, and subsequently a permanent rod is placed along the convexity.

A child's level of activity can also affect the longevity of an implant. In more active children, the components tend to loosen, so that screws back out of the pedicles. Although this was not a problem from a neurologic standpoint, some of the implants did become prominent, and a decision had to be made either to tolerate this effect or change the screw site on an outpatient basis. These were some of the reasons for additional surgeries.

Pelvic obliquity is seen primarily in patients with neuromuscular scoliosis. Flexible pelvic obliquity is best treated by carrying the growing screws low into the lumbar spine, to either L4 or L5. For more rigid pelvic obliquity, an anterior release may be necessary to gain flexibility. In that instance, a stronger construct is necessary to maintain correction, and iliac wing screws combined with S1 or S2 screws should provide sufficiently firm fixation to allow a fixed rod to be joined to a growing screw in the lower lumbar spine, attached to a cross connector or domino box, fixed to one rod with Allen setscrews, and allowed to slide along the rod on the opposite side. With the use of domino connectors on both the right and left sides, the pelvic obliquity can be controlled reasonably well and growth over time allowed.

One of the questions every practitioner of growth rod treatment raises is, What is the best thing to do for the patient at maturity? The experience that we have had

with Shilla rods is similar to that seen with distraction rod systems. The question at maturity is whether the rods should be left in place, replaced with permanent rods and fusion, or removed entirely. The most common option is removal of the growing rods and insertion of a permanent fused system that achieves a final correction at the time of the fusion. This technique is exemplified by the patient in ▶ Fig. 13.1, in whom a growing rod had been inserted during a period of active growth. After 2 years of activity, the rod had broken and sufficient maturity had been achieved to allow a permanent fusion and definitive correction of the residual deformity. Another option may be simply to remove the metallic device and allow the spine to maintain the alignment previously achieved through the growth guidance technique.

In summary, the Shilla procedure harnesses a child's inherent growth potential while avoiding the problems of premature fusion and ankylosis associated with the Luque trolley system. However, the placement of pedicle screws in small patients requires caution and can be challenging. The Shilla procedure does not require repeated trips to the operating room and allows a more normal childhood, free of bracing, casts, and repeated trips to the operating room, in which the patient is able to participate in most childhood activities, including many sports.

References

[1] Pehrsson K, Larsson S, Oden A et al. Long-term followup of patients with untreated scoliosis. A study of mortality, causes of death, and symptoms. Spine 1992; 17: 1091–1096

[2] Karol LA. Early definitive spinal fusion in young children: what we have learned. Clin Orthop Relat Res 2011; 469: 1323–1329

[3] Karol LA, Johnston C, Mladenov K, Schochet P, Walters P, Browne RH. Pulmonary function following early thoracic fusion in non-neuromuscular scoliosis. J Bone Joint Surg Am 2008; 90: 1272–1281

[4] McCarthy RE, Campbell RM Jr Hall JE. Infantile and juvenile idiopathic scoliosis. Spine: State of the Art Reviews 2000; 14: 163–180

[5] Cahill PJ, Marvil S, Cuddihy L et al. Autofusion in the immature spine treated with growing rods. Spine 2010; 35: E1199–E1203

[6] Sankar WN, Skaggs DL, Yazici M et al. Lengthening of dual growing rods and the law of diminishing returns. Spine 2011; 36: 806–809

[7] Flynn JM, Matsumoto H, Torres F, Ramirez N, Vitale MG. Psychological dysfunction in children who require repetitive surgery for early onset scoliosis. J Pediatr Orthop 2012; 32: 594–599

[8] Suk SI. Pedicle screw instrumentation for adolescent idiopathic scoliosis: the insertion technique, the fusion levels and direct vertebral rotation. Clin Orthop Surg 2011; 3: 89–100

[9] McCarthy RE, Sucato D, Turner JL, Zhang H, Henson MA, McCarthy K. Shilla growing rods in a caprine animal model: a pilot study. Clin Orthop Relat Res 2010; 468: 705–710

[10] Lee SM, Suk SI, Chung ER. Direct vertebral rotation: a new technique of three-dimensional deformity correction with segmental pedicle screw fixation in adolescent idiopathic scoliosis. Spine 2004; 29: 343–349

14 The Experts' View: A Narrative of the Great Debate

Colin Nnadi

14.1 Introduction

A debate between four of the world's leading experts in early onset scoliosis was held on September 8, 2011, in Christ Church, Oxford, United Kingdom. These experts were brought together to discuss their experiences and preferred methods of treatment for the very complex condition that is early onset scoliosis. The session was moderated by a professor of spinal surgery from the University of Oxford.

Growing rod treatment techniques are broadly classified into three categories—namely (1) distraction-based, (2) growth guidance, and (3) tethering- or tension-based systems. Each of the debaters has pioneered and championed at least one of these groups. The speakers shared their experiences with members of the audience and also presented reasons for their chosen modus operandi in handling some of the most difficult cases known to the spinal community.

The moderator of the debate was **Jeremy Fairbank**, **MA, MD,** Professor of Spinal Surgery of the Nuffield Orthopaedic Centre at the University of Oxford (▶ Fig. 14.1). He is also a past president of the British Scoliosis Society.

The presenters were as follows:

Behrooz Akbarnia, MD, is a past president of the Scoliosis Research Society and spearheaded the international Growing Spine Study Group. He was instrumental in pioneering conventional growing rod technology and led the development of the magnetic growing rod system (▶ Fig. 14.2).

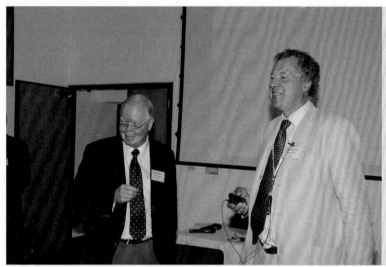

Fig. 14.1 Robert M. Campbell, Jr. *(left)* and Jeremy Fairbank.

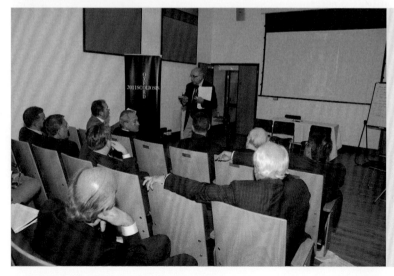

Fig. 14.2 Behrooz Akbarnia speaks.

Robert (Bob) M. Campbell, Jr., MD, is an attending surgeon and director of the Center for Thoracic Insufficiency Syndrome at the Children's Hospital of Philadelphia, Pennsylvania. He is best known for his work on thoracic insufficiency syndrome and is also the inventor of the vertical expandable prosthetic titanium rib device.

Richard (Rick) E. McCarthy, MD, is a professor of orthopedic surgery at the University of Arkansas for Medical Sciences College of Medicine, Little Rock, and a past president of the Scoliosis Research Society. He invented the Shilla technique, which is gaining prominence as a treatment option for patients with early onset scoliosis (▶ Fig. 14.3).

John Webb, MB, Apothecary to The Prince of Wales and his Household, is a former president of the British Scoliosis Society. He is known for his work on the Luque trolley technique (▶ Fig. 14.4).

What follows is the discussion presented during that 2011 debate. The presenters were supplied with the case report (Case Report Box (p. 112)). Discussion with the audience was also solicited. The roundtable format has been preserved, but the discussion has been edited for print and ease of reading.
–Colin Nnadi

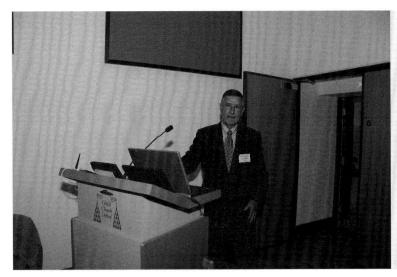

Fig. 14.3 Richard E. McCarthy.

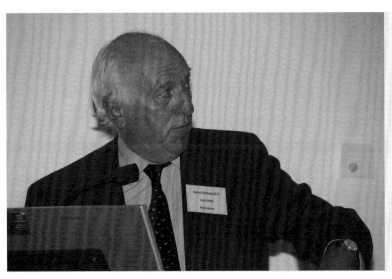

Fig. 14.4 John Webb.

14.2 The Great Debate

Case Report

A 3-year-old girl whose birth was a full-term, normal delivery has a left talipes deformity that was managed by splinting. In addition, she has a subluxing patella that is due for surgical treatment.

In June 2009, she had a 35-degree thoracolumbar curve convex to the left, which was treated with serial casting and bracing. The family believed that the casting did not work, but they thought the bracing was very good. Magnetic resonance (MR) imaging showed a normal neuraxis.

The first presenting chest radiograph was obtained when the child was 11 months of age. Lateral radiography was also performed at this time. The rib–vertebra angle difference is between 45 and 69 degrees, and the Cobb angle is 35 degrees. Another radiograph was obtained that revealed progression. Scoliosis is present when the child lies down. The sagittal balance is appropriate.

This year the curve has shown a fairly clear progression. The patient's developmental milestones are normal, and she is able to walk. What would you consider to be the best course of action for this patient?

14.2.1 Behrooz Akbarnia, MD

The classification of Skaggs grouped growth-friendly procedures into those based on distraction, guided growth, or tension. In principle, the four debaters today are talking about two systems in each of the first two groups. It is worth noting that only the vertical expandable prosthetic titanium rib (VEPTR) is approved in the United States; therefore, the debate can be one of two ways—namely, growth-guided vs. distraction-based or chest vs. spine, the latter being the most challenging if nonoperative treatment fails and if surgery is needed.

As health care professionals, we must do the following:

- Pay attention to the correction. The correction is not just about the Cobb angle; it is about a three-dimensional correction of the spine and thoracic deformity.
- Achieve spinal growth. We must define what is meant by growth and how growth is measured.
- Improve pulmonary function. A huge debt of gratitude is owed to Bob Campbell, MD, for his contributions in this area.
- Ensure that any intervention is safe and minimizes complications.
- Improve the health-related quality of life of the patient.

If we are referring to growing rods, we must define whether they are single or dual rods; the statistics and results are different, so it is important to be specific. For example, the growing rod technique has been established and is based on proximal and distal foundations. There are two rods, which may be magnetic or conventional.

The principle is to distract the two parts of the spine. *This is specific.* Elongation and growth should also be differentiated. When elongation is performed at the beginning of treatment, this is not growth; rather, growth starts from after the course of the initial surgery and goes on until the end of treatment. Curve correction and balance should also be noted. Pulmonary function in terms of actual improvement in function or lung volume is important. Consideration must be given to the impact of the diagnosis on outcomes because etiology does matter. Complications must be compared.

14.2.2 Literature Review

In my view, most of the currently available data are based on opinion, not on evidence. We need to have evidence-based data.

One of the earliest reports on the dual growing rod technique noted that up to 5 cm of elongation and 5 cm of growth could be subsequently achieved. The yearly average growth rate was reported to be 1.2 cm, and on average, more growth was observed per year in patients younger than 5 years of age than in their older counterparts. Thompson et al[1] looked at 28 patients and found a significant difference in the amounts of curve correction and in growth rates when single rod constructs were compared with dual rods. Another series revealed significantly better correction with dual rod constructs than with single rod constructs. A comparison of studies using the VEPTR technique and the Cobb angle as denominator noted that the maximal curve correction was 34%, which is still less than that shown with the dual rod technique.

There is a case report of a patient with Marfan syndrome who was almost 4 years of age when she started treatment. The patient continued treatment up to about the age of 13 years before definitive fusion took place, meaning that she received about 9 years of growing rod treatment. That is exactly the end point we want to see; the beginning of the correction right at the start was 50%, the curve stayed basically the same throughout the treatment period, and the patient's growth continues to increase.

Emans et al[2,3] looked at growth rates and found that average growth was 1.2 cm ± 0.9 each year following the initial VEPTR procedure, indicating a reasonably good growth.

Hasler et al[4] reported a 30% Cobb angle correction following the initial surgery and a 25% correction that was maintained at follow-up. A 40% complication rate was also noted, which was in line with the rate in other studies. The Philadelphia series[5] showed a mean Cobb angle correction of 34% and a complication rate of 33%. The correction rates when bracing and casting were used were 51% and 59%, respectively. The researchers reported that the casting group had a better correction rate than did the group that underwent VEPTR.

Does etiology matter? We looked at some of the patients in the larger groups (i.e., idiopathic, neuromuscular, congenital, syndromic). The idiopathic and congenital groups had more growth per year compared with the other larger groups, but those belonging to the congenital group had an increased loss of correction. This difference in etiology between the groups should be recognized so that we can begin to understand which group will do what. In an assessment of dual growing rods in 19 patients with congenital scoliosis, a 29% correction rate was seen and growth was almost 11 mm per year, which is relatively in line with the rate in the idiopathic group. Campbell et al[6] looked at the differential growth rates on the convex and concave sides of the curve and discovered that the rates were 8.3 mm and 7.9 mm per year, respectively. The growth rate was also found to be higher in children younger than 5 years of age ($p < 0.033$).[7]

So, are improvements in the anatomical volume of the lungs and the functional volume and capacity of the lungs important? Bob Campbell has put this topic on the map with his description of the thoracic insufficiency syndrome, which impresses upon us the need to pay attention to the chest and thorax.

Emans et al[2] studied eight patients who underwent preoperative and postoperative spirometry. They reported an increase in the forced vital capacity (FVC) and forced expiratory volume in 1 second, but this result was not statistically significant. The predicted FVC value did not significantly change between baseline and the last test, indicating that the increase was in line with growth of the lung volume rather than the actual effects of surgery.

Studies measuring the lung volume in three-dimensional reconstructions of computed tomographic (CT) scans have shown a 25 to 90% increase in lung volume based on analysis following VEPTR surgery. However, these lung volume measurements were not corrected for somatic growth. In addition, the static measurements of functional residual capacity were performed with patients in the supine position. Reports from Michigan showed that preoperative function in patients with scoliosis improved by 29%, but in data presented to the Scoliosis Research Society (SRS),[8] functional outcome in patients remained unchanged and no significant difference was seen between preoperative and postoperative values. In addition, no statistically significant difference was seen in complication rates or in pulmonary values, lung volumes, scoliosis angles, and SRS scores between patients in various sex, age, and disease categories.

Olson et al[9] performed experimental work on three different groups of animals (normal, simulated thoracic insufficiency syndrome, and simulated thoracic insufficiency syndrome with expansion thoracoplasty). The authors concluded that there was inconclusive evidence to support the concept that pulmonary hypoplasia is induced by thoracic insufficiency syndrome and controlled by expansion thoracoplasty.

With regard to lung volume and decreasing FVC rate, Redding and Mayer[10] showed that the benefits of VEPTR are stabilization of the thorax and improvement of respiratory mechanics, but they are measured in other ways.

Karol et al[11] researched early thoracic fusions. They reported that if the thoracic height from T1 to T12 is less than 18 cm, the incidence of severe pulmonary restrictive disease is 63%. As the height increases from 18 to 22 cm, the incidence decreases to 25%. Therefore, there is a correlation between thoracic height and the development of pulmonary problems.

We put this to the test. There were 51 patients involved in the study. Participants were younger than 10 years of age at index surgery, had undergone more than 3 lengthening procedures, and, per the inclusion criteria, had to have complete data sets. In terms of etiology, 20 patients had neuromuscular scoliosis, 10 idiopathic, 10 syndromic, nine congenital, and two thoracogenic scoliosis. The mean preoperative T1-T12 height was 152 mm, which postoperatively increased to 175 mm and was 205 mm at the latest follow-up ($p < 0.001$). These patients underwent growing rod treatment. After reviewing these results, the researchers concluded that a significant increase in thoracic height could be correlated with patient age at index surgery, number of lengthening procedures, and correction of scoliosis and kyphosis, as well as with correction and maintenance of the major curve.

14.2.3 Complications

Unwanted fusions may occur with growing rods and VEPTR. Problems may also occur at anchor points. Put simply, complications are comparable between the VEPTR and growing rod techniques. In the one study of the quality of life of patients treated with the VEPTR vs. the growing rod technique, physical function, parental burden, and total score results for the two treatment options were very close.

14.2.4 Future Treatment Options

I believe the future of growing rods is headed toward MAGEC (Ellipse Technologies, Irvine, California), which is a magnetically controlled growing rod. When MAGEC is compared with other systems, such as the standard growing rod, the amount of growth seen is very similar. Maintaining distraction means stimulating growth, which cannot be done with growth-guided systems. It is hoped that this technology will have fewer complications than its predecessors.

Many of the recent developments in growing rod technology can be attributed to the dedication and time of Bob Campbell. I acknowledge the tremendous work he has done over the last 30 years to help children around the world.

The treatment of early onset scoliosis involves a careful review of several aspects of the condition. The best outcomes are achieved by addressing the issues of deformity, growth, and pulmonary function and by minimizing complications. Currently practicing spine surgeons have the option of using nonoperative treatment techniques as well as various growth-sparing systems. We must be prepared to use the best possible treatment method for each patient.

Jeremy Fairbank, MA, MD: With regard to long-term follow-up, can you clarify whether the growth potential of these children is normal? In other words, if you look at the growth rate of the limbs, is the rate normal? Sometimes, we assume that people with congenital scoliosis tend to be rather short anyhow.

Behrooz Akbarnia, MD: Yes, we must look at the whole patient. I think we must also look at each diagnosis, not merely look at the spine and the chest for lengthening; rather, we should look at the patient with cerebral palsy or Morquio syndrome and begin thinking about it as a pediatric problem.

Robert (Bob) M. Campbell, Jr., MD: There is a sequence when the specific treatment for scoliosis is determined. Basically, we start with whatever we are taught in training, and then perhaps we sometimes grope at what is currently accepted in the literature and what is set as the current standard of care. Among those options, we ought to look at the one that best addresses each individual patient's acute and long-term disease concerns (▸ Fig. 14.5).

Differences are now noted between adult, juvenile, and infantile curves. I was taught during residency training that fusing both was an appropriate treatment option, but this is not true. That is why a great struggle exists with regard to growth-sparing techniques. It is worth noting that all of these techniques are brutal and expensive, and they have high morbidity rates. They are not good options, but they are not quite as horrible as natural history.

With that said, the goals of treatment should be these:
- Correcting the Cobb angle;
- Minimizing complications;
- Reducing costs;
- Minimizing morbidity rates;
- Improving operative long-term health over natural history.

As previously mentioned, spine deformity should be controlled while also allowing for growth. In some cases, this can be done with bracing or casting; however, if these options fail, then we must turn to options similar to what Dr. Akbarnia mentioned earlier. The Harrington rod was the original growing rod, which was then followed by growth guidance instrumentation and with tethering and tension techniques. Per the U.S. Food and Drug Administration (FDA), the VEPTR instrumentation is indicated for the treatment of thoracic insufficiency syndrome.

Dr. Akbarnia explained how well Harrington's goals have been defined. John Emans has also lectured on this topic and says that for patients with chest involvement, VEPTR is better than spinal growing rods. The concept seems rather simple until you look carefully and ask what this means. For example, should the VEPTR or a growing rod technique be used for a child on oxygen with Larsen syndrome?

Both techniques are appropriate if the anteroposterior (AP) radiograph is the only thing you look at; however, if you look at the CT scan, a problem of volume is present. In this scenario, which technique is more appropriate? Which is going to straighten it out, growing rods or VEPTR? (It is worth noting that the answer is unknown with growing rods because only AP radiographs have been used to analyze the results; CT scans have not.)

Therefore, the choice depends on the goals of the health care professional. Correcting the Cobb angle and minimizing complications are fairly standard options and are supported in the medical literature. But what is the evidence for these options? Although many series have been presented, all of them are small and are made up of heterogeneous populations and different syndromes. We are now discovering that the term *idiopathic* probably

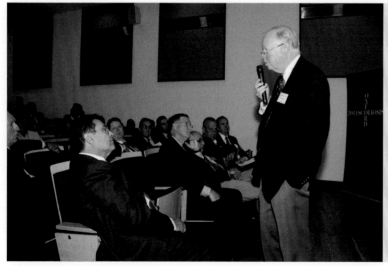

Fig. 14.5 Dr. Bob Campbell addressing delegates.

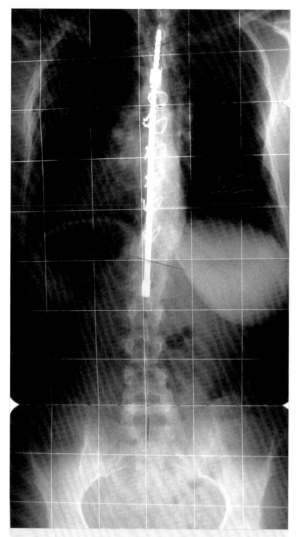

Fig. 14.6 Segmental fixation with Harrington-Luque technique.

covers many syndromic populations. VEPTR has the same problems—namely, heterogeneous populations and small clinical series. Both appear to function the same for correcting the Cobb angle and minimizing complications. It is not worth quibbling over 39% vs. 43% improvement rates for Cobb angles and then calculating Cobb angles up to three decimal points! Note that the measurement error is never mentioned; it is huge, and many of these children may be in the congenital group. For these, the measuring error is very high; among children in the idiopathic group, the error could be 5 degrees or more. Add in that figure and the statistics may become meaningless.

It is my hope that a large prospective clinical study of a homogeneous population that compares growth rods with VEPTR will be possible. Such a study would take a long time, it would be expensive, and I do not know who would pay for it, but its results might settle some of these issues. Comparing retrospective series is fine for debate, but it is not good science.

There is a lot of talk about morbidity rates between the two techniques, and basically, we have not done much better than Paul Harrington with these approaches. A two-point fixation can be seen, and there are many problems with that. A new approach, the Shilla technique, was taught to us in a way by the Luque trolley. The Shilla technique may be able to minimize costs and morbidity rates. It is only one operation, so patients are not taken back to the operating room. If you count the screws, there is also a three- or even an eight-point fixation; it is somewhat more segmental. However, additional operations may be required for complications, and there may be an unknown loss of thoracic spine growth because of the central fusion / anchor points. What is being traded off for this big central segment of spine fusion? There need to be long-term data to answer this question. The long-term complication rate is yet to be established. Everyone looks good at 5 years, but at 10 years is when we are likely to find out what has been going on.

What about growing rods vs. VEPTR, and what about self-expansion? Dr. Akbarnia mentioned that there might be less cost and lower morbidity rates. So what exactly is the long-term cost? The units will have to be replaced. Ultimately, how much are they going to cost when they come to the market for widespread distribution? There is still only a two-point fixation, and the so-called point of diminishing returns may be valid with the self-expansion as well as the manual extension devices.

Will the treatment work in the long term? In the case of devices extending extremities, many pulled out in the long term. The health care professional is likely to trade known complications for new ones when choosing the path of innovation.

Improving the patient's operative long-term health over his or her natural history is important because this goal is what treatment should really be all about. Very few data exist about the natural history of untreated scoliosis. Data from Scandinavia reveal that mortality rates are extremely high for untreated infantile scoliosis and very high for juvenile scoliosis, but not necessarily adolescent scoliosis. With regard to the morbidity rates of natural history, there is a higher risk for respiratory failure in patients with curves greater than 110 degrees. There is also a higher risk for cor pulmonale and cardiac issues in patients with severe curves. As Dr. Akbarnia mentioned, children with scoliosis and thoracic insufficiency syndrome have a worse quality of life than those who have scoliosis without thoracic insufficiency syndrome.

The mortality rates of the operative history are unknown for growing rods and the Shilla / Luque trolley technique. For VEPTR, a higher mortality rate was seen among patients in the hypoplastic cohort.

Very little pulmonary data exist on growing rods. VEPTR has been studied, but most of its pulmonary data

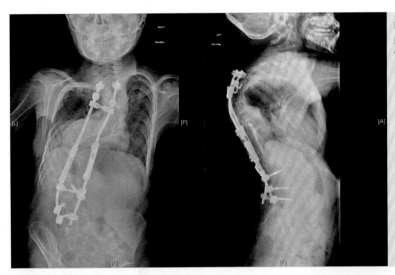

Fig. 14.7 Dual growing rod fixation. Note proximal junctional kyphosis at top of construct.

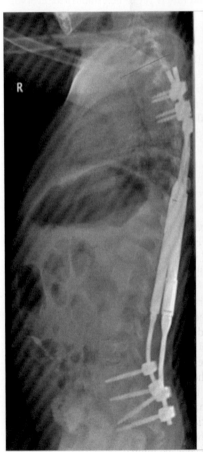
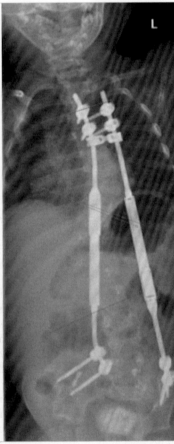

Fig. 14.8 Magnetic growth rods inserted from thoracic spine to pelvis.

are based on older children because we do not yet have the ability to measure these data in younger children. However, a decreased normal but stable vital capacity has been seen among patients with scoliosis and fused ribs operated on after the age of 2 years. It has been implied that because the vital capacity gets better and improves, then that result was negative. However, the rate has just been maintained and stabilized, which is a good thing. What is lethal is when vital capacity normal percentage decreases. So, how can the "best" option simply be to stabilize it? That option may change in the future, but it currently holds true now. Pulmonary data for Shilla are

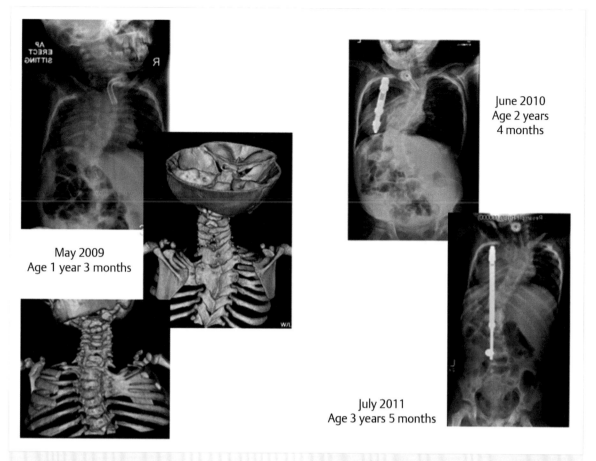

May 2009
Age 1 year 3 months

June 2010
Age 2 years
4 months

July 2011
Age 3 years 5 months

Fig. 14.9 Treatment of thoracic insufficiency syndrome with VEPTR.

currently unknown. This large hole in the data needs attention.

Cardiac morbidity rates are also unknown for all four techniques. These must be looked at systematically in the future.

Data on quality of life for the VEPTR have been submitted to the FDA; these data are what Dr. Mike Vitale has been looking at all these years. I believe that issues of quality of life tend to be dubious, subjective, and complicated, and I am unsure whether they have a real bearing on the world.

My philosophy on growth-sparing techniques is just as valid today, but it may change tomorrow. As Dr. Akbarnia previously mentioned, no data exist on them because the literature is composed mostly of opinion-based medicine. In my opinion, the safest and most logical position is to do whatever it takes to get the largest, most symmetric, most functional thorax by skeletal maturity, not to look at Cobb angles and available space for the lung.

For patients with congenital scoliosis, the VEPTR has a strong place. Dr. Emans has reviewed CT lung volumes as children grow up. Experiments on rabbits by Dr. Schneider revealed that lungs expanded with the VEPTR

approach seemed to have better viscology, but these results are very complex; more issues are being uncovered than are being solved. This new model is much more lethal, and it really does make the case for extrinsic lung disease.

In terms of early scoliosis, if a patient presents with a flexible curve and correction of the concave intercostal space is achieved with bending films and at either end there is a normal growing spine, I would consider growing rods. However, if hemithoracic insufficiency syndrome is present, then I would consider VEPTR but would continue to use growing rods on occasion because the issue is still open; the technique has not been proven by any prosthetic trial. I might also choose VEPTR with the possibility of growing rods when there has been limited correction of the concave intercostal space with bending films. For example, in a neuromuscular case, the intercostal space does not open up that much with bending films, suggesting that there is an intrinsic contraction of the entire thorax that I suspect needs to be addressed; I can push on the spine, but doing so is very difficult. I would treat this patient with an Eiffel Tower construct with VEPTRs. However, it is worth noting that improvements have been made on the dynamic MR images of the lungs by doing this, and in the future, perhaps these improvements will be seen with the growing rod.

If kyphosis is present that has not been emphasized yet, either growing rods or VEPTR I or II could be considered; however, neither instrumentation has been proven to address these issues. In a patient with severe scoliosis, many of us are likely to consider a halo and then try instrumentation. Kyphosis is an unsolved issue at this time.

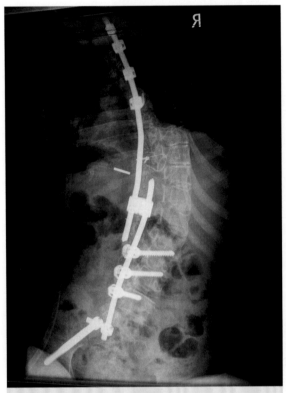

Fig. 14.10 Unilateral dual growing rod construct.

In the case of an 8-month-old child with a VEPTR II, I have been pushing the limits with him. Periodically, I bend up the flexible rods at the top of the VEPTR II to perform an extension moment. Will this technique work in the long term? I hope so, but I do not know yet. In 10 years I may have some decent results.

I think myelomeningocele is good for the VEPTR. The trouble with this technique is that the gibbous angle must be managed, but the chest must also be taken out of the pelvis to avoid secondary thoracic insufficiency syndrome. In my opinion, VEPTR is probably the best option because the health care professional stays out on each side and is not as centrally located as would be the case with spinal instrumentation. This is how to help these children—nurture them along until after they reach 10 years of age and then try something definitive.

In one patient with pelvic obliquity, I used growing rods. I could have just gone down with iliac bolts and attempted to treat the pelvic obliquity that started 2 years after the growing rod was put in, but instead I put in a VEPTR and straightened it out that way. We can cheat and use hybrids, so to speak.

14.2.5 Looking Toward the Future

In the future, I think there will be more types of growth-sparing instrumentation, but will these instrumentation techniques bring about better results or just different? There is a big difference. We need better surrogate outcome measures than the Cobb angle. We need rigorous clinical trials to settle current issues, and we should stop talking about retrospective series. Perhaps the only settings where those data can be taken seriously are at orthopedic meetings.

We also need long-term follow-up data to settle these issues and find out what our patients are doing 30 to 40 years later. We need to worry less about the hardware and more about why it is being used. We need the courage to

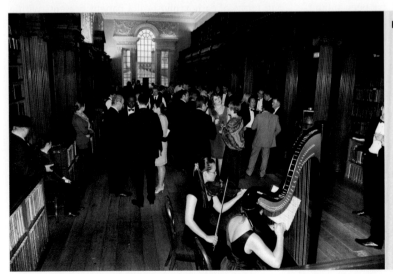

Fig. 14.11 Drinks reception.

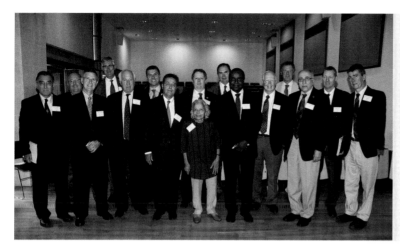

Fig. 14.12 Faculty. *Back row, left to right:* Evan Davies, James Wilson-MacDonald, Thanos Tsirikos, David Marks, Mike McMaster, Jeremy Fairbank, Gavin Bowden. *Front row, left to right:* Hussein Mehdian, Rick McCarthy, John Webb, Alain Dimeglio, Min Mehta, Colin Nnadi, Bob Campbell, Behrooz Akbarnia, Bob Crawford.

abandon many of our preconceived notions and look at the world a little differently and more critically. We need to go from a two-dimensional focus of scoliosis to more of a three-dimensional dynamic approach.

I think the issues are interesting to discuss, but not much progress has been made in the past 10 years. We now have better questions than we did 10 years ago. I think it is important to talk about the issues, but I cannot strongly defend VEPTR or any of the other techniques because they all have many shortcomings. As health care professionals, we must learn from what we are doing with our patients and move on to a better technique or treatment and critically test it.

14.2.6 Richard (Rick) E. McCarthy, MD

There are a variety of diagnoses that we deal with every day with regard to patients with early onset scoliosis, and the result is always the same: we see deformities, an impression of the chest, and compromised pulmonary function. We know that the scoliosis leads to an early death.

What is the future of scoliosis treatment? The currently available surgical options encourage an increase in thoracic height and an expansion of the pulmonary capacity, but at what cost? Distraction techniques are known to produce repeated trips to the operating room. Proximal junctional kyphosis is also a serious issue.

There is some loss of growth centers in all systems because the systems need to be fixed to the spine somewhere; otherwise, the growing rod systems slide. In the distraction systems, these are platforms. In the Shilla system, it is the apex. However, there must be an anchor somewhere. Stiffness of the chest wall seen in VEPTR is another important issue. There is now evidence that repeated trips to the operating room may lead to cognitive delays in learning among small children. Furthermore, skin issues, such as infection and scarring, can lead to the complications mentioned previously by Dr. Akbarnia.[12]

So, these issues beg the following questions:
- Should we direct the corrective forces toward the most curved portion of the spine?
- Should we place the fused anchor point at the apex?
- Should we correct the primary deformity in all planes?
- Should we utilize the normal growth and power of a child's spinal growth?

Well, the answer to these issues was discovered by Eduardo Luque when he discussed the concept of growth guidance. He described a trolley designed to slide apart, but the anchors were wrong, which caused premature fusion and ultimately inconsistent results.

Our current answer is growth guidance with the Shilla variety. (The term *Shilla* comes from the hotel I was staying in when I came up with the idea.) The concept was born of a desire to harness spinal growth and naturally guide that growth, to correct the apex in all planes and anchor the rods at the apex with limited fusion, and, probably most importantly, to let the child concentrate on the lessons of childhood (i.e., and not simply be a patient coming back to the hospital every 6 months). This technique does not involve a brace and requires only minimal hospitalization.

The evidence for the Shilla technique comes from the animal studies that my colleagues and I performed on goats. When the goats were sacrificed at 6 months, we found that all of the specimens showed consistent signs of growth. We see this now in our patients: they all grow. The system does not cause stenosis, as we were worried and suspected we might see. We saw none of that in the goats. Some metallosis was seen that was isolated to the local lymph nodes adjacent to the moving parts. I have also seen metallosis in VEPTRs.

The techniques are somewhat unique; a subperiosteal exposure at the apex alone is used, and Smith–Petersen osteotomies allow increased flexibility of the posterior elements. The growing screws are placed through the muscle with a Jamshidi needle or can be placed freehand; however, the muscle stays intact and the pedicle is seen only radiographically. It is tapped, and then a cannulated screw is placed.

When my colleagues and I began this study, a cap fixed to the top of the screw; however, because of the current restrictions imposed by the FDA, I have been performing the technique with a closed polyaxial screw. This screw allows the same fixation, captures the rod at the ends, and allows the rod to slide along with growth while staying fixed to the pedicle.

This type of growth guidance has been used for the last 7 years in patients with multiple diagnoses, including idiopathic scoliosis, spina bifida, and all forms of cerebral palsy and syndromic scoliosis. My colleagues and I presented some of this information at an SRS meeting, where we looked at our early results. We presented a typical case involving an 8-year-old child who played Little League baseball. The boy had an increase in the space available for his lung, and he had undergone one revision when he grew off the rods. Currently, he has had the rods in place for 5 years.

We presented information at the 2009 SRS meeting, where we showed that we had treated 22 patients with 26 additional procedures; yet, when we looked at those 26 additional procedures and compared that number with what the number of procedures would have been, the number for scheduled lengthening was much larger.

Furthermore, my colleagues and I again looked at our patient cohort in 2011 and found that we now had 40 patients at the 2-year follow-up point, and that there had been 52 wound and instrumentation problems, as well as other issues, that required a return to the operating theater. These results suggested to us that any trip to the operating room should be considered a complication, which is an issue that my fellow debaters have not addressed. Their complication rates are actually outrageous. In comparing these 52 procedures with the number of procedures that the children would have undergone for scheduled lengthening, we arrived at 250 cases.

Currently, my colleagues and I are now following up to 60 patients in Little Rock, Arkansas, and 30 patients in St. Louis, Missouri. The more I talk about the technique, the more I discover that other health care professionals are doing this around the world, in different locations, using a variety of techniques.

14.2.7 Tips on Technique

For a stiff curve, additional techniques, such as preoperative traction, may be necessary. I may use a temporary rod on the convexity and coronal benders to bring the spine over to the concave rods; in some cases, I will rescue the screws. For flexible curves, I use intraoperative rod rotation and direct vertebral derotation.

Pelvic obliquity and neuromuscular scoliosis are certainly issues. If pelvic obliquity is flexible, then my team carries the instrumentation down to L4 or L5. For rigid pelvic obliquity, we use the principles of Jean Dubousset —that is, we think of the pelvis as an intercalary vertebra, fix the children firmly to the pelvis, and then put a sliding device between the pelvis and the apex, essentially creating a side-to-side domino without the locking setscrews in so that the construct can slide apart.

What must be done with the rods after maturity is a critical issue. Originally, I thought we would no longer use metal and instead send the children into adulthood without it. However, upon further reflection, there are some cases that require further treatment. Once such borderline case was that of a 10-year-old child with early onset scoliosis. She was short, but her mother was tall. She presented with an operative curve, my team decided to use the growth guidance Shilla technique, and the rod broke. Her mother was not happy with the child's residual rotation at this point, so my team performed a definitive fusion.

As an aside, in my experience, all rods break. Any rod fixed in the body, which is moving, will eventually break. I do not consider breakage a complication; rather, it is an expected outcome.

Another young lady came to us with a spinal cord injury and progressive scoliosis. She had been treated with growth guidance, but when her rods started to break, we looked at her age and felt that she was very close to maturity. Her mother asked if we could remove all of her implants, which we did. Six months following the surgery, we hope the correction is maintained. We will continue to watch the patient, although it is possible that a definitive fusion will need to be performed in the future.

14.2.8 Conclusion

The Shilla procedure harnesses a child's inherent growth potential yet avoids the problems of the Luque trolley. It is worth noting that the placement of pedicle screws in small patients can be very challenging. The Shilla procedure does not require repeated trips to the operating room and avoids all of the potential problems that go along with repeated surgery. The procedure does allow the child a chance of experiencing a reasonable childhood, free of bracing or casts, and the ability to engage in some sports and participate in life.

14.2.9 John Webb, MB

My talk will specifically address issues among patients who present with early onset scoliosis within the first few years of life. The most difficult challenge is that these patients will die early.

A patient in whom a growing rod is placed has an operation every 6 months. Once a patient reaches 13 years of age, imagine how many operations they will have had! Unfortunately, there is a complication rate of 80%.

I knew Eduardo Luque well, and he introduced me to the Luque trolley. He visited my unit twice. I used the Luque trolley technique for patients with early onset scoliosis whose prognosis was not particularly good. In some of the best cases, the patients do grow.[13] In 1992, Lonstein and Bradford said that patients do not grow with the Luque trolley, but my own results and those of my colleagues suggest otherwise. Then, there is the spectrum of early onset scoliosis—the malignant type, in which patients grow very little (maybe only 20% with growing rods), and the more benign type, in which patients have about 70% of expected growth.

The problem with the Luque trolley is the Cobb angle, which deteriorates significantly when a Luque trolley is used alone. The worst aspect is that the Cobb angle was not as bad as the rib deformities, which were awful. How could we stop this? I decided to perform a convex epiphysiodesis, which has previously been described by many people. We did a bending film to identify the stiffer curve. We released this by taking the disks out, and then, only on the convex side, placed a small bar (fusion). Then, we went to lower levels and placed some laminar wires at each one. These grew off the *l* rods and started to deform again, so we went much longer—what I called the trombone—and much overlap could be seen to allow further growth. However, even those grew off and created problems. Ultimately, we used fixation at the top and bottom with long rods so that the patients would not develop kyphosis or deteriorate. These patients had a great deal of growth, and for almost the entire length of the construct, the rods overlapped.

The Cobb angles of the children we treated were all below 40 degrees, except for two malignant cases. Of course the Cobb angle is an important issue, and what we hope to achieve by the end of growth is a curve of less than 40 degrees with a reasonable chest. Some of the children did not reach this end point, but others did. One such child has not required any correction. He is now 25 years of age, and the rods are still in place. There are at least 25 to 30 people with these implants in them, who have virtually stopped growth. If a patient is not presenting with symptoms, should the rods be taken out? I suspect it would be technically very difficult; therefore, they carry on with their rods.

When other patients reached the end of their growth phase, they began to deteriorate. When they started to lose correction, I performed definitive fusion. They had had their rods since the age of 2 or 3 years and were now 13 years old. So, if these children were going to start losing correction, I surmised that it was better to take the rods out and perform fusion, which I have done in a number of cases. Similar to the last patient, these patients were not put in a brace. They were allowed to lead a normal life. I follow up with them once a year, and they play football if they want to. That is very important to me—namely, that they are not

coming back into the hospital every 6 months to have their rods lengthened.

A concerning issue with growing rods is that they do not address anterior growth problems; it is possible that one day the patient will get a rib deformity. Five years ago, I presented data at the SRS annual meeting. My team and I had 31 patients who had reached adulthood or were at least 18 years of age. Of these, 23 had reached 16 years of age, and 13 of them had needed a definitive fusion at the mean age of 14.5 years. The other 10 did not need any further surgery. The rods were put in when they were very young, and they have remained in situ.

Patients left without treatment until the rib–vertebra angle difference was much worse were the ones who tended to require further surgery in adolescence. In addition, the initial constructs were inadequate; the patients grew right off them, and then they would start to deform again. So, the original *l* construct of the Luque was not acceptable; hence, we performed the *u* construct, and the patients grew off some of those as well, so we went to the newer construct. Nine of our patients required definitive fusion because they were growing off in adolescence. They had grown off their rods. It is important to remember these were the initial *l* rods; therefore, when this started happening, we changed to the *u* rods. Some of the patients developed junctional kyphosis. The condition is not difficult to correct because definitive surgery with a couple of minor osteotomies posteriorly can be done to achieve normal sagittal alignment.

Because the patients grew off the *l* rods, they needed correction and definitive surgery. The patients with *u* rods were less likely to require further surgery, and we believe that those with the long rods will require even less revision surgery.

The big downside of this technique is the need for sublaminar wires in a child aged 2 to 3 years—that means many surgeries and significant risk. Surprisingly, however, this is not true if the health care professional is experienced at passing sublaminar wires! The procedure is not difficult in a 2-year-old child; the canal has a reasonable dimension. Only a certain number of patients require definitive surgery at adolescence. The child will commonly lead a normal life, no longer having to come in for surgery every 6 months, be admitted, and be given an anesthetic. Remember that the complication rate is 80%. A total of 90% of patients have complications, infections, or cutouts. At the present moment, this certainly is a very experimental procedure.

Interestingly, we have begun to re-review the data of our 27 patients in much more detail, and it is quite apparent that not all of them were straightforward cases of idiopathic early onset scoliosis. Many cases were syndromic. When we looked at them more closely, we discovered that they had different mild forms of syndromes. Of course, some of them had other obvious conditions. However, if we look at one patient whom we would consider to have had early onset idiopathic scoliosis, the preoperative Cobb angle was 56 degrees; by the end of growth, it was 19 degrees.

With this technique, we are attempting to achieve a spine that grows, maintains respiratory function, and has a cosmetically good outcome. When a child presented with a 19- to 20-degree curve at the end of growth and maintained a good height, that presentation indicated that we should look at respiratory function.

14.3 Question-and-Answer Session

Floor: The most important issue about coronal plane deformities is the sagittal alignment with the different techniques. Can you preserve the sagittal contour of the spine?

Richard (Rick) E. McCarthy, MD: Yes, I think that it is a critical issue. Whenever a distraction is present, proximal junctional kyphosis is likely to be produced. As we move into the next generation of growing rods, we must plan for proper sagittal alignment. You can do this with the Shilla rods, which is an essential component of this if it is contoured properly. If it is distracted, then kyphosis is produced.

Floor: At the bottom of your radiographs, you are creating lumbar lordosis. How does the bent rod pass through open screws? If there is a growth rod present and a bend is put in it, it will not lengthen because it catches.

Richard (Rick) E. McCarthy, MD: It will if the opening is left large enough.

Behrooz Akbarnia, MD: There is no scientific evidence that distraction is kyphogenic. For example, the development of sagittal balance in children is different from that in adults. There are studies that show how children develop normally. We don't really have a grasp of the sagittal balance in children aged 2 to 3 years and how that balance changes with age. There also is no evidence to show how sagittal balance is affected after each procedure. Unless we have full knowledge of what is normal and the changes that occur following instrumentation, we cannot really say. However, some evidence from biomechanical studies shows what happens to the intradiskal pressure in the anterior part of the spine in the growing rod construct. The intradiskal pressure decreases anteriorly. By contrast, if there were a kyphogenic effect, we would expect this pressure to increase.

Jeremy Fairbank, MA, MD: A group in Utrecht has been doing some longitudinal studies on the natural history, so there are people looking at it, but the follow-up is not long enough.

Floor: If you distract with the straight Harrington rod and you distract with a slightly contoured rod so the disk pressure in the anterior aspect increases, are we talking about similar mechanisms?

Behrooz Akbarnia, MD: I think there are so many factors involved in proximal junctional kyphosis. It's not just the distraction. For instance, there is the level of arthrodesis. Studies have identified optimal levels for arthrodesis. We are not sure whether to go to T2 or T3 or T4 and so on, and what construct to use or whether to use one at all. However, what I can say is that the number of patients with dual rod construction who are fused with four anchors at T2 and have proximal junctional kyphosis is small. I think one needs to realize the difference between these groups and, hence, the multifactorial involvement.

Floor: How do you measure the length?

Behrooz Akbarnia, MD: I measure the length by using the picture archiving and communications system as well as markings on the instrumentation.

Floor: Dr. Campbell, if you were going to use a VEPTR in this case, would you have to perform a chest wall release? We use it in congenital cases, of which I have some limited experience, and I think it is a fantastic device! But this is an entirely different situation; you have a child here with no congenital anomalies and no real problem with the deformity of the chest wall in association with the scoliosis. But doing an extensive chest wall release from front to back would worry me with this group of patients. Do you have to perform a full thoracostomy?

Robert (Bob) M. Campbell, Jr., MD: I disagree. I know the history of the child with a clubfoot on one side and also a hyperligamentous laxity on the other side. There may be an element of an Ehlers–Danlos type of syndrome. I want to point out that the radiographs are pretty much standard—that is, "Here's your AP X-rays, make your call." The last patient put in the cast with the ribs bent way down shows spinal deformity in the cast, so that will be a very rigid kind of deformity. Bending films would be nice to see before we make any decisions.

John Webb, MB: Let us assume that there is no problem with this child—that she is a relatively normal child and the investigations are normal. She has a standard curve that is what I would call normal for early onset scoliosis. In that scenario, what would you do? Would you use the VEPTR? I understand that you have indicated that in the case of thoracic insufficiency you might use it, and I have used it myself. However, for a standard, routine case like this, would you use the VEPTR or would you use another system?

Robert (Bob) M. Campbell, Jr., MD: With a 50-degree curve, good flexibility, no rotation, no rib hump, and normal respiratory function, you could use any of the techniques we discussed in that situation. The flexibility would play a prominent role in my decision making. If the chest wall opened out and it was an early intervention, then I might consider a variety of growing rods.

I started with this VEPTR project in 1987. By 1996, I was making a formal presentation to the chief of the FDA, and he asked me why I had not submitted it for premarket approval. I told him that most of the cases were mine, that I was the creator. I think we probably do a better job than most people, and I probably continue to be the most experienced VEPTR surgeon around. Most of us, however, will not be able to produce the same results.

Floor: I can't imagine you have any safety issues, but I think you have a very, very strong hand, and I know that you are interested in the chest. One thing about the VEPTR is that it is very effective at correcting the actual scoliosis and balancing the patient. I know you have written a paper on using the VEPTR for correcting curves with a big tilt of the head and the shoulders, and it is hugely effective at doing that. All of the other techniques would not even touch that, but yours corrects that which the others cannot do. These other techniques do not even have any effect on the actual chest. The ribs will carry on their merry way, and the humps get bigger. Your cases do not.

Alain Dimeglio (audience member): I think the future lies in the magnetic field. We can lengthen more frequently each year. In our growing rod program at Montpellier, we discovered that by gradual daily lengthening, we can obtain more than 1 cm of growth per year and in some cases more than 3 cm without neurologic damage. In the future, the concept of gradual lengthening will be of great advantage.

It is appropriate to measure the T1–S1 length, but we also need to be more rigorous in following up on results and surgical outcomes. For example, the patient at skeletal maturity had an almost normal trunk, but I would be very pleased to see the sitting height to compare that with an expected normal sitting height for that patient. What is the final weight? What is the normal vital capacity?

There is so much technology available now, but do we need all this just for a table to put the patient into the supine position and follow up with them every 6 months to measure trunk height? If you can obtain 2.5 cm of growth in the trunk every year before the patient is 18 years of age, as well as 3 to 4 cm of growth during puberty, then you are doing very well.

Jorge Mineiro (audience member): We hear people talking about the Luque trolley, and the good results are all from Nottingham. When you look at the literature, no one has reproduced good results; by contrast, some of the results have been rather disastrous. How can a procedure be successful if it is not reproducible?

John Webb, MB: You might well be right! I think it was an evolution because we had problems; the top wires cut out with the very first cases, so then we put in the double wire system, which is a very complicated wiring system, and that seemed to stop it. Then the rods were too short and they started to bend. So, in the beginning, we did have problems and the wires did break out at the top, but I ignored them.

Floor: When you put the Luque trolley in, it is such a massive exposure that it is difficult to believe they do not fuse.

John Webb, MB: Interestingly, if you go back in, they have a sheet of fine bone; however, if you look at the data, they grow in spite of that because the sheet of bone does not prevent spinal growth. It is not a thick fusion like what is seen in cases of scoliosis.

Floor: You are leaving the rods in—presumably most of them have fused—and the patients have had no problems with them, but alternatively, you explain that if they grow, that is great. However, I've noticed with some of the other growing rods in which you have to lengthen them, when I have been going in and revising to a final fixation, they have spontaneously fused with bone that has formed beneath the rods and they fuse themselves anyway. Those are the ones that have definitely grown. I have no doubt that by the time these patients are 17 or 18 years of age the sheet of bone will be thicker, but the patients have not come back to me.

Floor (another audience member): My team has been doing a very similar thing, and we have not seen any of the problems that others have had. I think the most impressive thing that I find is that these are two very different techniques; the effect on the child of multiple surgeries cannot be underplayed. I have had three patients with VEPTR in whom we have had to abandon treatment because the patient cannot come into the hospital any longer. Bringing these children back to the clinic has a huge effect on them.

John Webb, MB: Yes, this is an evolution, and I am not saying that people should do it now. The currently available data suggest that the best outcomes in early onset scoliosis occur if the procedure is performed in children at a very young age but the concept of lengthening the rods every 6 months until the children are 13 years old is unbelievably difficult to comprehend. I think that we have the ability to lengthen the rod with the MAGEC system and without the need for an operation; however, the follow-up is only 18 months.

Floor: I have a concern about the cases that Dr. McCarthy presented. Using the Shilla technique, he fused four levels at the apex, so essentially he removed growth from one-third of the thoracic column.

Richard (Rick) E. McCarthy, MD: It was three growth centers. I have tried using fewer screws, which has worked fine. On flexible curves I use four screws and a one-level fusion. I have to fix the rod in some place, so I will use as short an area as I can at the apex. The problem is that I am getting curves of 90, 110, and 130 degrees in my current patients, and I need to get all the fixation on that apex that I can. So I am worried about it pulling out if I use too few points of fixation.

The technique also depends on the ability of the surgeon, the quality of the bone, and the stiffness of the curve. Those factors will determine how much fixation and what you need to do to loosen up that apex so you can bring it around.

Floor: I think fixation is a very interesting idea and technique, but the critical screws you are putting in are the most difficult screws you are going to put into a construct when you are going to instrument every level. If you are instrumenting only two or three levels, the levels you choose to go into it are the most technically demanding. I would agree with you, but the general surgical population may put those screws in the wrong places.

Floor (another audience member): Cadaver sessions are sometimes run for residents in order to show them how to place a hook. John, will your technique die out if trainees are not shown how to place the wires?

John Webb, MD: It would be a great shame if that happens because when you have a difficult construct you may have to use sublaminar wires to attach the spine to the rod because you cannot get the screws in. I do not think it will die out because it is a technique you should have available.

Floor: I want to raise a historical problem with segmental instrumentation. One of the problems was that the Cobb angle did improve but the thoracic deformity was rather ugly, even at the end of growth. We know that double growing rods have slightly improved that aspect of the deformity. Will these two techniques enable us to see better results than what we have observed in the past?

John Webb, MD: Yes. I think the reality is that when we looked at early onset scoliosis in the past, we thought patients were purely nonsyndromic, and we would convert them back to a virtually straightened normal spine up to about 19 to 25 degrees with a good chest wall. These patients had a slightly increased lordosis, and you would notice that when they stood. But they looked like normal children for early onset starting at age 3 years. The syndromic cases are much more difficult, but they do not get a hump in their rib. They seem to reverse back to a normal spine. We have convincingly reversed that trend from a progressive to a resolving curve. But the syndromic cases are very different in that they do have the deformity, and they are the ones who are more difficult to treat.

14.4 Closing Statements

Robert (Bob) Campbell, Jr, MD: Two things have been absent from this technical discussion. Please consider pulmonary function studies. In children older than 6 years, let's study pulmonary function in them because it is not very expensive, it is easy to do, and it is noninvasive. We may have some way to compare this, perhaps in the same way imagine the thoracic height—22 cm should be the goal.

Richard (Rick) E. McCarthy, MD: Dual growing rods and Luque rods have been around for a long time. We have all been yearning for something different because

we have a sense that things are not right. They are not where they should be. A number of years ago, after placing a number of these dual rods, I decided that I was going to start out thinking about the ultimate goal of treatment. What should our next stage of treatment be? It should be something that allows a flexible spine in the end and allows the child to grow without going back to the operating room.

Maybe Shilla is part of the next generation; maybe you feel that it is not. But I would challenge the people in this audience to think on your own and be creative, come up with the next generation if this is not it. Somehow, we must move beyond where we are now.

Dr. Campbell has criticized me for some of the fixation points, and as stated earlier, the fixation points must be accurately and properly done so that they provide the fixation. And in his system, it is anchoring the ribs. Those little ribs often break, and so that and the chest wall stiffness pose a problem for me when considering the VEPTR.

However, at the same time, when I am faced with a child who has a chest wall deformity and an especially long, complex thoracic congenital scoliosis, I use a VEPTR. It is rare that I meet a patient who has a true double major curve in early onset, but I have encountered two in the last 5 years; in those cases, I used dual rods. So dual curves, dual rods. But in all of the other curves that I have encountered, I have been able to use the Shilla technique, and it works.

John Webb, MD: I think it is a criminal act to take a child back to the theater every 6 months for 10 years, particularly with such a high complication rate. I do not think it is an acceptable technique at the present time. If magnetic lengthening comes of age and we have good data, I think that is may be a very good option. I think that would be the future. I think my technique is an old technique that works well.

I think it is important to show that patients do have good respiratory function. At the moment, every paper I have read on growing rods suggests a high complication rate. They are experimental and should not be universally used throughout the world, but only in selected centers. We have not used them in our unit because we think the complication rate is too high.

Behrooz Akbarnia, MD: Unless we collect data prospectively, as we do now, the answer to what to do when you have a spinal fusion will remain unknown. It is exciting to see how much interest there is in this topic. With the exception of Dr. Campbell, it would appear that within the last 10 years there has been an ever-increasing interest in early onset scoliosis. I think there was a lot of concern about the lack of options to treat this condition in the past, but now options do exist to alter the patient's natural history.

Therefore, I think we need to develop prospective studies, and I think the format should be through study groups and meetings, such as those held by the SRS. It is obvious that we all want answers to these questions.

14.5 Commentary

It is obvious that this is a rapidly evolving field in which opportunities for exciting high-end research abound. However, the key points to emerge from my observations are as follows:

- This is a group of patients in which the etiology is so varied that it is often difficult to compare outcomes.
- Much of the current evidence is based on opinion; therefore, an urgent need exists for regulated and evidence-based research in this area.
- Treatment strategies should be planned in the realms of three dimensions.
- Focus should be given to pulmonary development and spinal growth.
- The abiding principle of treatment should be to improve the overall quality of life of these patients.
- A drive to minimize complications from any form of treatment should be paramount.
- Treatment strategies should be individualized to reflect patient characteristics and need.

–Colin Nnadi

References

[1] Thompson GH, Akbarnia BA, Campbell RM Jr. Growing rod techniques in early-onset scoliosis. J Pediatr Orthop 2007; 27: 354–361

[2] Emans JB, Caubet JF, Ordonez CL, Lee EY, Ciarlo M. The treatment of spine and chest wall deformities with fused ribs by expansion thoracostomy and insertion of vertical expandable prosthetic titanium rib: growth of thoracic spine and improvement of lung volumes. Spine 2005; 30 Suppl: S58–S68

[3] Emans JB, Ciarlo M, Callahan M, Zurakowski D. Prediction of thoracic dimensions and spine length based on individual pelvic dimensions in children and adolescents: an age-independent, individualized standard for evaluation of outcome in early onset spinal deformity. Spine 2005; 30: 2824–2829

[4] Hasler CC, Mehrkens A, Hefti F. Efficacy and safety of VEPTR instrumentation for progressive spine deformities in young children without rib fusions. Eur Spine J 2010; 19: 400–408

[5] Smith JR, Samdani AF, Pahys J et al. The role of bracing, casting, and vertical expandable prosthetic titanium rib for the treatment of infantile idiopathic scoliosis: a single-institution experience with 31 consecutive patients. Clinical article. J Neurosurg Spine 2009; 11: 3–8

[6] Campbell RM Jr Smith MD, Hell-Vocke AK. Expansion thoracoplasty: the surgical technique of opening-wedge thoracostomy. Surgical technique. J Bone Joint Surg Am 2004; 86-A Suppl 1: 51–64

[7] Campbell RM Jr Hell-Vocke AK. Growth of the thoracic spine in congenital scoliosis after expansion thoracoplasty. J Bone Joint Surg Am 2003; 85-A: 409–420

[8] Wilson PL, Newton PO, Wenger DR et al. A multicenter study analyzing the relationship of a standardized radiographic scoring system of adolescent idiopathic scoliosis and the Scoliosis Research Society outcomes instrument. Spine 2002; 27: 2036–2040

[9] Olson JC, Kurek KC, Melita HP, Warman ML, Snyder BD. Expansion thoracoplasty affects lung growth and morphology in a rabbit model: a pilot study. Clin Orthop Relat Res 2011; 469: 1375–1382

[10] Redding GJ, Mayer OH. Structure-respiration function relationships before and after surgical treatment of early-onset scoliosis. Clin Orthop Relat Res 2011; 469: 1330–1334

[11] Karol LA, Johnston C, Mladenov K, Schochet P, Walters P, Browne RH. Pulmonary function following early thoracic fusion in non-neuromuscular scoliosis. J Bone Joint Surg Am 2008; 90: 1272–1281

[12] Dede O, Motoyama EK, Yang CI, Mutich RL, Walczak SA, Bowles AJ, Deeney VF. Pulmonary and radiographic outcomes of VEPTR (Vertical Expandable Prosthetic Titanium Rib) treatment in early-onset scoliosis. J Bone Joint Surg Am 2014; 96: 1295–1302

[13] Luqué ER. Paralytic scoliosis in growing children. Clin Orthop Relat Res 1982; 163: 202–209

Further Reading

Corona J, Matsumoto H, Roye DP, Vitale MG. Measuring quality of life in children with early onset scoliosis: development and initial validation of the early onset scoliosis questionnaire. J Pediatr Orthop 2011; 31: 180–185

Dubousset J. [CD instrumentation in pelvic tilt] Orthopade 1990; 19: 300–308[Article in German]

Karol LA. Early definitive spinal fusion in young children: what we have learned. Clin Orthop Relat Res 2011; 469: 1323–1329

Mayer OH, Redding G. Early changes in pulmonary function after vertical expandable prosthetic titanium rib insertion in children with thoracic insufficiency syndrome. J Pediatr Orthop 2009; 29: 35–38

Pehrsson K, Larsson S, Oden A, Nachemson A. Long-term follow-up of patients with untreated scoliosis. A study of mortality, causes of death, and symptoms. Spine 1992; 17: 1091–1096

Roberts DW, Savage JW, Schwartz DG et al. Spinal Deformity Study Group. Male-female differences in Scoliosis Research Society-30 scores in adolescent idiopathic scoliosis. Spine 2011; 36: E53–E59

15 Complications of Growing Rod Treatment

Nima Kabirian and Behrooz A. Akbarnia

The growing rod technique is the prototype of posterior distraction-based growing spine procedures used for the surgical treatment of progressive early onset scoliosis that is not controlled with nonoperative care. The standard course of treatment includes an initial growing rod implantation with limited fusion at the foundations sites, distraction procedures at regular intervals to maintain or stimulate growth of the nonfused segments, and a definitive final spinal fusion at skeletal maturity.[1] Planned and unplanned revisions may be at times necessary to address implant- or patient-related complications.

The surgical treatment of early onset scoliosis with contemporary techniques is inherently prone to adverse events. Frequent operations, young age at initial surgery, associated medical conditions and malnutrition, and complex underlying spinal deformities place these patients at increased risk for complications. Depending on the etiology of early onset scoliosis, the number of surgeries, and the length of follow-up, complications after growing rod surgery have been reported variably in different studies. This chapter reviews the complications that commonly develop after growing rod treatment.

15.1 Review of the Literature

The complication rates reported in the earlier literature on the first generation of growing rods (i.e., subcutaneous Harrington or Moe rods) were unacceptably high. In 2002, Mineiro and Weinstein reported the results of subcutaneous rodding and repeated distraction procedures in 11 patients. The most common complication was rod failure, which occurred in more than half of patients. The subcutaneous placement of Harrington or Moe rods achieved acceptable deformity correction and variable spinal height gain, but with an average of 1.5 complications per patient.[2]

Klemme et al reviewed spinal instrumentation without fusion in 67 patients treated over a period of 21 years. They reported details of the complications, including implant-related problems, which occurred in 33 procedures in 25 patients (8%), and hook dislocations, which occurred on 21 occasions. Rod fracture was seen 12 times: seven times with Moe-modified Harrington rods, four times with Harrington rods, and one time with a pediatric Cotrel–Dubousset rod. Despite the frequency of the complications, the authors believed that instrumentation without fusion could be applied to a selected group of children with progressive scoliosis, but they also suggested that arthrodesis must be performed without delay in the event of suboptimal gain in length.[3]

In 2010, Bess et al published a comprehensive review of complications after growing rod surgery in 140 patients with early onset scoliosis.[4] Their landmark study described complications of the classic growing rod construct, which was introduced in 2000 by Akbarnia and Marks.[5] The authors reviewed 140 cases of index growing rod surgery, 633 lengthening procedures, and 74 unplanned procedures. The total numbers of surgeries and lengthening procedures per patient were 6.4 and 4.5, respectively. Of the 140 patients, 81 (57%) had at least one complication. A total of 177 complications occurred after 897 surgeries (20%). An unplanned surgical procedure was needed to manage 74 of the 177 complications (42%). The patients were divided into treatment groups based on type of growing rods (51% single vs. 49% dual) and location of implants (37% subcutaneous vs. 63% submuscular). The complications were categorized as implant-related (45% of all patients), wound-related (16%), alignment-related (7%), neurologic (3%), or general medical and surgical (12%) complications. There were 94 complications in 43 patients with a single growing rod and 83 complications in 38 patients with dual growing rods. Superficial wound infections were more common in the patients with dual rods, whereas hook dislodgments and unplanned procedures due to other implant complications were more common in the patients with a single rod. Implant complications more often led to unplanned surgical procedures in patients with a single rod (45%) than in those with dual rods (24%; $p < 0.05$). Three patients (2%) had neurologic complications. Fifty-one patients (37%) had subcutaneous growing rods, and 88 patients (63%) had submuscular growing rods. Subcutaneous rod placement was associated with more frequent complications per patient, more frequent wound complications, and more prominent implants than submuscular rod placement ($p < 0.05$). Survival analysis of all patients showed that the rate of complications increased after a given number of surgeries. The authors concluded that complications could be reduced by delaying the initial implantation of growing rods if possible, using dual rods, and limiting the number of lengthening procedures. Submuscular placement reduced wound complications and implant prominence and reduced the number of unplanned operations.[4]

15.2 Classification of Complications

Efforts have been made to classify complications after growth-friendly procedures and to reach a consensus for more efficient communication, the preparation of treatment guidelines, and prognostication. Smith et al recently developed a new, consensus-based classification system to report complications after growth-friendly procedures.[6] A complication was defined as an unexpected medical event that occurred during the course of treatment. Complications were classified as disease- or surgery-related and were graded according to severity. A surgery-related complication of severity grade I (SV-I) was defined as a complication that does not necessitate unplanned surgery. SV-II requires unplanned surgery: SV-IIA only one surgery and SV-IIB multiple surgeries. SV-III changes the course of planned treatment. A disease-related complication of SV-I does not necessitate hospitalization, but SV-II requires hospitalization for treatment. The authors tested the new classification system by using it to evaluate 65 patients from five centers with early onset scoliosis and at least 2 years of follow-up, including 14 with growing rods, 47 with a vertical expandable prosthetic titanium rod, and four with hybrid constructs. There were 57 surgery-related SV-I, 79 SV-IIA, 10 SV-IIB, and 6 SV-III complications. The authors concluded that although complications were common, only six were severe enough to change the course of planned treatment, and they suggested that this new system could be used to facilitate better communication among pediatric spine surgeons.

15.3 Implant-Related Complications

15.3.1 Rod Fracture

Rod fracture as a complication of nonfusion spinal instrumentation in the immature spine was first described by Moe et al.[7] Fracture of the longitudinal implants in a growing rod system is a common complication; however, its significance and effect on the ongoing care of a patient depend on the timing of the fracture and number of implanted rods. In our experience, if only one rod fractures and the patient is close to his or her next scheduled lengthening, the rod exchange can be planned at the next lengthening. However, if the patient has a single growing rod or a rod fractures soon after a lengthening procedure, unplanned revision should be performed so as not to lose curve correction and achieved spinal height gain.

Yang et al studied the risk factors for rod fracture after growing rod surgery. In a retrospective study of 327 patients who had undergone growing rod surgery, 86 rod fractures occurred in 49 patients (15%). The mean time to fracture after initial insertion was 25 ± 21 months, and it was 5.8 ± 3 months after the previous lengthening. Rod fractures occurred most commonly adjacent to tandem connectors and at thoracolumbar region (T11-L1). The incidence of rod fracture was highest in patients with syndromic early onset scoliosis (14%). Risk factors for rod fracture were prior rod fracture, single rod, stainless steel material, smaller diameter, proximity to the tandem connector (within 1 cm), short tandem connector, and

preoperative ambulatory status. Patients with a single growing rod had a higher rate of fracture than those with dual growing rods. The repeated fracture always occurred on the same side and within one vertebral level of the original fracture. The authors suggested the use of dual growing rods with a maximal diameter whenever possible and of gradual rather than focal bends. They also suggested exchanging the entire section of the construct if one rod breaks.[8]

David et al reviewed 413 lengthening procedures in every patient undergoing growing rod surgery at a single center from 1997 to 2012. They found 42 rod fractures in 22 patients (10%), with the first rod fracture occurring at a mean of 37 months after the primary surgery. Following a revision procedure combined with lengthening, there were 21 rod re-fractures (50%). In seven of the episodes (17%), the rod fractures were bilateral, requiring revision of both sides. Among fractures of a single rod in which revision on a single side was undertaken (n = 15), there were 8 re-fractures (53%), with a mean time to re-fracture of 17 months. When both sides were revised (n = 18) following failure of a single side, seven re-fractures occurred (39%; $p = 0.32$), with a mean time to re-fracture of 19 months. The majority of rod re-fractures (13 of 15) occurred on the same side as the initial fracture. In contrast to the usual belief, David et al advised against a bilateral exchange of rods in patients with a single-sided growing rod fracture.[9]

We have continued to change both rods if one rod breaks in order to prevent fatigue of the other rod and an early failure.

15.3.2 Anchor Failure

Anchor failure is the second most common growing rod complication after rod fracture (29%), with hook dislodgment in 21% and screw dislodgement in 3% (▶ Fig. 15.1).[5] Depending on the type and time of the anchor failure, treatment strategies are different. Unilateral anchor failure in a patient with no neurologic or vascular injury, an intact contralateral growing rod construct, and close to the next planned growing rod lengthening can be managed during planned revision at the next lengthening event.

Skaggs et al compared complications of hooks vs. screws in 247 patients who underwent growing rod treatment with a mean follow-up of 40 months. Among 896 pedicle screws, 22 complications (2.4%) were directly related to the screw, including acute loss of fixation (4), migration (14), breakage (1), skin breakdown (2), and unspecified loss of fixation (1). Among 867 hooks, there were 60 complications (6.9%), including acute loss of fixation (35), migration (22), and unspecified loss of fixation (3). There were no intraoperative pedicle screw–related issues, but two hooks plowed intraoperatively, resulting in bone damage. The average time to loss of fixation was 19 months for both implants. No complications involved

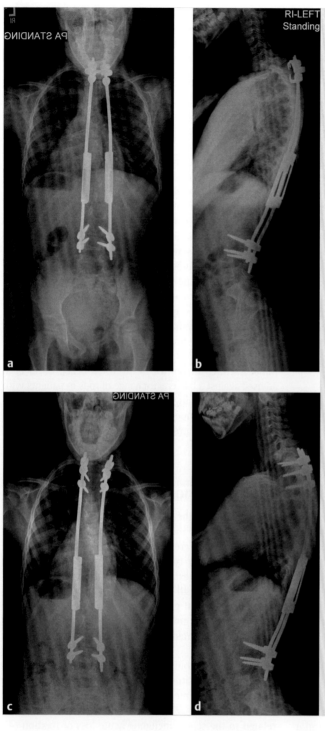

Fig. 15.1 Posteroanterior (**a**) and lateral (**b**) radiographs of a 6.5-year-old girl with idiopathic early onset scoliosis who underwent growing rod surgery at the age of 4 years showing anchor pullout at the upper foundation level 1 month before her planned sixth lengthening procedure. Posteroanterior (**c**) and lateral (**d**) radiographs of the same patient after planned revision of the upper foundation and a change from laminar hooks to pedicle screws. Because the patient was close to her next lengthening procedure, the revision was postponed for a month to be performed at the same time as the lengthening procedure.

neurologic or vascular injury directly related to hooks or screws.[10]

The use of spine anchors on the proximal ribs as fixation points has recently received attention as an alternative growing rod technique, commonly referred to as a hybrid growing rod technique. Skaggs et al reviewed the result of the hybrid growing rod technique in 28 patients (23 with a single growing rod and five with dual growing rods) over a mean follow-up of 37 months. The mean primary coronal curve (measured by the Cobb method) at the time of index surgery was 69 degrees, which was corrected to 19 degrees, and the correction was maintained through the latest follow-up. The mean increase in T1-S1 length at the latest follow-up was 49 mm, with a mean increase of 13 mm per lengthening procedure. Complications occurred in seven patients (24%), all with congenital scoliosis. A nonsignificant trend was observed for complications to be associated with a younger age and a larger Cobb angle at index surgery. Patients who had complications included two with wound issues, nine with loss of fixation of the rib anchors, and one rod breakage. There were no neurologic complications. No loss of fixation occurred in any construct that had a proximal foundation of at least four up-going hooks on ribs, and no complications occurred in dual constructs.[11]

Akbarnia et al compared the biomechanical properties of the four bilateral proximal anchors commonly used in growing rod technique in an in vitro porcine model and found that claw-fashioned rib hook constructs had a significantly higher load to failure compared with bilateral laminar hooks and bilateral transverse process–laminar hooks, but not with pedicle screw constructs. The authors suggested that rib anchors may serve as an alternative upper foundation in growing rod technique.[12]

15.3.3 Surgical Site Infection

Surgical site infection is one of the least desirable complications in any surgery, and specifically in growth-friendly procedures in the pediatric population. The classic approach to treating deep surgical site infection in orthopedic surgery is to explore and copiously irrigate the wound, débride the infected tissues, and remove metallic implants in cases of intractable infection to interrupt the biological environment for seeding, biofilm formation, and further survival of the microorganisms.

Hedequist et al, in a study of 1,771 patients with a mean age of 15 years who underwent spinal fusion for a wide variety of diagnoses, found that all patients with delayed deep surgical site infection (26) eventually underwent implant removal, with an average of 1.7 operations (range, 0–14) before removal. No patient had a recurrence of infection; however, six patients (23%) required revision and re-instrumentation because of progressive deformity. The authors found that the financial burden was proportional to the timing of implant removal.[13] Ho et al reported an 8.5% incidence of deep surgical site infection in 622 patients with a mean age of 14.3 years who underwent posterior spinal fusion and instrumentation for scoliosis. The authors stated that retention of implants was the single most important predictor of further surgery.[14] In growth-friendly procedures, however, removing all implants means losing all or most of the spinal growth and curve correction already achieved in young patients who still have a few years remaining before skeletal maturity.

Kabirian et al reviewed 379 patients who had early onset scoliosis and underwent growing rod surgery with a minimum of 2 years of follow-up. Of these, 42 patients (25 boys and 17 girls; 11.1%) had at least one deep surgical site infection. The mean age of the patients at initial growing rod surgery was 6.3 years, and the mean interval between the initial surgery and the first deep surgical site infection was 2.8 years. The authors found that the incidence rates of

deep surgical site infection after initial growing rod surgery and lengthening procedures were 2.6% and 7.7%, respectively. Implant material, ambulatory status, and number of revisions before the first infection were found to differ significantly between the patients with and those without deep surgical site infection. Also, a neuromuscular etiology, nonambulatory status, and lower body mass index (BMI) increased the possibility of implant removal after deep surgical site infection. The authors reported that 22 patients (52.4%) underwent implant removal (13 complete and nine partial) to control their infection. Of those who underwent partial implant removal, growing rod treatment was terminated in 22%, whereas it was terminated in about half of the patients (46%) who underwent complete implant removal. The authors concluded that if implant removal to treat infection is inevitable, partial removal with at least one stable longitudinal member in place should be considered so as to continue the course of lengthening until skeletal maturity.[15]

15.3.4 Neurologic Deficit

The incidence of neurologic deficits after both index and lengthening growing rod procedures is very low. Sankar et al reviewed 782 growing rod surgeries performed in 252 patients from a multicenter study group database. The authors found that 92% of the primary growing rod surgeries, 69% of the growing rod exchanges, and 61% of the lengthening procedures had been performed with neuromonitoring. The single clinical injury noted in their series resulted in an injury rate of 0.1% (1 of 782). This deficit occurred during an implant exchange while pedicle screw placement was being attempted, and it resolved within 3 months. The authors reported two neuromonitoring changes during 231 primary implant surgeries (0.9%), one change during 116 implant exchanges (0.9%), and one neuromonitoring change during 222 lengthening procedures (0.5%). They concluded that the rates of neuromonitoring change during primary growing rod implantation (0.9%) and implant exchange (0.9%) justify the use of intraoperative neuromonitoring during these surgeries. Because no neurologic events occurred during 361 lengthening procedures in patients with no previous neurologic events, the question may be raised as to whether or not intraoperative neuromonitoring is necessary for simple lengthening procedures in these patients.[16]

Currently, we use neuromonitoring for all growing rod surgeries, including index surgery, surgical lengthening, planned and unplanned revisions, and final fusion.

15.4 Sagittal Spinal Profile and Junctional Kyphosis

Concern over the kyphogenic properties of distraction-based growth friendly procedures has arisen over the last few years; however, the true incidence and etiology of kyphogenesis have not been studied in detail. The effects of serial growing rod lengthening procedures on sagittal balance, thoracic kyphosis, lumbar lordosis, and pelvic parameters have been reviewed by Shah et al in 43 patients who underwent a mean number of 6.4 lengthening procedures. An initial decrease in maximal thoracic kyphosis after the index surgery was followed by a significant increase over the course of lengthening. A nonsignificant increase in lumbar lordosis and a nonsignificant minimal change in pelvic parameters were noted over the treatment period. Significant improvement in sagittal imbalance was observed both in patients with positive and those with negative sagittal imbalance. The study showed no significant effect of the number of lengthening procedures (< 5 or ≥ 5) on maximal thoracic kyphosis, lumbar lordosis, and proximal and distal junctional kyphosis.[17]

Some investigators have measured proximal junctional kyphosis from one level cephalic to the upper instrumented vertebra to one level caudal to the upper instrumented vertebra. Skaggs et al used two levels cephalic to the upper instrumented vertebra, and with this new method, they found a 56% rate of proximal junctional kyphosis in 32 patients who had previously undergone growing rod surgery. Of 18 patients with proximal junctional kyphosis, eight (44%) had upper anchor failure, with seven requiring unplanned operations to revise the failed implants. In comparison, five of 14 patients (36%) without proximal junctional kyphosis had upper anchor failure; however, the difference between the two groups was not statistically significant. Of the four patients with proximal junctional kyphosis who underwent final fusion, three (75%) needed fusion and instrumentation to levels cephalic to the growing rod construct. Proximal junctional kyphosis was more common in patients with dual than in those with single growing rods (5 of 13; 38%), and it was more common in those with spine-to-spine constructs (10 of 17; 59%) than in those with hybrid constructs, such as upper hooks on ribs (5 of 12; 42%).[18]

Mahar et al examined the biomechanical properties of posterior distraction forces and their effects on the anterior column of the spine in the growing rod technique. Posterior distraction forces resulted in anterior disk separation (distraction), and the distraction forces were distributed evenly across multiple levels rather than delivered to the disk immediately adjacent to the foundation site. Constructs with upper foundation pedicle screws resulted in greater distraction forces in comparison with hooks, possibly because of hook motion during distraction. This distribution pattern of posterior distraction did not strongly support the kyphogenic properties of the growing rod construct, as is commonly believed.[19]

To avoid proximal junctional kyphosis, attention should be paid to appropriate rod contouring at the level of the thoracic kyphosis. The interspinal ligaments should be kept intact as much as possible. Short instrumentation should also be avoided, and the upper foundation usually needs to be extended to the upper thoracic spine to reduce the risk for proximal junctional kyphosis. This is especially true in children with nonidiopathic early onset scoliosis.

15.5 Autofusion

The true incidence, timing, and pathophysiology of autofusion during growing rod treatment are still unclear. The most objective yet retrospective way in which to diagnose autofusion is with close observation at the time of final surgery. With improved and less invasive surgical techniques, which limit surgical dissection to the foundation sites only, autofusion is expected to occur less commonly; however, other factors (i.e., surgical distraction, physiologic factors, and tissue–implant interaction) probably play a role in this phenomenon as well.

In a review of patients undergoing growing rod treatment until final fusion surgery, Cahill et al found that autofusion had occurred in eight of nine patients (89%) at the time implant removal during final fusion surgery. They noted a mean of 11 autofused vertebrae in each patient, and each patient underwent a mean of 7 Smith–Petersen osteotomies to correct the spinal deformity. The authors stated that autofusion does not preclude spinal growth, similar to the phenomenon described by Campbell and Hell-Vocke in which length is achieved through distraction in patients with congenital scoliosis, including those with a unilateral unsegmented bar. The authors proposed immobilization, disturbance of the paraspinal musculature, and the natural tendency of the immature periosteum to produce bone rapidly as causative factors. The younger the patient and the longer the treatment, the higher the rate of autofusion will be.[20,21]

15.6 How to Minimize Complications in Growing Rod Surgery

An awareness of growing rod complications, an understanding of what can be expected from any particular treatment, and education are as important as the physician's approach to management in minimizing complications. General recommendations to decrease the risk for undesirable outcomes in growing rod surgery include, but are not limited to, the following:

- Individualize your treatment. Idiopathic early onset scoliosis diagnosed in a 5-year-old ambulatory patient without malnutrition is different from neuromuscular early onset scoliosis in a 3-year-old wheelchair-bound patient with a low baseline respiratory reserve.

- Assess the patient's nutritional status and the physiologic reserve of the vital organ systems (pulmonary and cardiovascular), and treat preoperatively if indicated.
- Depending on the rate of progression and underlying etiology, start growing rod surgery at an appropriate age. The younger the patient, the higher the risk for complications.
- Whenever feasible, use dual rods in a submuscular fashion. Avoid smaller-diameter rods, short instrumentation, and short tandem connectors. Use enough anchors, and secure your foundation sites.
- Avoid unnecessary soft tissue dissection, and pay extra attention to soft tissue coverage and handling.
- Whenever feasible, use neuromonitoring for all growing rod surgical procedures.
- Avoid the overdistraction of growing rods.
- Avoid acute correction of the sagittal deformity, especially if it is stiff.
- Monitor the growth of the spine.
- Be aggressive in treating surgical site infections.
- Be proactive in planning how to revise your anchors if they fail.

15.6.1 Risk of Anesthetic Exposure

Current evidence on the neurotoxicity of repeated exposure to anesthetic agents in early life is inconclusive. Preclinical evidence in rodent and nonhuman primate studies has shown that the anesthetics in common clinical use are neurotoxic to the developing brain in vitro and can cause long-term neurobehavioral abnormalities.

Zhu et al investigated the effects of repeated exposure to isoflurane on cognition and neurogenesis in juvenile and mature animals. Postnatal day 14 rats as well as adult rats were anesthetized with isoflurane for 35 minutes daily for 4 days successively. Object recognition and reversal learning were significantly impaired in isoflurane-treated young rats, whereas adult animals were unaffected, and the deficits became more pronounced as the animals grew older. These findings show a previously unknown mechanism of neurotoxicity causing cognitive deficits in a clearly age-dependent manner.[22] Two large-scale clinical studies are currently under way in the United States to address this issue further.

15.6.2 Risk of Ionizing Radiation Exposure

Exposure to ionizing radiation is known to have detrimental effects on human tissues, depending on the dose, duration of exposure, and type of tissue. The treatment of early onset scoliosis with growing rods necessitates serial radiographic assessments of the deformity and the surveillance of spinal growth. Mundis et al reviewed all spine-related imaging studies done with ionizing radiation in 24 consecutive patients at a single center. They

showed a significant inverse correlation between the mean age of the patients at initial exposure to radiation and the total mean dose of ionizing radiation. The total mean dose of ionizing radiation was 3.4 times greater than the estimated background radiation dose (2.4 millisievert [mSv] per year) during the study. Patients who underwent revision surgery at least once had a higher level of exposure to ionizing radiation than did patients who did not undergo revision surgery. The mean total dose of ionizing radiation from the initial radiographic study to the first postoperative year was highest in patients with congenital scoliosis, followed by patients with syndromic, idiopathic, and neuromuscular scoliosis. Nearly 90% of the radiation dose was attributed to plain X-ray studies.[23]

A company known as EOS imaging Inc. (Paris, France) has developed a new slot-scanning imaging technique that shows promise in significantly decreasing exposure to ionizing radiation from conventional and digital radiography in patients with adolescent idiopathic scoliosis. Yaszay et al compared exposure to ionizing radiation in patients undergoing conventional radiography with exposure in those undergoing EOS imaging and showed that the mean total annual dose of radiation per patient and per etiology was smaller with the new imaging system.[24]

15.7 Conclusion

Complications in the course of any growth-friendly procedure, including growing rod surgery, are inevitable. Patients and their families must be informed of this reality, and the treating physicians have to be ready for appropriate management. The treatment of some surgery-related complications can be deferred until the next planned lengthening procedure, whereas others require an earlier intervention with an unplanned surgery. Efforts should be made not to lose the spinal growth and deformity correction that have been achieved early in the course of treatment. Previous studies have shown that the spinal height gain will decrease and the complication rate will increase after a specific number of surgeries.[5,15,25]

Premature final fusion is the last resort to abort the cycle of repeated complications in a patient who has failed different treatments or who is close to the skeletal maturity. Extensive research is under way to classify complications, evaluate the outcome of current and novel treatments, and foresee the natural history of the disease should planned routine care have to be completely changed.

References

[1] Akbarnia BA, Marks DS, Boachie-Adjei O, Thompson AG, Asher MA. Dual growing rod technique for the treatment of progressive early-onset scoliosis: a multicenter study. Spine 2005; 30 Suppl: S46–S57
[2] Mineiro J, Weinstein SL. Subcutaneous rodding for progressive spinal curvatures: early results. J Pediatr Orthop 2002; 22: 290–295

[3] Klemme WR, Denis F, Winter RB, Lonstein JW, Koop SE. Spinal instrumentation without fusion for progressive scoliosis in young children. J Pediatr Orthop 1997; 17: 734–742

[4] Bess S, Akbarnia BA, Thompson GH, Sponseller PD, Shah SA, El Sebaie H et al. Complications of growing-rod treatment for early-onset scoliosis: analysis of one hundred and forty patients. J Bone Joint Surg Am 2010; 92: 2533–2543

[5] Akbarnia BA, Marks DS. Instrumentation with limited arthrodesis for the treatment of progressive early-onset scoliosis. tate of the Art Reviews 2000; 14: 181–189

[6] Smith JT, Johnston CE, Skaggs DL, Flynn J, Vitale M. A new classification system to report complications in growing spine surgery. A multicenter consensus study. J Child Orthop 2012; 6: 439–459

[7] Moe JH, Kharrat K, Winter RB, Cummine JL. Harrington instrumentation without fusion plus external orthotic support for the treatment of difficult curvature problems in young children. Clin Orthop Relat Res 1984: 35–45

[8] Yang JS, Sponseller PD, Thompson GH, Akbarnia BA, Emans JB, Yazici M et al. Growing Spine Study Group. Growing rod fractures: risk factors and opportunities for prevention. Spine 2011; 36: 1639–1644

[9] David M, Gardner A, Jennison T, Spilsbury J, Marks D. The impact of revision of one or both non-fusion spinal rods on the re-fracture rate and implant survival following rod fracture. J Child Orthop 2012; 6: 439–459

[10] Skaggs DL, Myung KS, Johnston CE, Akbarnia BA and Growing Spine Study Group. Pedicle screws have fewer complications than hooks in children with growing rods. J Child Orthop 2010; 4: 481–501

[11] Skaggs DL, Myung KS, Yazici M, Diab M, Noordeen HH, Vitale M et al. Hybrid growth rod using spinal implants on ribs. J Child Orthop 2010; 4: 481–501

[12] Akbarnia BA, Yaszay B, Yazici M, Kabirian N, Blakemore LC, Strauss KR et al. Biomechanical evaluation of 4 different foundation constructs commonly used in growing spine surgery: are rib anchors comparable to spine anchors? Spine Deformity 2014; 2: 437–443

[13] Hedequist D, Haugen A, Hresko T, Emans J. Failure of attempted implant retention in spinal deformity delayed surgical site infections. Spine 2009; 34: 60–64

[14] Ho C, Skaggs DL, Weiss JM, Tolo VT. Management of infection after instrumented posterior spine fusion in pediatric scoliosis. Spine 2007; 32: 2739–2744

[15] Kabirian N, Akbarnia BA, Pawelek JB, Alam M, Mundis GM Jr, Acacio R et al. Deep surgical site infection following 2344 growing-rod procedures for early-onset scoliosis: risk factors and clinical consequences J Bone Joint Surg Am 2014; 96: e128

[16] Sankar WN, Skaggs DL, Emans JB, Marks DS, Dormans JP, Thompson GH et al. Neurologic risk in growing rod spine surgery in early onset scoliosis: is neuromonitoring necessary for all cases? Spine 2009; 34: 1952–1955

[17] Shah SA, Karatas AF, Dhawale AA, Dede O, Mundis GM Hr, Holmes L Jr et al. The effect of serial growing rod lengthening on the sagittal profile and pelvic parameters in early-onset scoliosis. Spine 2014; 39: E1311–1317

[18] Skaggs DL, Myung KS, Lee CI. Proximal junctional kyphosis in distraction-based growing rods. J Child Orthop 2011; 5: 387–401

[19] Mahar AT, Kabirian N, Akbarnia BA, Flippin M, Tomlinson T, Kostial P et al. Effects of posterior distraction forces on anterior column intradiscal pressure in dual growing rod technique. J Child Orthop 2010; 4: 481–501

[20] Cahill PJ, Marvil S, Cuddihy L, Schutt C, Idema J, Clements DH et al. Autofusion in the immature spine treated with growing rods. Spine 2010; 35: E1199–E1203

[21] Campbell RM Jr Hell-Vocke AK. Growth of the thoracic spine in congenital scoliosis after expansion thoracoplasty. J Bone Joint Surg Am 2003; 85-A: 409–420

[22] Zhu C, Gao J, Karlsson N et al. Isoflurane anesthesia induced persistent, progressive memory impairment, caused a loss of neural stem cells, and reduced neurogenesis in young, but not adult, rodents. J Cereb Blood Flow Metab 2010; 30: 1017–1030

[23] Mundis G, Nomoto EK, Hennessy MW, Pawelek JB, Yaszay B, Akbarnia BA. Longitudinal analysis of radiation exposure during the course of growing rod treatment for early-onset scoliosis. Presented at: 19th International Meeting on Advanced Spine Techniques (IMAST); July 18–21, 2012; Istanbul, Turkey

[24] Yaszay B, Kabirian N, Mundis GM, Pawelek J, Bartley CE, Akbarnia BA. EOS-imaging system is available for early onset scoliosis patients and can reduce their ionizing radiation exposure. J Child Orthop 2012; 6: 439–459

[25] Sankar WN, Skaggs DL, Yazici M, Johnston CE, Shah SA, Javidan P et al. Lengthening of dual growing rods and the law of diminishing returns. Spine 2011; 36: 806–809

Part 5

Neuromuscular Scoliosis

16 The Natural History of Neuromuscular Scoliosis

Vivienne Campbell

The aims of this chapter are the following:
- Explore what is meant by the term *neuromuscular scoliosis*;
- Critique the published literature regarding the natural history of neuromuscular scoliosis in specific conditions;
- Consider whether the term *neuromuscular scoliosis* is helpful in predicting the natural history of scoliosis.

16.1 What Do We Mean by *Neuromuscular?*

The 10th Revision of the International Classification of Diseases (ICD-10), approved by the 43rd World Health Assembly in May 1990, codes neuromuscular scoliosis as follows: M41.4, Neuromuscular scoliosis. Scoliosis secondary to cerebral palsy, Friedreich's ataxia, poliomyelitis, and other neuromuscular disorders.

The 28th edition of *Stedman's Medical Dictionary* (© 2006, Lippincott Williams & Wilkins) defines *neuromuscular* as follows: "Referring to the relationship between nerve and muscle, in particular to the motor innervation of skeletal muscles and its pathology (e.g., neuromuscular disorders)."

16.2 Looking at Specific Conditions

If we accept this definition of *neuromuscular*, it is clear that the term can be applied to a large variety of disorders, the physical effects of which change with the growth and development of a child and young person over time. In addition, the phenotype of each condition may vary considerably. McCarthy, in his article "Management of Neuromuscular Scoliosis," expands on the range of conditions classified as neuromuscular scoliosis by the Scoliosis Research Society.[1] The purpose of this chapter is to consider the evidence base for the natural history of scoliosis in specific conditions listed in ICD-10.

16.3 Cerebral Palsy

The published evidence of the natural history of the spine in cerebral palsy (CP) relies heavily on retrospective series of adults in residential settings. CP is defined as a group of permanent disorders of the development of movement and posture that are attributed to non-progressive disturbances that occurred in the developing brain. Where evidence is taken from cohorts of patients with learning disability there is no guarantee that these individuals would meet this diagnostic criteria.[2] The increased availability of neuroimaging and advances in the genetic diagnosis of alternative conditions mean that, in pediatric practice at least, many of the subjects who were assumed to have a diagnosis of CP in historical papers would today be classified as having a specific or syndromic condition. In addition, changes in nutritional, orthopedic, and medical management mean that the cohort of more severely affected children and young people surviving into adulthood are possibly very different today. The management of scoliosis has changed to favor a consideration of spinal surgery in children and young adults with severe disability, so that contemporary data about the natural history of CP may be less easily available.

16.3.1 Systematic Review

Loeters et al performed a systematic review of the risk factors for the emergence and progression of scoliosis in severe CP.[3] They identified 10 papers published between 1966 and 2009 (two prospective studies, four cross-sectional studies, and four retrospective studies) that they felt to be of sufficient quality to be included in a systematic review. The authors excluded papers in which an intervention, such as bracing or intrathecal baclofen (ITB), was the main focus; these interventions are discussed later in the chapter.

Their findings were stark, highlighting the fact that little quality evidence exists to predict the emergence and progression of scoliosis in children with severe CP. Specifically, no paper that these authors included in their review gave a clear indication as to why CP had been diagnosed in the cohort that was the subject of the paper. Five studies drew on information from institutionalized patients who had a learning disability, with the potential for many alternative diagnoses by today's standards. The authors concluded that they could find only weak evidence for an association between the presence of scoliosis and the severity of CP, hip dislocation, and pelvic obliquity. No systematic associations were found between the type of CP and scoliosis, or the age, type, and location of the curve and the progression of scoliosis.

As well as questioning the methodologic quality of the published evidence available, this review highlighted differences in the literature pertaining to the definition of scoliosis (which varied from "clinically apparent" to an increased Cobb angle; angles larger than 10 degrees and angles larger than 45 degrees were both used as cutoff values for scoliosis). Recorded measurements of physical ability also varied—for instance, from ambulant vs. non-ambulant or bedridden to use of the Gross Motor Function Classification System (GMFCS; Palisano) in later papers.[4] Despite their limitations, individual papers within the aforementioned systematic review are often referenced as predictors of the development of scoliosis. I was pleased to note, however, that since 2009, Persson-Bunke et al have reported their series of 666 children, which are discussed at the end of this section.[5] A few examples of the literature before 2009 are summarized below.

Saito et al[6]

This was a retrospective study in a residential unit for patients with severe psychosomatic disorders. Of the 108 residents identified, 79 were felt to have spastic quadriplegia, and 54 had a scoliotic curve with a Cobb angle of more than 10 degrees. Of the 54 with a Cobb angle of more than 10 degrees, 37 had had radiographic surveillance of their scoliosis from before 15 years of age, with a mean follow-up of 17.3 years (range, 10–25 years). Of these, six were ambulatory, 24 could sit, and seven were classified as bedridden (i.e., could not sit). The strength of this paper is that the subjects did not receive any intervention, in keeping with views at the time, and their follow-up from childhood to final radiograph was well into adulthood (mean age, 25.1 years; range, 15–36). The authors found that when scoliosis started before the age of 10 years, it progressed rapidly during the adolescent growth period, continuing to increase after this growth period ended. They published the finding that a curve with a Cobb angle of more than 40 degrees before 15 years of age was associated with a significantly worse progression over time. Of their 37 patients, 20 required increased amounts of nursing time to complete various activities of daily living. The average Cobb angle for those 20 patients was 73 degrees, where it was 34 degrees in those patients who did not require increased assistance.

Majd et al[7]

The authors clinically assessed the 240 residents of an institution for patients with severe physical and/or learning disability, identifying 56 adult residents who had reached skeletal maturity (defined as Risser stage 5). These adults were followed both radiographically and clinically to detect functional decline in abilities over time and whether decline correlated with the progression of scoliosis. Functional deterioration was observed in 10 adults over time; the Cobb angle of curves changed from a mean of 41.1 to 80.6 degrees in the group with functional decline, as opposed to a change from 33.9 to 56.5 degrees in the group without decline. The authors then extrapolated these statistically significant data to estimate that the yearly deterioration of a curve ranged from 3 degrees (in the stable population) to 4.4 degrees (in the group with deterioration).

Subjects were also divided into groups depending on whether their curve was s-shaped, c-shaped, or kyphotic, and they further subdivided patients within these groups based on the location of the primary curve or on the presence or absence of scoliosis if the curve was kyphotic. The authors then described progression in each of these subgroups and were unable to show statistically significance differences between the groups in terms of progression rate or size of the initial curve. For instance, 40 patients had long c-shaped curves and the initial curve averaged 32 degrees (range, 15–85), with an average progression rate of 3.5 degrees (range, 0–13 degrees) per year. Given that these were adults who were skeletally mature, the range in this subset is so large as to be meaningless in trying to use the data to predict an individual patient's likelihood of deterioration.

Thometz and Simon[8]

In this institution-based retrospective study, 51 adults were followed for between 4 and 40 years (mean, 16 years) after skeletal maturity. They were among 900 adults in the institution, 180 of whom were felt to have CP; of these, 110 had scoliosis. Only patients for whom radiographs were available 4 years after skeletal maturity were included; 10 were excluded because an intervention (arthrodesis or brace) had been used to treat their scoliosis.

As in the sample of Majd et al, the variation between subjects was huge.[7] The authors reported that thoracic curves at the time of skeletal maturity were 46 degrees (range, 18–115), thoracolumbar curves were 54 degrees (range, 19–143), and lumbar curves were 63 degrees (range, 20–120). All radiographs were taken with the patients in the supine position to avoid the effect of gravity. Grouping their data together, the authors were able to show a difference in the mean annual rates of curve progression at skeletal maturity, which were 0.8 degrees if the Cobb angle was less than 50 degrees and 1.4 degrees if it was more than 50 degrees. Looking at their data retrospectively, they showed that a curve that developed before age 10 was likely to progress, but the development of a curve after 10 years did not protect against progression.

The authors provide useful information about the degree of change and range of curves in this population. However, whether their data can be used for a "degree of deterioration" measurement is of questionable relevance in predicting the clinical course of an individual child or young person.

Kalen et al[9]

In their prospective study of institutionalized adults with learning disabilities, Kalen et al attempted to find differences between the incidence rates of decubiti, highest functional levels achieved, degrees of functional loss, levels of oxygen saturation, and pulse rates in patients who had CP with untreated scoliosis greater than 45 degrees and the incidence rates in those with mild or no curves.

Their sample included 62 adult patients with a mean age of 39 years (range, 29–67) who were described as having CP: 54 with spastic quadriplegia, six with diplegia, one with hemiplegia, and one unclassified. Although the authors found no differences in the health of the two groups as described above, it is interesting to note that average oxygen saturation values of 80% (i.e., significantly low) were recorded in both groups. These levels feel uncomfortable by the standards of health one would expect even in these particularly vulnerable subjects, and such results would today raise questions about the health needs of both populations.

Senaran et al[10]

This prospective study compared 23 children who had scoliosis and unilateral hip dislocation with a control group of 83 children who had scoliosis and no hip dislocation. The mean age at the diagnosis of scoliosis in the group with scoliosis and a dislocated hip was 10.4 years (range, 4–16), and the mean follow-up was 3.6 years (range, 2–8). In the group with scoliosis alone, the average age at diagnosis was 10.5 years (range, 3–18), and the mean follow-up was 4 years (range, 2–11). The aim of this study was to look at the effect of untreated unilateral hip dislocation on the emergence of scoliosis, and the authors found that pelvic obliquity was more of a marker than the hip dislocation per se. They reported pediatric progression at a mean of 12.2 degrees per year in the control group and of 12.9 degrees per year in the group with unilateral dislocation. This is the only study included in this systematic review to indicate the deterioration seen during the childhood growth spurt. Again, no clear diagnostic criteria were mentioned.

16.3.2 Papers Excluded from the Systematic Review

Gu et al[11]

In a study published after the systematic review of Loeters et al, Gu et al looked at 110 children younger than 18 years of age who were reported as having CP; all but one had a GMFCS level of 5 and resided in a pediatric nursing home. The first radiograph was taken when scoliosis became a clinical concern, and a thoracolumbosacral orthosis (TLSO) was worn by the 38 subjects for whom it was prescribed (there is no account of whether this was worn during subsequent radiographs). The authors were able to demonstrate that Cobb angles larger than 40 degrees by the age of 12 years were more likely to increase with age when taking the whole group together. The range of scoliosis evident at first assessment was large, although the quoted initial mean Cobb angle for the group was 20.7 degrees, the range was 0 to 92 degrees on radiograph. Equally, the mean Cobb angle on the last X ray was 39 degrees—the range was 4 to 120 degrees.

Persson-Bunke et al[5]

This paper addresses the prevalence of scoliosis in a total population of children with CP, with the objective of analyzing the relation between scoliosis, gross motor function, and CP subtype, and of describing the age of patients at the time of a diagnosis of scoliosis. The authors reported a prospective epidemiologic follow-up study based on information from their CP register, in which 98.5% of the children with identified CP were included. Between 1995 and 2008, information about the results of spinal examination and investigation in 666 children between the ages of 4 to 18 years was identified.

The authors were able to demonstrate that in their population, the risk for the development of scoliosis increased with age and the GMFCS level (but not the subtype of CP), and they showed that in most children, scoliosis was diagnosed after 8 years of age. Children with a GMFCS level of 4 or 5 had a 50% risk for having moderate to severe scoliosis on clinical examination, with a moderate curve defined as a curve seen in both an extended position and on forward bending and a severe curve defined as a pronounced curve preventing upright positioning without external support. The authors also noted that their data stopped at 18 years of age, so that this 50% risk did not take into consideration possible deterioration into adulthood. The purpose of the surveillance was to optimize hip management in the cohort, and the authors mention that there may be a causal link between the aggressive management of hip dysplasia and the incidence of scoliosis.

These conclusions will be of no surprise to spinal surgeons working in the field. However, it is striking that this is the only prospective study of the development of scoliosis in a well-defined population of children with CP in which a definite attempt is made to identify and include only children in whom CP is a definable diagnosis.[5]

16.3.3 Studies of Interventions

Bracing

It is debated whether bracing makes any change to the natural history of scoliosis in a physically disabled person, with unsatisfactory evidence to either support or refute the premise. One of the often-quoted papers refuting the use of bracing is that of Miller et al.[12] Assuming that a brace will not change the natural history of scoliosis significantly, then can we use studies aiming to describe bracing or other interventions to help us describe more accurately the natural history of scoliosis?

Miller et al compared 22 patients who had no interventions with 21 patients treated with a Wilmington custom-moulded orthosis for 23 hours a day. They retrospectively reviewed the available charts of patients who were known to their service between 1979 and 1991 and who were quadriplegic, recording that the majority were nonambulatory. Whether children were braced or not depended on their physician's opinion of bracing as useful or not, leading to unacceptable bias by today's standards. No information is given about the ages of the children and young people other than that data were available before skeletal maturity. The mean age at which the curve reached 50 degrees was the end point of the study. This paper is often quoted as evidence that bracing is not helpful in altering the rate of curve progression in CP. One would have to question whether the paper does in fact supply any evidence useful to this debate (because of both the methodology and the lack of clarity of the diagnosis). However, it does provide a snapshot of the cases observed; for instance, 28 of the 43 subjects had a long c-shaped curve, and curvature was seen to accelerate coincidentally with the age at which one would expect an adolescent growth spurt. The average age at which 50 degrees was reached was 12.7 years, with no range given. Perhaps the most useful observation from their data (assuming that the orthoses made no difference to the overall progression of the curves) is that curve progression in 22 patients with spinal rotation of 2 degrees or less (Nash and Moe) was 12.6 degrees per year, and if spinal rotation was more than 2 degrees, curve progression was 25.3 degrees per year.[13]

Terjesen et al reported their retrospective study of 86 patients treated with a spinal orthosis, identified from records between 1982 and 1996.[14] They drew this cohort from 99 young people who were identified between 1982 to 1996 and were recorded as having a diagnosis of CP and a learning disability; the authors did not include the other 13 patients because their radiographs were insufficient, or they could walk independently, or kyphosis was their main presenting difficulty.

All were described as having severe spastic quadriplegia and a learning disability and were nonambulant. Spinal orthosis was prescribed if the curve measured 25 degrees or more or if the patient had problems with sitting. The ages of the patients at the start of the study were between 5 and 33 years (mean, 13.6). The mean duration of follow-up was 6.3 years (range, 2 to 14). Curve progression was measured in stratified age groups, with mean yearly progression recorded at the following ages: younger than 10 years (6.6 degrees per year), 10 to 14 years (4.7 degrees per year), 14 to 19 years (2.1 degrees per year), and older than 20 years (0.8 degrees per year); however, these differences were not statistically significant. Although the use of bracing may signify that this was not strictly a natural history cohort, the numbers do seem to fit with clinical experience in children and adolescents.

Intrathecal Baclofen: Can We Draw Information about the Natural History of Scoliosis?

Papers comparing the rates of scoliosis in children who are receiving ITB with the rates in those who are not are also a source of information on natural history. It is likely that these more recent studies, in which neurologic high tone is treated by neurosurgical means, will show greater concordance with studies in a population of children who have a positive diagnosis of CP.

Shilt et al[15]

This analysis included 50 patients receiving ITB and 50 controls. The controls were from the authors' spasticity database (i.e., they did not necessarily have preexisting scoliosis, as opposed to the group of Senaran et al[10]; see below). The control children were aged 9.7 years (range, 3–17), and 87% were defined as quadriplegic. The control group were followed for 3 years (range, 0.3–6.9). The initial Cobb angle on radiography was 12.7 degrees (range, 0–67). The final Cobb angle was 27 degrees (range, 2–91). The mean rate of progression was 5 degrees per year (range, –4 to 27). Incidentally, there was no statistically significant difference between the mean change in the Cobb angle of patients treated with ITB (6.6 degrees per year) and the mean change in the matched controls (5.0 degrees per year; $p = 0.39$).

The children in the ITB group received their implants between 2000 and 2005. Although no time period is stated for the control group, they were age-matched to within 12 months, so it is assumed that they were contemporaneous. In addition, the matched group were recorded as "with spasticity," assuming a far tighter match with a diagnosis of CP. The individual variations were still significant, however, and a degrees-per-year measure extrapolated from them might not benefit individual patients.

Senaran et al[10]

Senaran compared a similar group after ITB with a control group matched for age, sex, and functional ability (measured by the GMFCS). The focus of the study was to compare the group of children with spastic CP who either had preexisting scoliosis or went on to develop scoliosis following ITB between 1997 and 2003. Of the 107 patients undergoing ITB treatment for a minimum of 2 years, 26 patients subsequently developed or had progression of scoliosis. There were 25 children in the control group, who had a mean age of 11.6 years (range, 5–18) and were followed for a mean of 4 years (range, 2–11); of these, 3 were GMFCS level 4 and 22 were GMFCS level 5. The mean curve magnitude at diagnosis was a Cobb angle of 28 degrees (range, 0–64), and at follow-up it was 73 degrees (range, 24–113), with a progression of 16.1 degrees per year. As before, the variation in scoliosis adds value; however, the extrapolation of degrees per year may not.

16.3.4 Cerebral Palsy: Conclusions

The natural history of scoliosis in CP is not well evidenced as described in the published literature. More striking to a pediatrician is that the diagnosis of CP is not explicit, and that much of the data presented may not be from individuals who would be given this diagnosis today. The challenge will be to define the population accurately so as to be able to answer questions about natural history in the future.

16.4 Friedreich Ataxia

Friedreich ataxia (FA) is a progressive, degenerative, autosomal recessive condition caused by a deficiency of frataxin. This multisystem disorder affects the central and peripheral nervous systems, heart, skeleton, and endocrine pancreas.

Frataxin is a mitochondrial protein. In FA, a homozygous guanine–adenine–adenine (GAA) trinucleotide repeat expansion on chromosome 9q13 causes a transcriptional defect of the frataxin gene. In unaffected individuals, the GAA repeat occurs seven to 22 times, whereas in FA it occurs over and over again, hundreds and even thousands of times. The genetic basis of the condition was described in the 1990s, with the phenotype of early presentation, severe clinical illness, and death in young adult life associated with long expansions of the GAA repeat and a more benign course with shorter expansions. Before genetic confirmation, the diagnosis was clinical, and patients were described based on their neurologic phenotype as typical, presenting before 20 years of age, or atypical (presenting past 20 years of age).

16.4.1 The Spine in Friedreich Ataxia: Is the Curve Neuromuscular and Due to Weakness, or Is It Idiopathic with Its Own Unique Properties?

Historical papers that described the natural history of scoliosis in what was then termed typical FA were describing the more severe phenotype. Furthermore, early studies were based on cohorts of patients presenting for spinal surgery, and it was assumed that all cases had severe and unrelenting deterioration of the spine.

Although they did not recognize this in their clinical experience, Labelle et al in 1986 (before genetic confirmation, and so relying on phenotype) studied a cohort of 56 people with typical FA and excluded those with atypical FA. The patients were followed for an average of 9 years (range, 1–16 years), with the age at last follow-up being between 8 and 33 years.[16] The authors found that this severely affected group of patients could be divided into three roughly equal subgroups with respect to their spinal profile. One-third had a clearly relentless progression of scoliosis to a Cobb angle of more than 60 degrees. The second subgroup had scoliosis; however, this remained under 40 degrees without progression, and given that the follow-up of these patients was reported at 10 years after skeletal maturity, this would seem to be a robust finding. The third subgroup also had scoliosis that was under 40 degrees; however, at the time of publication, these patients had not been followed for 10 years after skeletal maturity, and the authors felt that they could not predict that progression would not occur. With these findings, the authors felt that they were in a position to be able to question the previously held belief that the scoliosis in FA was relentlessly progressive. A second assumption that the same group questioned was the role of muscle weakness in the pathogenesis of the curve—that is, did the curve behave like a neuromuscular curve or like an idiopathic curve with individual variation?

In 1995, Beauchamp et al, in the same group, published a study examining strength in their population of patients with typical FA.[17] A physiotherapist assessed 33 people with FA. The investigators were not able to demonstrate a decrease in strength over the time when either the subjects were losing their ability to walk or their curves were progressing, increasing their belief that the curves were idiopathic.

In the meantime, the availability of genetic confirmation with a range of trinucleotide repeats both expanded the phenotype and led investigators to work in which they tried to predict the clinical course based on the number of trinucleotide repeats. La Pean et al. looked to determine what would predict the clinical course of a child with FA.[18] They looked at a number of factors—for instance, the genotype (number of repeats), age of the patient at presentation, and age at which a wheelchair was used, either by choice or necessity. They found a correlation between the number of GAA repeats and deterioration (with a greater number of repeats leading to a worse phenotype) and also that the age at which a child had to use a wheelchair was as good a predictor of deterioration in walking ability as the genotype.

So, does this help us to predict the course of scoliosis in a patient with FA? The presence of scoliosis was noted in this cohort, but sadly no detailed information was taken correlating its progression with either functional ability or genotype. La Pean et al have confirmed that this information is lacking and may form part of cohort descriptions in the future (August 2011).

16.4.2 Friedrich Ataxia: Conclusions

The natural history of the spine in FA is likely to be of an idiopathic or syndromic nature and is not necessarily aggressive. At the present time, therefore, we cannot use the genotype or indeed the phenotype to predict the natural history of the spine.

16.5 Duchenne Muscular Dystrophy

The relentless progression of scoliosis in boys with Duchenne muscular dystrophy (DMD) after loss of ambulation is often referenced and used to influence surgical management.[19] Some cohorts would suggest that a far less aggressive progression is seen in a proportion of boys, whose natural history differs from that described and may vary in curve type, curve progression, and management. The pros and cons of early planned surgery vs. conservative management have led to spirited debate. Rather than focus on the historical data, which have influenced management for decades, it is perhaps more interesting to focus on new or emerging developments that may alter the natural history of scoliosis in boys and young men affected with DMD.

16.5.1 Maintaining Ambulation with Knee–Ankle–Foot Orthoses

A steady deterioration in the spinal curve is seen when boys become wheelchair-dependent. Rehabilitation into a knee–ankle–foot orthosis at the beginning of loss of ambulation has been found to prolong the time that boys remain ambulant by about 2 years and is standard practice.[20] It is suggested that maintaining the ability to stand and walk may help to prevent the rapid progression of scoliosis in DMD.[21]

16.5.2 Steroids

Kinali et al looked at 123 boys who were known to their service and who in 2007 were 17 years of age or older.[22] Of these, 78% had been rehabilitated into a knee–ankle–foot orthosis at loss of ambulation and 30% had been treated with steroids for a varied length of time ranging from 2 months to 9 years (median, 1 year). The authors were able to demonstrate a strong association between both older age of loss of ambulation and length of steroid use and delay in the onset of scoliosis, with older age at loss of ambulation associated with lesser curves.

In previous decades, steroid use in North America was considerably greater than that in the United Kingdom. In 2007, King et al, via a retrospective chart review of 143 boys and young men recruited from 2000 to 2003, reported the orthopedic outcomes of daily corticosteroid use in DMD.[23] The decision to treat with steroids was based on parental choice and tolerance of adverse effects. The treated group (53%) took steroids for more than a year. Those who took steroids for less than 6 months or not at all were labeled as untreated (47%). The group treated with steroids ranged in age from 5 to 18 years. The spread of boys' and men's ages was large at the beginning of the study. The mean age of the treated group

was 16.9 years (range, 6–30), and the mean age of the nontreated group was 14 years (range, 1–39). The development of scoliosis was reported only after 9 years of age and was defined as the presence of a curve of 10 degrees or more on a radiograph.

The mean number of degrees of scoliosis in the untreated group was 33.15 ± 29.98 and was 11.58 ± 15.65 in the treated group ($p < 0.0001$). Of the patients in the nontreated group age 9 years or older, 91% had a scoliosis curve of 10 degrees or more, whereas 31% of the treated group had a scoliosis curve of 10 degrees or more.

16.5.3 Degrees of Scoliosis by Cohort

Alman et al and Biggar et al published their prospective cohort studies from Toronto, Canada, looking specifically at children and young men in their second decade.[24,25]

Alman et al reported the use of steroids and the development of scoliosis in DMD. Two groups of boys, aged 7 to 10 years and able to walk, were enrolled in a nonrandomized comparative study to determine the effect of deflazacort (a derivative of prednisone) on muscle strength and pulmonary function. Again, parental choice dictated the use of steroids. The 30 patients in the treatment group received deflazacort, and the 24 patients in the control group did not. Follow-up was to a mean age of 16 years (range, 15–18) in both groups. The mean duration of follow-up was 7.3 years (range, 5–8) in the series as a whole.

A curve of more than 20 degrees developed during the follow-up period in 16 of the 24 patients in the control group (67%) and in five of the 30 patients in the treatment group (17%). Of the 24 patients in the control group, 15 underwent spine surgery at a mean age of 13 years (range, 11–17); at the time of surgery, the mean curve magnitude was 35 degrees (range, 20–60). In contrast, of the 30 patients in the treatment group, five underwent spine surgery at a mean age of 15 years (range, 11–17); the degree of scoliosis in these patients was not given.

In 2006, Biggar et al, as part of the same group, expanded the above cohort to include 74 boys who were known to the center between 1990 and 2004 and who had been monitored between the ages of 10 and 18 years. Again, treatment was started based on parental choice, tolerance or fear of adverse effects, and whether steroids were routinely offered (i.e., after 1993). The boys in the treatment group started deflazacort between 6 and 8 years of age and continued taking deflazacort for at least 2 years.

By 18 years of age, 30 of 34 boys (90%) not treated had developed a spinal curve of 20 degrees and had undergone surgery, whereas four of 40 treated boys (10%) had developed a curve larger than 20 degrees and had undergone surgery.

Both centers highlight that although they have shown that steroid treatment slows the development of scoliosis, they have not been able to determine whether the decrease in scoliosis seen at that point of time was due to the older age of the patients at loss of ambulation or to the prevention of decrease in strength afforded by the use of steroids. Furthermore, they were not able to say if the development of scoliosis was delayed rather than avoided.

16.5.4 The Future: Exon-Skipping "Antisense Oligonucleotides"

Although this is encouraging evidence for a change in the natural history of the spine in DMD, unlike in CP and FA, there is the possibility of a change in the natural history of the disease itself. DMD is caused by mutations in the dystrophin gene. At a molecular level, the boys have a bit of a gene present (an exon), which interferes with their ability to make dystrophin. New therapies are directed at skipping over these exons, so that a greater amount of dystrophin is produced. The first phase 2 trial of this therapy was published in August of 2011. Cirak et al describe six boys with DMD who were given increasing doses of an exon 51–targeting phosphorodiamidate morpholino oligomer (or an antisense oligonucleotide), and an increase in dystrophin was seen.[26]

16.6 Conclusion

The three diagnoses included in the ICD-10 definition of neuromuscular scoliosis have been considered. The natural history of scoliosis is poorly served by the published evidence in CP, in which defining the condition itself will have huge impact. There is a reasonable understanding of the course of scoliosis in FA; however, we fall short of being able to use this as a predictive measure for individual patients, particularly because the phenotype is expanding. Perhaps it is where the evidence of the natural history of scoliosis is most robust, in DMD, that we are going to see the most exciting changes, as disease modification is clearly changing the natural history.

References

[1] McCarthy RE. Management of neuromuscular scoliosis. Orthop Clin North Am 1999; 30: 435–449, viii

[2] Rosenbaum L, Paneth N, Leviton A, Goldstein M, Bax M. The definition and classification of cerebral palsy. Dev Med Child Neurol 2007; 49: 8–14

[3] Loeters MJB, Maathuis CGB, Hadders-Algra M. Risk factors for emergence and progression of scoliosis in children with severe cerebral palsy: a systematic review. Dev Med Child Neurol 2010; 52: 605–611

[4] Palisano RJ, Rosenbaum PL, Walter SD, Russell DJ, Wood EP, Galuppi BE. Development and reliability of a system to classify gross motor function in children with cerebral palsy. Dev Med Child Neurol 1997; 39: 214–223

[5] Persson-Bunke M, Hägglund G, Lauge-Pedersen H, Wagner P, Westbom L. Scoliosis in a total population of children with cerebral palsy. Spine 2012; 37: E708–E713

[6] Saito N, Ebara S, Ohotsuka K, Kumeta H, Takaoka K. Natural history of scoliosis in spastic cerebral palsy. Lancet 1998; 351: 1687–1692

[7] Majd ME, Muldowny DS, Holt RT. Natural history of scoliosis in the institutionalized adult cerebral palsy population. Spine 1997; 22: 1461–1466

[8] Thometz JG, Simon SR. Progression of scoliosis after skeletal maturity in institutionalized adults who have cerebral palsy. J Bone Joint Surg Am 1988; 70: 1290–1296

[9] Kalen V, Conklin MM, Sherman FC. Untreated scoliosis in severe cerebral palsy. J Pediatr Orthop 1992; 12: 337–340

[10] Senaran H, Shah SA, Presedo A, Dabney KW, Glutting JW, Miller F. The risk of progression of scoliosis in cerebral palsy patients after intrathecal baclofen therapy. Spine 2007; 32: 2348–2354

[11] Gu Y, Shelton JE, Ketchum JM et al. Natural history of scoliosis in nonambulatory spastic tetraplegic cerebral palsy. PM R 2011; 3: 27–32

[12] Miller A, Temple T, Miller F. Impact of orthoses on the rate of scoliosis progression in children with cerebral palsy. J Pediatr Orthop 1996; 16: 332–335

[13] Nash CL Jr, Moe JH. A study of vertebral rotation. J Bone Joint Surg Am 1969; 51: 223–229

[14] Terjesen T, Lange JE, Steen H. Treatment of scoliosis with spinal bracing in quadriplegic cerebral palsy. Dev Med Child Neurol 2000; 42: 448–454

[15] Shilt JS, Lai LP, Cabrera MN, Frino J, Smith BP. The impact of intrathecal baclofen on the natural history of scoliosis in cerebral palsy. J Pediatr Orthop 2008; 28: 684–687

[16] Labelle H, Tohmé S, Duhaime M, Allard P. Natural history of scoliosis in Friedreich's ataxia. J Bone Joint Surg Am 1986; 68: 564–572

[17] Beauchamp M, Labelle H, Duhaime M, Joncas J. Natural history of muscle weakness in Friedreich's ataxia and its relation to loss of ambulation. Clin Orthop Relat Res 1995: 270–275

[18] La Pean A, Jeffries N, Grow C, Ravina B, Di Prospero NA. Predictors of progression in patients with Friedreich ataxia. Mov Disord 2008; 23: 2026–2032

[19] Wilkins KE, Gibson DA. The patterns of spinal deformity in Duchenne muscular dystrophy. J Bone Joint Surg Am 1976; 58: 24–32

[20] Bakker JPJ, de Groot IJ, Beckerman H, de Jong BA, Lankhorst GJ. The effects of knee-ankle-foot orthoses in the treatment of Duchenne muscular dystrophy: review of the literature. Clin Rehabil 2000; 14: 343–359

[21] Rodillo EB, Fernandez-Bermejo E, Heckmatt JZ, Dubowitz V. Prevention of rapidly progressive scoliosis in Duchenne muscular dystrophy by prolongation of walking with orthoses. J Child Neurol 1988; 3: 269–274

[22] Kinali M, Main M, Eliahoo J et al. Predictive factors for the development of scoliosis in Duchenne muscular dystrophy. Eur J Paediatr Neurol 2007; 11: 160–166

[23] King WM, Ruttencutter R, Nagaraja HN et al. Orthopedic outcomes of long-term daily corticosteroid treatment in Duchenne muscular dystrophy. Neurology 2007; 68: 1607–1613

[24] Alman BA, Raza SN, Biggar WD. Steroid treatment and the development of scoliosis in males with Duchenne muscular dystrophy. J Bone Joint Surg Am 2004; 86-A: 519–524

[25] Biggar WD, Harris VA, Eliasoph L, Alman B. Long-term benefits of deflazacort treatment for boys with Duchenne muscular dystrophy in their second decade. Neuromuscul Disord 2006; 16: 249–255

[26] Cirak S, Arechavala-Gomeza V, Guglieri M et al. Exon skipping and dystrophin restoration in patients with Duchenne muscular dystrophy after systemic phosphorodiamidate morpholino oligomer treatment: an open-label, phase 2, dose-escalation study. Lancet 2011; 378: 595–605

17 Assessing Outcomes in Neuromuscular Scoliosis

Michael Grevitt

"Would you tell me, please, which way I ought to go from here?"
"That depends a good deal on where you want to get to."
"I don't much care where —"
"Then it doesn't matter which way you go."
–Lewis Carroll, Alice in Wonderland

This chapter examines the outcomes of surgery for neuromuscular scoliosis and the methodologic problems inherent in defining a "good" result. An examination of retrospective case series highlights reasons for inconsistencies in the reported outcomes of scoliosis surgery and caregiver satisfaction rates. The concept of "cognitive dissonance" is introduced as a possible explanation for the dichotomy between published outcomes and the lack of substantial postsurgical functional gains. Improved cosmesis as an aspect of parental or caregiver perception are also discussed. As a counterpoint to the results of retrospective studies, a prospective report is highlighted. Finally, some suggestions for future research and outcomes assessment are made. Total-involvement spastic cerebral palsy is used as an exemplar for the group.

17.1 Background

Surgery for neuromuscular scoliosis has reflected the evolution of spinal surgery in general. Harrington first applied his rod to the treatment of deformity arising from paralytic poliomyelitis. However, it was the instrumentation developed by Eduardo Luque that ushered in the era of segmental correction, stable fixation, higher fusion rates, and the avoidance of prolonged postoperative immobilization or reliance on external orthosis (▶ Fig. 17.1). When the importance of pelvic obliquity in contributing to pain

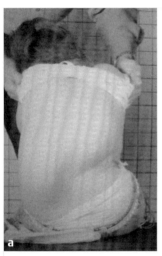
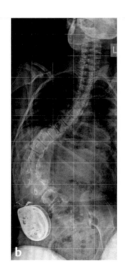
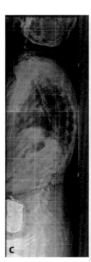
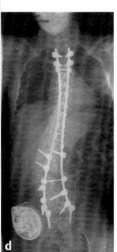
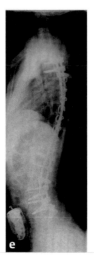

Fig. 17.1 (a) A 13-year-old girl with total-involvement cerebral palsy. Note the asymmetric sitting posture, weight concentrated on the left buttock, and need for assistance. (b) Posteroanterior whole-spine radiograph shows typical features of pelvic obliquity, costopelvic impingement, and significant lumbar scoliosis. A baclofen intrathecal pump is in situ. (c) Lateral radiograph shows thoracic hyperkyphosis. Although it is not evident on this radiograph, these children have significant problems with sagittal imbalance if not secured. Previous surgery on the hips is also demonstrated. (d) Post-operative frontal radiograph shows correction of scoliosis and pelvic obliquity with a balanced spine. "Hybrid" instrumentation of pedicle screws and sublaminar wires. Reduced thoracic kyphosis and improved sagittal profile.

and disability was recognized, further elaborations, such as the Galveston pelvic fixation technique and the unit rod, were introduced. The often-stated objectives of surgery for neuromuscular deformity can be summarized as follows:

1. Reduced pain and improved health-related quality of life;
2. Correction of pelvic obliquity and costopelvic impingement;
3. Spinal balance in the frontal and sagittal planes;
4. Solid arthrodesis;
5. Minimal complications.

17.1.1 High Rates of Caregiver Satisfaction

Many papers dating back to the early 1980s have documented high rates of caregiver satisfaction with the results of surgery. Comstock et al noted that 85% of parents or caregivers were very satisfied with the results of surgery and noted a beneficial impact on the patient's ability to sit, physical appearance, ease of care, and comfort.[1]

Using a questionnaire given to parents and caregivers, Tsirikos et al noted that caretakers did not recognize the effects of scoliotic deformity on patients' head control, hand use, or feeding ability.[2] Both parents and caregivers reported a very positive impact of surgery on patients' overall function, quality of life, and ease of care. Parents had more appreciation of the beneficial effects on their children's appearance, whereas educators and therapists were more likely to acknowledge improvement in gross and oral motor function. Most parents (95.8%) and caretakers (84.3%) said they would recommend spine surgery.

Bohtz et al used a modified version of the Caregiver Priorities and Child Health Index of Life with Disabilities (CPCHILD) questionnaire to assess patients' outcomes via their parents or caregivers.[3] A significant improvement in health-related quality of life was noted after the operation. The patients' rate of satisfaction with the outcome of surgery was 91.7%.

17.1.2 Significant Complication Rates

The problem with spinal surgery in this patient group is the high complication rate. Lonstein et al reported 83 early complications in 54 patients, for an early complication rate of 58%. Reoperation during the initial hospitalization was required in two patients (1.1%): one for infection and one for proximal hook cutout and proximal junction kyphosis. There were 81 late complications in 44 patients (47%). Most of the complications were minor (i.e., the patient did not require additional care or surgery). Pseudarthrosis developed in seven patients (7.5%), presenting at an average of

30 months postoperatively. Late complications in eight patients required nine procedures: five for repair of a pseudarthrosis, three for removal of a prominent iliac screw, and one for superior junctional kyphosis.[4]

In the series of Master et al, there were 46 major complications in 37 patients (28% prevalence), including two deaths. Non-walking status and a larger preoperative curve magnitude were associated with an increased prevalence of major complications. Nonambulatory patients were almost four times more likely than ambulatory patients to have a major complication. A preoperative major curve magnitude of more than 60 degrees was the most accurate indicator of an increased risk for a major complication.[5]

Even in the era of pedicle screw instrumentation (in which there is theoretical advantage of less intraoperative blood loss than in the Luque–Galveston technique), complication rates are significant. Modi et al reported a 32% rate of major complications in their series, most of them pulmonary. There were two perioperative deaths, and one patient developed neurologic deficit due to screw impingement in the spinal canal, which resolved after removal.[6]

17.1.3 Lack of Demonstrable Functional Benefit

A further problem is a dearth of papers that show significant functional improvement following surgery in neuromuscular scoliosis. Modi et al[6] retrospectively examined 32 patients at a mean of 3 years after surgery. Using a modified Ranchos Los Amigos Hospital functional rating system, in which grade 1 indicates an independent ambulator and grade 5 indicates a bed-bound patient, they demonstrated that 42% of the patients had gained functional improvement of one grade or more. For those who were non-walkers, the health gain was either improvement to independent sitting or conversion from a bed-bound state to some form of secured seating arrangement.

Watanabe et al[7] noted that functional improvements after surgery seemed limited, with improved sitting balance the most noteworthy (93%). Nonetheless, 8 to 40% of patients perceived their surgical results as an improvement, with an overall satisfaction rate of 92%.

The study of Bohtz et al[3] demonstrated no significant correlation between degree of scoliosis correction and parents' or caregivers' subjective rating of change in health-related quality of life. Of interest was the lack of correlation between the occurrence of complications or changes in health-related quality of life and the rate of satisfaction with the outcome of an operation.

Mention has already been made of the high satisfaction rate reported by Comstock et al.[1] It is therefore of note that there was a high rate of late complications. At a median follow-up of 4 years (range, 2–14), late progression of scoliosis, pelvic obliquity, and decompensation were noted in more than 30% of the patients. More than 75% of the patients with late progression were skeletally immature at the time of surgery and underwent a posterior procedure only. Disease progression necessitated a revision procedure in 21% of the patients.

In summary, despite the often high rates of complications after surgical treatment in patients with spastic neuromuscular deformity, the rates of parental and caregiver satisfaction are high. Moreover, there is limited evidence for significant functional gain in the majority of reports and no correlation between radiologic improvement (in scoliosis or pelvic obliquity) and reported satisfaction. Potential explanations for these apparent inconsistencies are discussed below.

17.2 Retrospective Studies

The literature on the outcomes of surgery in patients with neuromuscular deformity consists largely of retrospective series from single centers. In the majority, no validated outcome instruments or questionnaires are used. The inherent methodologic problems are illustrated by the study of Watanabe et al,[7] in which 84 patients with spastic cerebral palsy were evaluated at a mean of 6.2 years postoperatively (range, 2–16). In addition to radiologic evaluations, the investigators used a questionnaire that sought to determine aspects of pain, function, appearance, and other health-related quality-of-life issues specific to this patient group:

1. Expectations (1 question);
2. Cosmesis (2);
3. Function (6);
4. Patient care (3);
5. Quality of life (3);
6. Pulmonary issues (2);
7. Pain (1);
8. Comorbidities (1);
9. Self-image (1);
10. Satisfaction (3).

The authors demonstrated that after surgical treatment, the majority of patients (or more appropriately their parents and caregivers) were satisfied. Those patients who were less satisfied with their outcome had more postoperative complications and less correction of the major curve Cobb angle.

However, closer scrutiny of the paper reveals fundamental flaws. Because of severe learning difficulties, only four of the 84 patients (5%) answered the questionnaire; for the remaining patients, the caregivers or parents completed the questionnaire. Furthermore, the preoperative status and postoperative status for each functional domain were included in the same question. Thus, the validity of the results may be called into question because of recall bias (especially over a 16-year follow-up period in some cases) and third-party reporting (when a

patient's experience is given by proxy). Finally, the value of an outcomes instrument in which no explanations of internal consistency, construct validity, or test–retest reliability are included must be queried.

17.3 Cognitive Dissonance

An apparent paradox has been observed in which a surgical intervention that has a high complication rate and provides little or no functional gain to the patient is viewed very positively by the parents, with high satisfaction rates. This may be explained by the concept of cognitive dissonance and the complex dynamics of the patient–parent–surgeon troika.

Cognitive dissonance is a popular theory in social psychology that is used to describe the feelings of unease, anxiety, or guilt that an individual may experience when simultaneously holding two or more conflicting "cognitions" (e.g., ideas, beliefs, or values). One of the central tenets of the theory is that affected individuals seek to reduce emotional discord (or "dissonance") in one of three ways: downgrading the importance of one of the discordant factors, adding consonant elements, or changing one of the dissonant factors. An example is cigarette smoking. A smoker has to reconcile the desire to live a long, healthy life and enjoyment of the habit with its well-publicized adverse health risks. Thus, the smoker may deny the evidence linking smoking to lung cancer, concluding that only a few smokers become ill, that only very heavy smokers become ill, or that if smoking does not kill him or her, something else will.

17.4 Effort Justification Paradigm in Scoliosis Surgery

An aspect of cognitive dissonance theory that is highly relevant to decisions regarding surgical intervention and subsequent views of outcomes is the "effort justification paradigm." Effort justification is an individual's or a group's tendency to ascribe a greater value (usually abstract worth, status, or a feeling of well-being) to an outcome that requires effort to acquire or achieve. Dissonance is generated whenever individuals voluntarily engage in an unpleasant activity to achieve some desired goal. Dissonance can be reduced by exaggerating the desirability of the goal. In one of the earliest classic experiments in this field, individuals, to become members of a group, had to undergo either a severe or a mild initiation ceremony. In the severe initiation ceremony, the individuals had to engage in a highly embarrassing activity. In the mild initiation ceremony, the task was more mundane. In the event that the activities of the group that the individuals aspired to join proved dull and uninteresting, those who underwent the severe initiation ceremony evaluated the group activities as more interesting than did those who underwent the mild initiation scenario. The former test group, whose initiation process was more difficult (embarrassment equaling effort), had to increase their subjective value of the group to resolve the dissonance.

How does all this apply to neuromuscular scoliosis? In the scenario of neuromuscular scoliosis, parents and caregivers are likely to experience cognitive dissonance when faced with a situation in which a child's deformity is progressing but the potential solution to the disability (i.e., surgery) is likely to entail a significant risk for complications. Notwithstanding any eventual postoperative problems or lack of functional gain in the aftermath, the effort justification paradigm makes it more likely that the reported outcome satisfaction rates will be good. In this case, the emotional investment in the decision for surgery and the time spent in the hospital supporting a child during an inpatient stay are a proxy for effort.

17.5 Cosmesis

Before improved cosmesis in patients with neuromuscular deformity is specifically addressed as a factor in caregiver satisfaction, it is necessary to consider the same issue in adolescent idiopathic scoliosis, in which improved cosmesis is an established objective of surgery. More importantly, the otherwise healthy adolescent is an independent witness to any perceived reduced quality of life as a result of scoliosis and can voice opinions about the effect of surgery.

17.5.1 Data from Surgery in Adolescent Idiopathic Scoliosis

Bridwell et al[8] noted that parents' concerns about cosmesis were greater than those of their affected children and that the parents' expectations of surgery were higher. Sanders et al,[9] using a validated outcomes questionnaire (the Walter Reed Visual Assessment Scale), rated rib hump deformity and shoulder imbalance more severe than did adolescents. Rinella et al[10] asked both patients and parents to complete the Scoliosis Research Society (SRS 24) questionnaire. The parents' overall scores, as well as their scores for improved cosmesis and care satisfaction, were consistently higher than those of their children. These papers demonstrate that parental perceptions about rib hump and adverse cosmesis are worse than those expressed by their children.[10] Smith et al[11] also noted poor agreement between parents' and children's ratings of appearance after surgery.

17.5.2 Cosmesis in Neuromuscular Scoliosis

The situation in neuromuscular scoliosis is more complicated in that the child may have very severe learning difficulties and therefore cannot express an opinion on any apparent change in cosmesis after an operation to correct a deformity. Given the above, caregivers and parents are likely to project significant concerns about a child's overall appearance; together with a perception of increased pain, these concerns may push them toward a decision for surgery.

Furthermore, having a child be able to sit upright and be better able to engage with the surrounding environment is a very obvious benefit of successful spinal surgery. This aspect alone is a powerful validation of the decision for surgery. Such psychologically positive reinforcement may be as important in the perception of outcome as any functional gain achieved with a straighter spine after surgery. In cognitive dissonance theory, the improved cosmesis of a child sitting upright in a wheelchair, with a reduced need for adaptations, moulded seating, or restraining straps or supports, is a powerful "consonance" factor.

These factors seem to be borne out by the few studies that comment on cosmesis after surgery in patients with scoliosis secondary to cerebral palsy. Tsirikos et al[2] reported results from questionnaires, which indicated that parents were more like to appreciate an improved appearance after surgery, whereas therapists were more likely to describe improvements in gross and oral motor function. Watanabe et al[7] reported that 94% of parents perceived a significant postoperative improvement in their child's appearance. Better truncal cosmesis was also a significant factor in the high satisfaction rate reported by Comstock et al.[1]

17.6 Prospective Studies

The previous sections dealt with retrospective surveys of the caregivers or parents of patients with total-involvement cerebral palsy who underwent surgery to correct spine deformity. High satisfaction rates are demonstrated, but these are subject to retrospective and other forms of bias. Therefore, any study that seeks to evaluate the effect of surgery prospectively with validated outcome instruments deserves especial scrutiny. Unfortunately, there are few such published reports.

Jones et al used the Pediatric Orthopaedic Society of North America (POSNA) outcomes questionnaire (▶ Table 17.1), which was prospectively administered to the parents of a consecutive series of patients with total-involvement cerebral palsy before spinal fusion, 6 months after spinal fusion, and 1 year after spinal fusion.[12] The parents of 20 consecutive patients completed preoperative questionnaires. Questionnaires were completed for 10 of these patients at both 6 months and 1 year postoperatively, and seven more questionnaires were completed only at 1 year postoperatively.

The preoperative parental assessments indicated the expectedly high prevalence of comorbidities. Parental

Table 17.1 Pediatric Orthopaedic Society of North America MODEMS questionnaire[12]

Category		No. of questions	Example question
General patient well-being	Happiness	5	During the past week, has your child been very happy, somewhat happy, not sure, somewhat un-happy, or very unhappy with his/her looks?
	General health	4	During the past week, was your child energetic most of the time, some of the time, a little of the time, or none of the time?
	School absence	1	On average, over the past 12 months, how often did your child miss school (day care, camp, etc.) because of his/her health?
Parent satisfaction	Expectations	9	As a result of your child's treatment, do you definitely, probably, uncertainly, probably not, or definitely not expect your child to be able to perform activities at home?
	Satisfaction	1	If your child had to spend the rest of his/her life with his/her bone and muscle condition as it is right now, would you be very satisfied, somewhat satisfied, neutral, somewhat dissatisfied, or very dissatisfied?
Global function	Upper extremity function	8	During the past week, was it easy, a little difficult, very difficult, or impossible for your child to button buttons?
	Sports participation	12	During the past week, has it been easy, a little difficult, very difficult, or impossible for your child to bicycle or tricycle?
	Transfers/basic mobility	11	Does your child never, sometimes, approximately half the time, often, or always need help from another person for sitting and standing?
	Comfort (freedom from pain)	3	Has your child had very severe, severe, moderate, mild, very mild, or no pain during the past week?
Additional scales	Comorbidities	15 (3 parts each)	Has your child ever had asthma? Has your child ever received treatment for asthma? Are your child's activities limited by asthma now?
	Caretaker health	2	In general, would you say your health is excellent, very good, good, fair, or poor?

Abbreviation: MODEMS, musculoskeletal outcomes data evaluation and management system.

postoperative ratings indicated no significant changes between preoperative and postoperative physical function, school absence, comorbidities, and parental health. However, impressions of their child's pain, happiness, and frequency of feeling sick or tired improved significantly by 1 year postoperatively. Also, all but the ratings for pain and happiness were significantly improved by 6 months postoperatively. The presence of complications did not significantly affect questionnaire results.

Although this study is an erstwhile attempt at capturing relevant prospective data regarding the effect of surgery in a group with severe physical handicap and learning difficulties, it has major methodologic flaws. The most obvious problem is that the number of patients enrolled in the study is small, and the completion rate for the 6-month questionnaires was very poor. The potentially significant alpha error reduces the chance of finding meaningful differences between the preoperative and postoperative time points. The multiple-domain comparisons of the questionnaires also render a type II error probable, especially when the p value is little greater than 0.05. The lack of a Bonferroni correction to adjust for these multiple comparisons weakens the interpretation of the results.

It has to be questioned whether the POSNA questionnaire is really applicable to this group of patients. As the authors acknowledged in their discussion, this group of patients' mean global function score was more than 2.5 SD higher than that of children with other musculoskeletal complaints, in whom the questionnaire was validated.

For instance, questions regarding being able to do up buttons, participate in sports, and self-transfer are wholly inappropriate in the context of a child with total-involvement cerebral palsy, severe learning difficulties, and dependency. With these considerations in mind, it is possible that "ceiling" or "floor" effects are in operation when the construct validity of the questionnaire in the tested group is dubious.

Putting aside the above criticisms, the study did reinforce the findings of previous retrospective studies (i.e., high rates of parental satisfaction). Parental expectations were achieved in most cases. Of particular note was the parents' expectation that surgery would make their child look better. The dramatic alteration in trunk shape and sitting posture that modern surgery provides is perhaps the greatest demonstrable benefit, and this positive reinforcement and justification of effort as prime reasons for parental satisfaction is discussed above.

What is less understandable is the parents' perception of the child's "happiness" after surgery. The happiness score was calculated from five questions asking how happy the patients are perceived to be about their looks, body, health, and ability to wear clothes and perform the same activities as those of their peers. Clearly, such questions are more a reflection of parental perceptions rather than of any relevant feedback from the child.

In summary, this prospective study confirms previous retrospective data indicating high levels of parental satisfaction. However, the validity of the POSNA questionnaire in this group has to be questioned, and the small numbers make meaningful statistical interpretation difficult.

17.6.1 Need for More Objective Outcome Measures

From the preceding discussion, it is clear that the assessment of outcomes is heavily reliant on parental and caregiver perceptions and the "agenda" set by their expectations. The latter include altered cosmesis and abstract concepts, such as happiness, which are difficult to validate given the severe learning difficulties in this patient population. These "soft" outcome measures should be contrasted with the fact that even after successful surgery for spine deformity, the health status of this population is often precarious.

Asher et al[13] treated 117 patients who had neuromuscular spinal deformity with primary posterior instrumentation and arthrodesis. Subsequent spine surgery and death, and the time interval from surgery, were identified. Factors possibly influencing survivorship were studied. Reoperation and life survival statistics were available for 110 patients (94%) at an average follow-up of 11.9 ± 5.3 years (range, 2–20.9). The children in the younger half of the series at operation (< 13.75 years) were significantly more likely to have one or more perioperative complications ($p = 0.0068$). Twelve patients (11%) underwent subsequent spine surgery. Survival rates after subsequent spine surgery were 91% at 5 years, 90% at 10 and 15 years, and 72% at 20 years. Between 4 and 20 years postoperatively, 22 patients (20%) died. Life survival rates were 98% at 5 years, 89% at 10 years, 81% at 15 years, and 56% at 20 years. The only variable associated with life survival was the occurrence of one or more perioperative complications ($p = 0.0032$). In summary, life survivorship began to decline 4 years postoperatively and was significantly associated with the occurrence of one or more perioperative complications.

Tsirikos et al also documented the rate of survival among 288 pediatric patients severely affected with spastic neuromuscular scoliosis who underwent spinal fusion.[14] The mean age at surgery was 13 years and 11 months. Kaplan–Meier survival analysis demonstrated a mean predicted survival of 11 years and 2 months after spinal surgery. The Cox proportional hazards model was used to assess predictive factors, such as sex, age at surgery, walking and cognitive function, degree of coronal and sagittal plane spinal deformity, intraoperative blood loss, days in the intensive care unit, and length of inpatient hospital stay. The number of days in the intensive care unit after surgery and the presence of severe thoracic hyperkyphosis preoperatively were the only factors affecting survival rates. This study demonstrated statistically significant predictive factors for decreased life expectancy after spinal fusion in children with cerebral palsy.

Given these facts, it can be argued that more emphasis must be placed on identifying subsets of patients in whom surgery is likely to be beneficial in prolonging longevity or at least improving health-related quality of life. More objective measures of outcome, such as those listed below, may go some way in providing evidence for major surgery in a group of patients who cannot act as their own advocates. The following are some suggested objective measures of outcome after neuromuscular scoliosis surgery:

1. Nutrition and weight gain;
2. Nocturnal oxygen saturation;
3. Respiratory infection rates;
4. Sitting tolerance;
5. Decubitus ulcer rates;
6. Epileptiform seizure frequency;
7. Number of inpatient admissions.

References

[1] Comstock CP, Leach J, Wenger DR. Scoliosis in total-body-involvement cerebral palsy. Analysis of surgical treatment and patient and caregiver satisfaction. Spine 1998; 23: 1412–1424, discussion 1424–1425

[2] Tsirikos AI, Chang WN, Dabney KW, Miller F. Comparison of parents' and caregivers' satisfaction after spinal fusion in children with cerebral palsy. J Pediatr Orthop 2004; 24: 54–58

[3] Bohtz C, Meyer-Heim A, Min K. Changes in health-related quality of life after spinal fusion and scoliosis correction in patients with cerebral palsy. J Pediatr Orthop 2011; 31: 668–673

[4] Lonstein JE, Koop SE, Novachek TF, Perra JH. Results and complications after spinal fusion for neuromuscular scoliosis in cerebral palsy and static encephalopathy using luque galveston instrumentation: experience in 93 patients. Spine 2012; 37: 583–591

[5] Master DL, Son-Hing JP, Poe-Kochert C, Armstrong DG, Thompson GH. Risk factors for major complications after surgery for neuromuscular scoliosis. Spine 2011; 36: 564–571

[6] Modi HN, Hong JY, Mehta SS et al. Surgical correction and fusion using posterior-only pedicle screw construct for neuropathic scoliosis in patients with cerebral palsy: a three-year follow-up study. Spine 2009; 34: 1167–1175

[7] Watanabe K, Lenke LG, Daubs MD et al. Is spine deformity surgery in patients with spastic cerebral palsy truly beneficial?: a patient/parent evaluation. Spine 2009; 34: 2222–2232

[8] Bridwell KH, Shufflebarger HL, Lenke LG, Lowe TG, Betz RR, Bassett GS. Parents' and patients' preferences and concerns in idiopathic adolescent scoliosis: a cross-sectional preoperative analysis. Spine 2000; 25: 2392–2399

[9] Sanders JO, Polly DW Jr Cats-Baril W et al. AIS Section of the Spinal Deformity Study Group. Analysis of patient and parent assessment of deformity in idiopathic scoliosis using the Walter Reed Visual Assessment Scale. Spine 2003; 28: 2158–2163

[10] Rinella A, Lenke L, Peelle M, Edwards C, Bridwell KH, Sides B. Comparison of SRS questionnaire results submitted by both parents and patients in the operative treatment of idiopathic scoliosis. Spine 2004; 29: 303–310

[11] Smith PL, Donaldson S, Hedden D et al. Parents' and patients' perceptions of postoperative appearance in adolescent idiopathic scoliosis. Spine 2006; 31: 2367–2374

[12] Jones KB, Sponseller PD, Shindle MK, McCarthy ML. Longitudinal parental perceptions of spinal fusion for neuromuscular spine deformity in patients with totally involved cerebral palsy. J Pediatr Orthop 2003; 23: 143–149

[13] Asher MA, Lai SM, Burton DC. Subsequent, unplanned spine surgery and life survival of patients operated for neuropathic spine deformity. Spine 2012; 37: E51–E59

[14] Tsirikos AI, Chang WN, Dabney KW, Miller F, Glutting J. Life expectancy in pediatric patients with cerebral palsy and neuromuscular scoliosis who underwent spinal fusion. Dev Med Child Neurol 2003; 45: 677–682

18 Surgical Treatment and Outcomes

S.M.H. Mehdian and Nasir Quraishi

Neuromuscular disorders comprise a very diverse group of conditions. The most common myopathic form is Duchenne muscular dystrophy, and the most common neurogenic form is spinal muscular atrophy (SMA). The majority of patients with early onset neuromuscular scoliosis have SMA, which is an autosomal recessive disorder presenting in early childhood (homozygous mutation of survival motor neuron gene 1 on chromosome 5 and predominant skipping of survival motor neuron gene 2). Patients with SMA exhibit degeneration of the anterior horn cells of the spinal cord. The diagnosis is based on a combination of clinical features (hypotonia and absent reflexes), an electromyogram showing fibrillation and muscle denervation, muscle biopsy, and DNA genetic testing with polymerase chain reaction (PCR), which is a conclusive method for diagnosing the condition.[1]

This disorder has been classified into four types based on the age of the patient at presentation. Type 1 develops before the age of 6 months, type 2 at 6 to 18 months, and type 3 after the age of 18 months. Type 4 is benign and has an onset after 30 years. Scoliosis is present in more than 70 to 80% of patients with SMA. More specifically, all patients with type 2 SMA develop scoliosis by the age of 3 years, and by the age of 10, they develop significant curves of more than 50 degrees. Therefore, surgical intervention is at some time indicated for all children with type 2 SMA.[2]

SMA, like Duchenne muscular dystrophy, can have an effect on several systems, so that multidisciplinary evaluation and treatment are required. Progressive muscular weakness can result in pulmonary restriction, usually joint contractures, and nutritional disorders. The development of severe curves at a very young age poses unique challenges, and attempts at prophylactic or early bracing have not prevented curve development and progression. An immediate effect of this is difficulty breathing and restricted growth of the chest wall in the longer term. The spinal deformation is mostly a progressive, *c*-shaped thoracolumbar curve with the development of pelvic obliquity. An increase in either kyphosis or thoracic lordosis can be part of the deformity. The consequences of the deformity are loss of sitting balance, shortening of the trunk, and compression of the heart and lungs. The mobility of the ribs is reduced by rotation and deformation of the trunk; as a result, the breathing capacity is further decreased.

In this chapter, we describe our approach to the management of patients with early onset neuromuscular scoliosis (SMA in particular). Our discussion includes the preoperative assessment, our operative preference for self-growing rods, and the postoperative care required by this group of very delicate patients.

18.1 Indications for Surgery

Studies have shown that bracing is ineffective in preventing the progression of spinal deformity in patients with neuromuscular disorders. Spinal surgery is considered the primary treatment option for correcting severe scoliosis in neuromuscular disorders. It can improve the patient's cardiopulmonary function, sitting balance, appearance, and quality of life. However, in this population, surgery is considered a major intervention associated with high risk. A careful preoperative evaluation is necessary, and this should not be restricted to the spinal deformity itself; it must also include anesthetic management, pediatric cardiopulmonary care, postoperative intensive care, and postoperative rehabilitation.

We believe that surgery is indicated for those patients who have early onset neuromuscular scoliosis with rapidly progressing curves, which includes all children with type 2 SMA. We favor surgical treatment with growing constructs, to provide early correction of progressive curves and allow guided growth of the spine. This should, in theory, protect lung function and improve daily care of the children, including their mobilization with use of a wheelchair.

18.1.1 Preoperative Assessment

Preoperatively, respiratory function should be assessed in regard to both the timing of surgery and possible postoperative complications. The relationship between preoperative pulmonary function and postoperative complications is a little vague.[2] Wang et al have considered this issue at length, and their recommendations include preoperative sleep studies and closely monitored postoperative care, with extubation to noninvasive bi-level positive airway pressure therapy in patients who have marginal respiratory function.[3]

Attention should also be given to nutrition, bowel and bladder function, contractures, blood coagulation, and medication during the preoperative phase. A decision about resuscitation should be discussed with the parents, as well as the possibilities of a need for ventilation and/or tracheostomy. Patients and parents should be well informed about all aspects of the treatment, including the aims of surgery, and possible adverse events and their consequences in regard to daily functioning.

18.1.2 Perioperative Management

We recommend hypotensive anesthesia, the use of cell salvage and tranexamic acid, hemodilution, hemodynamic monitoring, and careful positioning of a nasogastric tube and a Foley catheter or indwelling urinary tract catheter. It is also important to maintain normothermia to prevent hemorrhagic complications and clotting problems. The use of anticholinergic agents should be avoided. Throughout the surgery, we use both somatosensory evoked potential (SSEP) and transcranial motor evoked potential (Tc-MEP) spinal cord monitoring.

18.1.3 Postoperative Management

The postoperative care should be conducted by an experienced multidisciplinary team of specialists: surgeons, a pediatric intensive care team, and rehabilitation specialists. The patient is admitted to the pediatric intensive care unit, especially as the threat of respiratory insufficiency requires intensive monitoring. A physiotherapist can coach the child in respiratory techniques and coughing.

The rehabilitation specialist verifies that adequate care is provided at home and coordinates the adaptation of facilities. The (electric) wheelchair may need to be adapted to support a position in which sitting and head balance can be maintained with the least effort on the child. Finally, in consultation with the general practitioner, temporary home care may need to be organized.[2] We do not recommend postoperative spinal braces because modern instrumentation is well suited to provide the required stability.

18.2 Surgical Options

As we have already mentioned, surgical treatment options for early onset neuromuscular scoliosis include both spinal fusion and growth-sparing techniques. Fusion techniques, however, inhibit spine and thoracic growth, and it is well-known that pulmonary development is not complete at birth. Thus, the thoracic deformity caused by scoliosis may adversely affect lung maturation up to the age of 8 years by inhibiting growth of the alveoli and pulmonary arterioles. Spinal growth peaks during the first 5 years of life and then diminishes from 5 to 10 years before increasing again.[4] Therefore, the early treatment of progressive curves without fusion becomes important to improve respiratory and visceral development and to normalize spinal growth as much as possible.

A surgical solution includes posterior spinal stabilization with growing rods. Dual growing rod techniques involve short fusion at the foundation sites and the placement of rods spanning the deformity. However, the rods need to be lengthened approximately every 6 months, with definitive spinal fusion performed after maximal spinal growth has occurred.[5] We have used a self-growing construct system over the last 20 years, which precludes the need for rod lengthening every 6 months. There is no doubt that the one procedure with general anesthesia used for this definitive self-growing rod construct is preferable to the multiple procedures with anesthesia used for the application of other systems.

18.2.1 Surgical Technique for the Self-Growing Rod Construct

Luque and Cardoso developed segmental spinal instrumentation to avoid the need for prolonged bracing while allowing further spinal growth in infantile or juvenile onset scoliosis.[6] Their initial report on a sample of 50 patients (mean follow-up, 23 months) showed Cobb angle correction from 73 to 22 degrees, and mean instrumented segment growth was 2.6 cm over 2 years. A subsequent report on paralytic scoliosis showed maintained correction and continued growth. Further reports on the Luque trolley in paralytic scoliosis secondary to poliomyelitis and in other types of scoliosis describe some problems of spontaneous fusion, modest spinal growth, loss of correction, and rod fracture.

Our self-growing rod construct is based on the Luque principles. After the patient is placed in a prone position and appropriately draped and prepared with padding at all pressure points, we perform a midline incision spanning the segment of the spine to be instrumented. Fixed spinal anchors (pedicle screws) and gliding spinal anchors (sublaminar wires free to travel along the rods) are then inserted. At the fixed proximal and/or distal anchorage points, a classic subperiosteal dissection is performed because these segments are to be fused. At the apex of the deformity, gliding anchors in the form of sublaminar wires are placed for maximal apical translation and deformity correction. We carefully perform midline laminotomies, partially remove the ligamentum flavum, and insert the sublaminar wires. Two double-stranded, short, closed-loop sublaminar wires are used in conjunction with the simple instrumentation designed by the senior author [SHM] at each level. These double-stranded looped wires, each measuring 1 mm, are available in three different lengths for different areas of the spine. The technique of wire passage and the modified instrumentation are detailed elsewhere.[7] The dissection at the gliding anchors is kept to a minimum by using extraperiosteal techniques (and muscle-sparing techniques to a degree) to avoid spontaneous fusion. Two pairs of 5-mm titanium rods are positioned, and the wires are tightened over in a standard fashion. A classic apical translation reduction maneuver is performed to correct the deformity.

We looked at the results of the use of self-growing rod constructs[8] at our institution between 1998 and 2010. From 1998 to 2006), we used the *h*-bar construct (n = 6). Two *l*-shaped rods are connected with two *h*-bars at the proximal and distal ends and secured to the spine with sublaminar wires (▶ Fig. 18.1). In this construct, spinal growth is provided at the proximal part of the fixation by migration of the *h*-bars cephalad (▶ Fig. 18.2). The rectangular shape created by the *h*-bars controls rotational

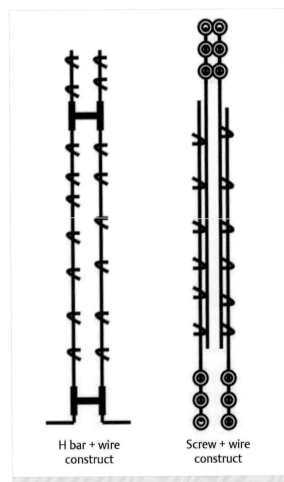

H bar + wire
construct

Screw + wire
construct

Fig. 18.1 Schematic representation of the self-growing H bar construct (group 1) and the four-rod self-growing rod construct (group 2).

forces and maintains the correction, yet allows spinal growth. In this first group of patients, a sufficient length of the rods was left free proximally to allow future spinal growth. We feel that fixation to the pelvis is preferable in all patients because it reduces the chance of loss of correction of sagittal and coronal balance in the long term.

From 2006 to 2010, we used a new hybrid self-growing rod (n = 10). This consists of a combination of screws, four rods, and sublaminar wires. In this construct, two contoured rods are secured to the proximal and distal screws on each side, proximally and distally. The distal rods are also fixed to the pelvic screws directly. The middle section of the spine between the proximal and distal screws is secured by sublaminar wires.

Fixation to the pelvis (including S1 and the ilium) was performed in all cases in both groups. The mean age of the patients in our series was 7 years (range, 5–8; ▶ Fig. 18.3 and ▶ Fig. 18.4). The new construct had the advantage of sound fixation proximally and distally, and this strong foundation could prevent proximal and distal junctional kyphosis and also provide a long space for spinal growth between screws. This is, we feel, advantageous in young children with a great deal of growth potential. The diagnoses in our series were type 2 SMA (n = 6), type 3 SMA (n = 3), hypotonia (n = 2), muscular dystrophy (n = 4), and cerebral palsy (n = 1). The mean follow-up period for group 1 was 11 years and for group 2 was 2 years.[8]

18.3 Surgical Outcome

In our study, the average measurements for scoliosis preoperatively were 68.9 degrees (range, 40–92) in group 1 and 68.28 degrees (range, 55.7–110) in group 2. At final follow up, they were 17.5 degrees (range, 7.8–41.3) in group 1 and 17.66 degrees (range, 7–30) in group 2. The

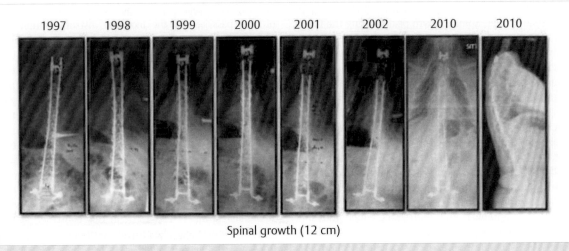

| 1997 | 1998 | 1999 | 2000 | 2001 | 2002 | 2010 | 2010 |

Spinal growth (12 cm)

Fig. 18.2 Case illustration of migration of the h-bar cephalad over time.

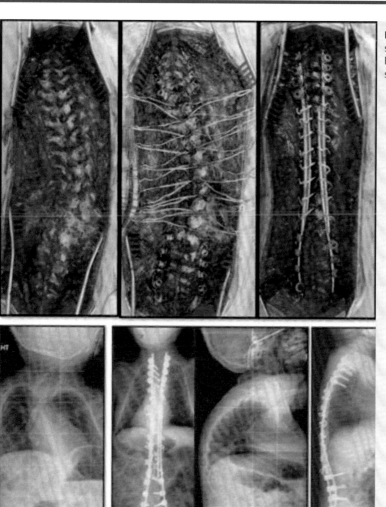

Fig. 18.3 Case illustration of the four-rod self-growing rod construct showing excellent correction of the deformity in both the sagittal and coronal planes.

improvement at 2 years was significant ($p = 0.002$). The chest area increased from 98.66 cm^2 (range, 86–114) to 172.4 cm^2 (range, 172–206; $p = 0.001$), and the forced vital capacity (FVC) was stable at 67% in group 2 (it was not reliably measured in the earlier patients in group 1). The average yearly spinal growth was 1.04 cm in group 1 and 1.17 cm in group 2. Complications included two cases of loss of fixation requiring revision in group 1 and one case of superficial wound infection in group 2.

Our retrospective analysis of 16 patients with early onset neuromuscular scoliosis shows that segmental self-growing rod constructs can control and maintain the correction with very low rates of operative morbidity and need for repeated surgery in children.[8] A comparison of the two constructs showed no significant differences in degree of correction and spinal growth, but the *h*-bar growing construct had less favorable proximal and distal fixation. In our experience, control of the head is partially obtained with surgery, but in the long term, this control is lost and patients need a head support to be adjusted to their wheelchair. We have also found that hand function is better in most patients following surgery. This, we opine, is a result of the spinal stability that surgery provides; the hands are not needed as much to support the body in the sitting position and thus are freed and can function with maximal capacity. The length of hospital stay in our series was similar to that of patients with idiopathic early onset scoliosis, but the pediatric intensive care unit stay was slightly longer in the patients with SMA. This was thought to be related to their already low FVC. These patients, in turn, require a more thorough preoperative assessment. No patient in our series required permanent fusion.

Lung area and chest wall size also improved significantly in both of our patient groups postoperatively, and this improvement was sustained during the

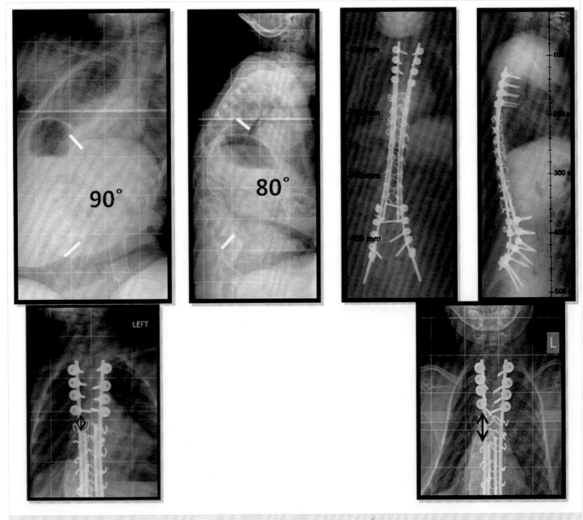

Fig. 18.4 Case illustration of a 5-year-old patient with spinal muscular atrophy undergoing treatment with the four-rod self-growing rod construct. At 3-year follow-up, 30 mm of growth was noted (*black arrows*).

follow-up years. Additionally, chest function improved significantly immediately postoperatively. This improvement decreases in the following 2 years as the disease progresses, but the self-growing rod construct protects lung function and volume and prevents further collapse of the chest wall. These results are comparable with those reported for growing rod constructs. However, rib collapse in patients with SMAs is very common; it is not possible to determine the exact cause of collapse, but intercostal muscle dysfunction may have an important role in rib collapse and in the shape of the thorax. Loss of coronal balance in some patients with SMA in the long term is related to the crankshaft phenomenon, which is more common in young patients. In our series, significant loss of coronal balance occurred only in one patient but did not significantly affect sitting balance.

In our opinion, pelvic fixation is almost always indicated in children with early onset neuromuscular scoliosis and long c-shaped curves because the patients are generally already confined to a wheelchair. Extension of the instrumentation from T2 to the pelvis not only corrects pelvic obliquity but also prevents failure of distal fixation because it reduces the chance of loss of correction of sagittal and coronal balance in the long term.

As we have already stated, early fusion in these patients limits trunk height and may exacerbate the pulmonary difficulties that are already a primary concern. This dilemma raises questions about the best method of controlling large curves during an extended period of growth. Depending on the patient's age and degree of skeletal maturity, definitive fusion carries risks for the development of the crankshaft phenomenon and restrictive pulmonary disease due to diminished thoracic cavity.

Several other methods of surgical treatment are available for patients with early onset neuromuscular scoliosis, including the rib distraction device (VEPTR), growing rods, and growth guidance growing rods (Shilla technique). Each of these systems has potential complications and requires repeated surgery in very unfit children. Recently, magnetic growing rods have been introduced that do not require reoperation and can be cost-effective. However, follow-up is very limited, and they could prove to have inadequate mechanical strength resistance for long-term distraction. Regardless of which system is used, the high complication rates, need for multiple procedures in growing children, and small relative gains in radiographic parameters still challenge proof of the efficacy of all such treatment methods. Much work remains to be done to identify the structural correlates of respiratory insufficiency and develop effective strategies for altering these.

White et al, in their small study of 14 patients with VEPTR and standard spinal implants for thoracic insufficiency syndrome, found that early preservation (minimum of 24 months of follow-up) of spinal growth and control of spinal deformity with a VEPTR system in combination with a conventional spine implant system as a spine-to-spine growing construct yielded results similar to those with growing rods previously reported by others.[9] The short follow-up mandates continuing assessment of these children to maturity. The VEPTR, when used for noncongenital scoliosis as a purely growing rod technique, does not control spinal deformities well (final Cobb angle correction of only 20%),[9] but it controls spinal deformity in patients with congenital scoliosis and chest wall abnormalities.[10]

Growing rod constructs not only allow continued trunk and lung growth (with better lung function) but also control and maintain correction of the deformity and pelvic obliquity.

The literature on growing rods is expanding. Akbarnia et al[5] reported a 54% correction of the initial curve in children with infantile or juvenile idiopathic scoliosis and an average T1-S1 growth of 1.2 cm per year. Their complication rate was 48%, with two deep infections, four superficial wound problems, two rod fractures, two hook dislodgments, one screw pullout, one case of crankshaft phenomenon, and one case of junctional kyphosis.

McElroy et al,[11] in a retrospective study, compared growing rods in 15 patients with SMA (follow-up of 54 ± 33 months) and in 80 patients with infantile or juvenile idiopathic scoliosis (follow-up of 43 ± 31 months). From time before surgery to latest follow-up, primary radiographic measurements in the patients with SMA improved as follows: curve, from 89 ± 19 degrees to 55 ± 17 degrees; pelvic obliquity, from 31 ± 14 degrees to 11 ± 10 degrees; and space available for lung ratio, from 0.86 ± 0.15 to 0.94 ± 0.21. T1-S1 length grew 8.7 ± 3.2 cm. Rib collapse continued despite growing rod treatment in the patients with SMA but not in those with infantile or juvenile idiopathic scoliosis. Hospital stays for lengthening procedures were longer for SMA than for infantile or juvenile idiopathic scoliosis ($p = 0.01$) and trended to be longer for initial surgery ($p = 0.08$) and final fusion ($p = 0.06$). The complication rates in patients with SMA and those with infantile or juvenile idiopathic scoliosis were, respectively, 0.5 and 1.1 major complications per patient ($p = 0.02$).

The authors concluded that growing rods improved trunk height and the space available for lung ratio while controlling curve and pelvic obliquity in young patients with SMA and severe scoliosis, but they did not halt rib collapse. Hospital stays were longer for patients with SMA than for those with infantile or juvenile idiopathic scoliosis, but the rate of major complications was lower. Another limitation is that this study does not account for the possibility that some of the differences in bone growth between the patients with SMA and those with idiopathic scoliosis might have been attributable to the propensity for the SMA population to be nonambulatory, whereas the patients with idiopathic scoliosis were all ambulatory. Finally, it is worth pointing out that the complication rate in the infantile or juvenile idiopathic scoliosis group was close to 100% (with 53 of 79 complications due to growing rod instrumentation), whereas it was 53% in the SMA group (6 of 8 due to growing rod instrumentation). The growing rod instrumentation accounted for most of these.

The apparent benefits of growth with the use of growing rods (and VEPTR) are achieved at the cost of additional multiple surgeries. In comparison, self-lengthening techniques require a substantially smaller number of additional surgeries (but possibly at the cost of less achievable growth). Growing rods and the VEPTR require on average an additional 6.6 and 7.1 surgeries per patient, respectively, whereas self-lengthening techniques such as the Shilla and modern Luque trolley require less than one (on average 0.5 and 0.6 additional procedure, respectively) per patient.[12]

Segmental self-growing rods provide a permanent solution to the correction of spinal deformity in these patients, and the length of hospitalization, number of repeated surgeries, and morbidity are reduced. Our team has been using segmental self-growing rods to treat early onset neuromuscular scoliosis for almost 13 years, and for the last 4 years, the hybrid system has been used. The rationale behind the change of system is that much younger children have greater growth potential, and the four-rod construct provides sufficient space between the two rods for increasing growth and also creates a good foundation at the proximal and distal parts in order to prevent failure. The senior author has acquired vast experience in the application of sublaminar wires during the last 25 years. However, users must be aware of the potential risks. Sublaminar wiring can be a time-consuming technique, with a risk for neurologic complications, but in the hands of experienced surgeons such complications are infrequent. Furthermore, it has been shown that wires do not cause spinal canal stenosis.

Complications rates with growing rod constructs vary from 8 to 80%. The most common complications are pneumonia, implant failure, and wound infection, either deep or superficial. In our series, we experienced two hardware failures in the patients in group 1 but none in the patients in group 2. We also had one superficial wound infection in group 1 that was treated conservatively with antibiotics.[8]

The severity of SMA varies considerably, and the natural history is thus difficult to predict, given the lack of a definable starting point. Changes in outcome with improvements in care will be similarly difficult to document, and the possibility of an increase in the proportion of more severely affected individuals exists if those who previously succumbed in infancy survive into childhood. The likelihood is that the population of children with early scoliosis that is uncontrolled by external bracing early in the growth years will increase substantially.[12]

Finally, we would advise that surgery in patients with early onset neuromuscular scoliosis be performed in a specialist center where the volume of procedures is high. A good medical support staff, including experienced pediatric anesthesiologists, physiotherapists, and nurses, is essential in dealing with these significantly handicapped children.

References

[1] Rutkove SB, Shefner JM, Gregas M et al. Characterizing spinal muscular atrophy with electrical impedance myography. Muscle Nerve 2010; 42: 915–921

[2] Mullender M, Blom N, De Kleuver M et al. A Dutch guideline for the treatment of scoliosis in neuromuscular disorders. Scoliosis 2008; 3: 14

[3] Wang CH, Finkel RS, Bertini ES et al. Participants of the International Conference on SMA Standard of Care. Consensus statement for standard of care in spinal muscular atrophy. J Child Neurol 2007; 22: 1027–1049

[4] Dimeglio A, Canavese F. The growing spine: how spinal deformities influence normal spine and thoracic cage growth. Eur Spine J 2012; 21: 64–70

[5] Akbarnia BA, Marks DS, Boachie-Adjei O, Thompson AG, Asher MA. Dual growing rod technique for the treatment of progressive early-onset scoliosis: a multicenter study. Spine 2005; 30 Suppl: S46–S57

[6] Luque ER, Cardoso A. Treatment of scoliosis without arthrodesis or external support: preliminary report. Orthop Trans 1977; 1: 37–38

[7] Mehdian H, Eisenstein S. Segmental spinal instrumentation using short closed wire loops. Clin Orthop Relat Res 1989: 90–96

[8] Mehdian SMH, Arealis G, Clamp J, Boreham B, Hammett T, Quraishi NA. Management of early onset neuromuscular scoliosis with segmental self-growing rod constructs. Eur Spine J 2012. In press

[9] White KK, Song KM, Frost N, Daines BK. VEPTR™ growing rods for early-onset neuromuscular scoliosis: feasible and effective. Clin Orthop Relat Res 2011; 469: 1335–1341

[10] Hasler CC, Mehrkens A, Hefti F. Efficacy and safety of VEPTR instrumentation for progressive spine deformities in young children without rib fusions. Eur Spine J 2010; 19: 400–408

[11] McElroy MJ, Shaner AC, Crawford TO et al. Growing rods for scoliosis in spinal muscular atrophy: structural effects, complications, and hospital stays. Spine 2011; 36: 1305–1311

[12] Ouellet J. Surgical technique: modern Luqué trolley, a self-growing rod technique. Clin Orthop Relat Res 2011; 469: 1356–1367

19 Best Surgical Strategies for Sitting Comfort

Robert Crawford

Children with neuromuscular disorders are often unable to walk and depend on wheelchairs for mobility. It is therefore doubly unfortunate for them that these disorders are also a potent cause of spinal deformity, which can make sitting comfortably in a wheelchair almost impossible. Untreated, they typically sit with a tilt to one side, requiring lateral support or the use of their arms to remain upright. The spine is scoliotic and often hyperlordotic or hyperkyphotic; this results in restriction of the chest and abdominal capacity, with the lower costal margin impinging painfully on the pelvis. The pelvis is tilted, causing an uneven and painful distribution of pressure in the weight-bearing areas, and the hips are asymmetrically positioned, with one or both often dislocated, causing further discomfort (▶ Fig. 19.1).

The main aim of treatment for neuromuscular scoliosis in wheelchair-dependent children is to improve their sitting comfort. The components of this treatment are the following: positioning the center of gravity of the trunk in the stable zone within the four corners of the sitting position, which are the ischial tuberosities and the posterior aspect of the thighs; making the trunk sufficiently straight that the thoracic and abdominal cavities can maintain a physiologic capacity; and positioning the pelvis and hips in relation to the spine so that the sitting pressure is distributed evenly.

The surgical strategy to achieve these aims requires a careful assessment of every aspect of the child's condition and lifestyle, how they are affected by the spinal deformity, and how this is likely to change in the future. The assessment should be carried out by the spinal surgeon in collaboration with the other physicians and other health care professionals who are usually already involved in the child's care. An understanding needs to be reached by all concerned, in particular the caregivers and in so far as is possible the child, of what is the best outcome of treatment that can be hoped for, what is the likelihood of achieving it, and what risks are involved. The surgery typically requires the correction of severe and stiff deformities of the spine and spinopelvic junction. It is technically demanding with a risk for significant complications, and it is seldom possible to achieve a perfect correction of the spinal curvature or a perfect sitting position. Nonetheless, with an appropriate preoperative assessment involving a multidisciplinary team, and with careful patient selection and surgical planning and execution, it is usually possible to improve the basic requirement of these children to be comfortably seated and to prevent or lessen the worsening of their sitting position that usually accompanies growth.

19.1 Natural History of Neuromuscular Scoliosis

The neuromuscular conditions that affect children are highly likely to cause scoliosis. Polio, now almost eradicated worldwide, has left a legacy of neuromuscular spinal deformity and loss of walking ability in countries where it was until recently endemic. In developed countries, cerebral palsy is the condition most commonly underlying neuromuscular deformity, although several other early onset neuromuscular conditions—for example, spinal muscular atrophy, Duchenne muscular dystrophy, and spinal dysraphism—cause similar problems, each with its own characteristics.

In general, the more severe the neurologic problem, the more likely it is that scoliosis will develop. This was demonstrated by Saito et al in 1998[1] in a review of 79 untreated, institutionalized patients with cerebral palsy in whom the progression of scoliosis was monitored with serial radiographs. Scoliosis affected 68% of these patients,

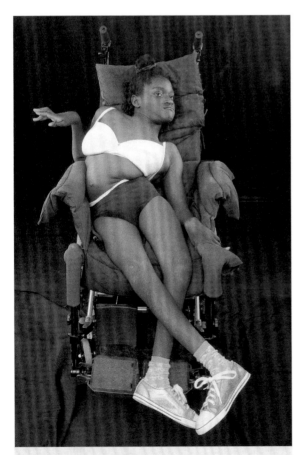

Fig. 19.1 Wheelchair-bound patient with cerebral palsy.

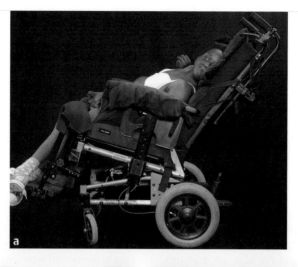

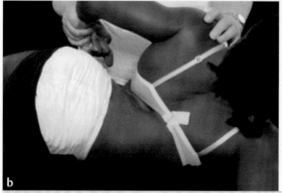
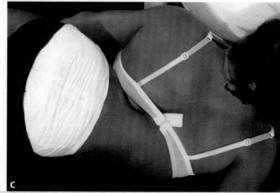

Fig. 19.2 (a–c) Severe scoliosis in a wheelchair-bound patient.

and it was found that the progression of spinal deformity correlated with the severity of their condition, as assessed by their ambulatory ability. No patients who were able to walk developed curves of more than 60 degrees; in contrast, 29% of those who were wheelchair-bound developed curves of more than 60 degrees, and all did who were bedridden (▶ Fig. 19.2). These findings were very similar to those of McCarthy et al,[2] who in 2006 found an overall incidence of scoliosis of 20% in patients with cerebral palsy but of 62% in nonwalkers (▶ Fig. 19.3).

Several publications have shown that musculoskeletal problems in children with cerebral palsy, such as scoliosis and hip dislocation, are becoming more common in developed countries, where the improved medical care of preterm neonates is increasing their survival. Although the incidence of cerebral palsy in babies of normal birth weight remained constant from 1980 to 1998, at between 2 and 3 per 1,000 births,[3] the survival of low birth weight and premature infants, in whom cerebral palsy is much more common, increased markedly during this same time.[4]

Typically, children with cerebral palsy have low muscle tone at birth and no deformity or joint contractures. However, the muscles affected by the neurologic injury

become hypertonic at an early age, and joint contractures, including spinal deformity, often develop between 5 and 10 years. The typical spinal deformity involves the whole spine in a single long c-shaped curve with an associated tilt of the pelvis and deformities of the hips, one or both of which often dislocate. This makes sitting (and for those able to, standing and walking), increasingly difficult.

19.1.1 Duchenne Muscular Dystrophy and Spinal Muscular Atrophy

In Duchenne muscular dystrophy, the progressive nature of the muscle weakness leads to a loss of ambulation around the age of 8 to 10 years, and respiratory compromise starts to become apparent at about 12 years. In spinal muscular atrophy, similar considerations apply, although the different subtypes progress at different rates. The purpose of surgery for children with these two progressive conditions, like scoliosis surgery for other wheelchair-bound children, is first to optimize sitting balance and free the arms from providing trunk support,

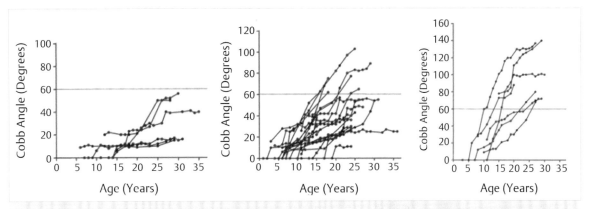

Fig. 19.3 (a–c) Cobb angle progression in patients with scoliosis due to cerebral palsy of different degrees of severity.[1] (Reprinted from The Lancet, 351(9117), Saito N, Ebara S, Ohutsuka K, Kumeta H, Takaoka K, Natural history of scoliosis in spastic cerebral palsy, 1687-92, 1998, with permission from Elsevier.)

allowing hand function, and second to protect lung capacity from the effects of spinal collapse, thus improving quality of life and increasing life expectancy.

The timing of surgery is ideally during the surgical window when bone growth has been sufficient to allow secure spinal fixation but the child has not yet reached the point of serious (> 50%) loss of vital capacity. In Duchenne muscular dystrophy, this is usually around age 12, when the Cobb angle is small and pelvic obliquity has not yet become an issue. The advantages of operating at this age rather than later are that the distal extent of fixation can be kept at L5 rather than the pelvis, and the operative time, blood loss, complications, and hospital stay are all reduced.[5,6]

19.1.2 Myelomeningocele

Scoliosis and hyperkyphosis are common in patients who have myelomeningocele, with the more proximal lesions resulting in more severe neurologic loss and a higher incidence of spinal deformity. More than 80% of patients with a thoracic lesion have a spinal deformity, whereas in those with a lumbar or sacral lesion, the incidence is about 20%.[7] As in most children with a neuromuscular spinal deformity, the severity increases with growth. Pelvic tilt in both the coronal and sagittal planes often accompanies the spinal deformity, and in addition, there may be developmental abnormalities of the pelvis itself. The effect of the deformity on seating is compounded by the associated numbness of the saddle area. Together with urinary and fecal incontinence, this numbness makes skin care a lifelong problem.

Hyperkyphosis, typically in the thoracolumbar or lumbar spine, results in forward tilting of the pelvis and forward displacement of the distribution of sitting pressure. Correction is made more difficult by the presence of scarring from the myelomeningocele and any closure surgery that may have been performed. Scarring, together with anesthetic skin, makes for problems with wound healing.

The technique requires shortening of the spine, either by posterior subtraction osteotomy at multiple levels or by excision of the apical vertebrae (kyphectomy), usually accompanied by transection and ligation of the thecal sac. Even in experienced hands, these operations are demanding and carry significant risks.[8,9]

19.2 Assessment of Spinal Deformity Problems in Wheelchair-Dependent Children

Wheelchair-dependent children with neuromuscular scoliosis have by definition an underlying condition that often results in complex pathology affecting multiple body systems. A systemic assessment should be done routinely so that important aspects of both the spinal and nonspinal problems are not overlooked by the surgeon, who may be preoccupied with the technical challenge of correcting the deformity. A technically satisfactory operation is pointless if, for example, swallowing difficulties lead to fatal postoperative inhalation pneumonia.

The various aspects of the child's condition should be assessed and managed by a multidisciplinary team that includes specialists from these fields:
- *Pediatric medicine* is responsible for the overall medical care of the child and the coordination of specialist services; the assessment of general health, chest and abdominal function, and nutritional status; and the coordination of hospital care with parents, caregivers, and community services.
- *Pediatric neurodisability medicine* ensures optimal control of spasticity and seizures. If an intrathecal baclofen pump has been placed, this has significant effects on the surgical assessment (ability of the pump to withstand magnetic resonance imaging) and

management (likelihood of catheter division or re-moval during surgery).

- *Neurodisability physiotherapy* assesses and monitors musculoskeletal function and maintains, as far as possible, joint mobility in the face of progressive spasticity.
- *Occupational / play therapy* assesses upper limb function and the extent to which it is affected by the sitting position. The inability to sit without using the upper limbs for support prevents the hands from being used for more creative purposes.
- *Pediatric orthopedics* is responsible for the treatment of limb deformity. Ideally, it should be possible for the lower limbs to be positioned in a 90–90–90 position. Scoliosis and pelvic obliquity are frequently accompanied by hip subluxation or dislocation, most commonly on the raised side of the pelvis. It is intuitive that scoliosis and pelvic tilt would predispose to hip dislocation, but evidence suggests that, at least once subluxation has started, hip dislocation will progress irrespective of whether scoliosis and pelvic obliquity have been corrected.[10] Hip subluxation and dislocation tend to occur earlier than severe scoliosis, so they are usually addressed first. However, if a child presents with both, reduction of hip dislocation is made difficult by the pelvic obliquity, so correction of the scoliosis usually takes precedence. The decision is also influenced by whichever deformity is causing the most discomfort.
- *Orthotics*, such as Lycra body suits, are effective in reducing spinal deformity in young children with mild deformity and low muscle tone, but they should not be persisted with if it becomes obvious that they are not working and the deformity is progressing. Rigid brace treatment has little place in these children because of the aggressive nature of the deformities and the discomfort that such a brace causes when used in a sitting position.
- *Pediatric nursing* ensures that the basic needs of the child are met, including the management of bowel function and micturition, and ensures the full involvement of parents and caregivers in decision making.
- *Nutritionists and speech and language therapists* assess swallowing and feeding difficulties. These may be exacerbated postoperatively, leading to a risk for reflux and aspiration pneumonia as well as undernourishment. Nasogastric or percutaneous endoscopic gastrostomy tube feeding may be necessary.
- *Wheelchair services* can provide moulded seat inserts, which promote sitting comfort by spreading the distribution of pressure and applying gentle corrective forces. Lateral pads may also be effective for controlling sideways tilt, and waist and shoulder straps may be necessary. Arrangements should be made for a postoperative reassessment because of the change in body shape. Spinal deformity correction can have adverse as well as advantageous consequences, such as difficulty in maintaining balance because of increased truncal height. The postoperative change in the seating position

may cause pressure problems in areas of skin subjected to weight bearing.
- *Social services, patient liaison, and support groups.*

19.3 Evolution of Surgery for Neuromuscular Spinal Deformity

The polio epidemic in the 1950s brought a surge in the number of patients presenting with neuromuscular scoliosis following the acute illness. At that time, the accepted surgical treatment for scoliosis consisted of preoperative curve correction with a turnbuckle cast, posterior spinal fusion through a window in the back of the cast, and continued postoperative cast immobilization. However, it became apparent that these devices, which were cumbersome at best, were impossible to use in patients with post-polio paralysis because of the additional respiratory problems they caused.

It remains the case today that braces, even when made from modern lightweight materials, have little place in the management of children with neuromuscular spinal deformity. This is particularly so when the children are bound to a wheelchair because of the further encumbrance that such orthoses create when the children are seated. Lycra suits, however, are often helpful in controlling truncal position in younger children with low tone.

The need to be able to treat neuromuscular scoliosis without casts was in part responsible for the development of the first commonly accepted internal spinal fixation systems, which were the Harrington rod in the 1960s and the Luque system in the 1970s. The advantage of the latter system, particularly for neuromuscular scoliosis, was the stronger fixation achieved by attaching the spine to the rods at all levels with sublaminar wires. Subsequently, more sophisticated methods of attaching the spine to the rods by means of multiple hooks and screws improved the strength of fixation, thereby allowing greater deformity reduction.

However, in the many patients with severe neuromuscular deformity involving both pelvic tilt and hip dislocation, it was recognized that it was not possible to improve the sitting position without addressing these two components of the deformity, as well as the spine. Correcting pelvic tilt in relation to the spine by attaching the spinal fixation system to the pelvis is now usually done as part of the spinal procedure. The surgical treatment of hip problems usually requires the release of contracted muscles and realignment osteotomy of the hip to allow stable reduction.[10]

Because pelvic obliquity and tilt are common components of severe neuromuscular disease in children, the fixation of scoliosis instrumentation to the pelvis is probably required in the majority of those who are wheelchair-bound. In response to the challenges posed by this problem, various methods of fixation to the pelvis have been developed.

Extending scoliosis fixation to the sacrum by means of wires, hooks, or screws proved inadequate to allow the forceful maneuver of correcting pelvic obliquity, and it was realized that fixation to the ilium is required. The method that initially proved most successful was the Galveston technique, described by Allen and Ferguson in 1984.[11] The Galveston technique modified the Luque method of segmental spinal instrumentation by introducing a bend in each rod at its lower end so that a rod could be inserted into the ilium via the posterior iliac crest on each side. The technique has since been further modified so that large iliac screws are used and attached to the rods by a variety of specifically designed connectors, which allow freedom of the screw trajectory in the ilium. Tsuchiya et al in 2006[12] demonstrated that this modified technique provides control of pelvic obliquity equivalent to that of the Galveston technique while avoiding the need for complex rod bending. Also, the superior fixation provided by screws compared with smooth rods results in less loosening within the ilium than the Galveston technique does.

Another method of inserting screws into the ilium, across the sacroiliac joint, was described by Chang et al in 2009.[13] Their method avoids the need for dissecting out to the posterior iliac crest and for lateral connecting bars between the rod and the iliac screws. However, the trajectory of the screw from this insertion point is more difficult to judge than it is with a posterior iliac crest insertion, and for this reason the iliac crest technique probably remains the most commonly used.

Neuromuscular scoliosis is often severe and stiff by the time a patient presents for surgery, so the intraoperative reduction of curves that are already severe is a significant issue. Various methods of reducing scoliotic curves both intraoperatively and preoperatively have been used. Preoperative reduction with halo gravity and halo–femoral traction, usually for 1 to 2 weeks, has been shown to be effective, although patients who have neuromuscular conditions are likely to have a range of multisystem disorders and may have difficulty tolerating this treatment. Intraoperative reduction as described by Takeshita et al,[14] by means of halo traction counterbalanced with unilateral femoral traction (on the side on which the pelvis is tilted up), avoids this problem. However, high traction forces are needed, so that care must be taken by means of intraoperative radiography and spinal cord monitoring to avoid a distraction injury to the cervical spine. Cranial nerve palsy, most commonly palsy of the abducens nerve, is also a recognized complication of forceful cervical traction, particularly in children, and cranial nerve function should therefore be assessed postoperatively in patients when this is used.

19.4 Outcome Evaluation

Sitting comfort and functional capacity are the all-important features in assessing treatment outcomes in wheelchair-bound individuals, but their assessment is difficult and often depends on an evaluation by parents or caregivers. A number of assessment tools have been developed for this purpose. These vary from general health instruments, such as the Klein–Bell Activities of Daily Living Scale,[15] to condition-specific questionnaires, such as the Shriners Pediatric Instrument for Neuromuscular Scoliosis.[16] Structured observation of a child's ability to perform various activities can also be used, such as with the Functional Mobility Scale described by Graham and Harvey in 2007.[17]

Quantifiable radiologic features are often used as surrogate measures for this assessment. The most obvious of these are the Cobb angle and pelvic obliquity in the coronal plane, and the sagittal Cobb angle and pelvic tilt in the sagittal plane. The distribution of sitting weight, measured by pressure-sensitive pads, would appear useful, but it has not been found to correlate well with radiologic correction of the spinal deformity or with the postoperative development of skin ulceration. This may be partly because the creation of a lengthened, rigid spine can negate the benefit of improved balance achieved by the surgery.[18,19]

Most studies of the results of spinal deformity surgery in these patients have used a combination of health questionnaires, as referred to above, and radiologic parameters. Watanabe et al reviewed 84 patients with cerebral palsy after scoliosis surgery, using a modification of the Scoliosis Research Society questionnaire.[20] They found an overall satisfaction rate of 92%, with poor results related to significant residual deformity and complications. Their findings demonstrate that a good technical outcome does correlate with a satisfactory clinical outcome.

19.5 Conclusion

As a consequence of the increasing number of infants with severe neuromuscular conditions who are now surviving, more wheelchair-bound children are presenting with spinal deformities and associated sitting problems. The surgical management of these children is often difficult because of the severity of their deformities and the other problems stemming from their underlying condition. However, improvements in medical and surgical care have made it possible to help more of these children by surgically treating their deformities.

The surgical strategy should aim for the following: ensure an even pressure distribution in order to optimize comfort and skin care; restore sitting height, thereby improving chest and abdominal function; restore sitting balance, so that the head is held in a normal position and the arms are freed from providing truncal support. Accomplishing these goals will allow the children a better interaction with their environment.

References

[1] Saito N, Ebara S, Ohotsuka K, Kumeta H, Takaoka K. Natural history of scoliosis in spastic cerebral palsy. Lancet 1998; 351: 1687–1692

[2] McCarthy JJ, D'Andrea LP, Betz RR, Clements DH. Scoliosis in the child with cerebral palsy. J Am Acad Orthop Surg 2006; 14: 367–375

[3] Sellier E, Surman G, Himmelmann K et al. Trends in prevalence of cerebral palsy in children born with a birthweight of 2,500 g or over in Europe from 1980 to 1998. Eur J Epidemiol 2010; 25: 635–642

[4] Wilson-Costello D, Friedman H, Minich N, Fanaroff AA, Hack M. Improved survival rates with increased neurodevelopmental disability for extremely low birth weight infants in the 1990s. Pediatrics 2005; 115: 997–1003

[5] Duport G, Gayet E, Pries P et al. Spinal deformities and wheelchair seating in Duchenne muscular dystrophy: twenty years of research and clinical experience. Semin Neurol 1995; 15: 29–37

[6] Sengupta DK, Mehdian SH, McConnell JR, Eisenstein SM, Webb JK. Pelvic or lumbar fixation for the surgical management of scoliosis in duchenne muscular dystrophy. Spine 2002; 27: 2072–2079

[7] Glard Y, Launay F, Viehweger E, Hamel A, Jouve JL, Bollini G. Neurological classification in myelomeningocele as a spine deformity predictor. J Pediatr Orthop B 2007; 16: 287–292

[8] Nolden MT, Sarwark JF, Vora A, Grayhack JJ. A kyphectomy technique with reduced perioperative morbidity for myelomeningocele kyphosis. Spine 2002; 27: 1807–1813

[9] Keessen W, van Ooy A, Pavlov P et al. Treatment of spinal deformity in myelomeningocele: a retrospective study in four hospitals. Eur J Pediatr Surg 1992; 2 Suppl 1: 18–22

[10] Senaran H, Shah SA, Glutting JJ, Dabney KW, Miller F. The associated effects of untreated unilateral hip dislocation in cerebral palsy scoliosis. J Pediatr Orthop 2006; 26: 769–772

[11] Allen BL Jr Ferguson RL. The Galveston technique of pelvic fixation with L-rod instrumentation of the spine. Spine 1984; 9: 388–394

[12] Tsuchiya K, Bridwell KH, Kuklo TR, Lenke LG, Baldus C. Minimum 5-year analysis of L5-S1 fusion using sacropelvic fixation (bilateral S1 and iliac screws) for spinal deformity. Spine 2006; 31: 303–308

[13] Chang TL, Sponseller PD, Kebaish KM, Fishman EK. Low profile pelvic fixation: anatomic parameters for sacral alar-iliac fixation versus traditional iliac fixation. Spine 2009; 34: 436–440

[14] Takeshita K, Lenke LG, Bridwell KH, Kim YJ, Sides B, Hensley M. Analysis of patients with nonambulatory neuromuscular scoliosis surgically treated to the pelvis with intraoperative halo-femoral traction. Spine 2006; 31: 2381–2385

[15] Dahlgren A, Karlsson AK, Lundgren-Nilsson A, Fridén J, Claesson L. Activity performance and upper extremity function in cervical spinal cord injury patients according to the Klein-Bell ADL Scale. Spinal Cord 2007; 45: 475–484

[16] Flanagan A, Gorzkowski M, Altiok H, Hassani S, Ahn KW. Activity level, functional health, and quality of life of children with myelomeningocele as perceived by parents. Clin Orthop Relat Res 2011; 469: 1230–1235

[17] Graham HK, Harvey A. Assessment of mobility after multi-level surgery for cerebral palsy. J Bone Joint Surg Br 2007; 89: 993–994

[18] Ouellet JA, Geller L, Strydom WS et al. Pressure mapping as an outcome measure for spinal surgery in patients with myelomeningocele. Spine 2009; 34: 2679–2685

[19] Lampe R, Mitternacht J. Correction versus bedding: wheelchair pressure distribution measurements in children with cerebral palsy. J Child Orthop 2010; 4: 291–300

[20] Watanabe K, Lenke LG, Daubs MD et al. Is spine deformity surgery in patients with spastic cerebral palsy truly beneficial?: a patient/parent evaluation. Spine 2009; 34: 2222–2232

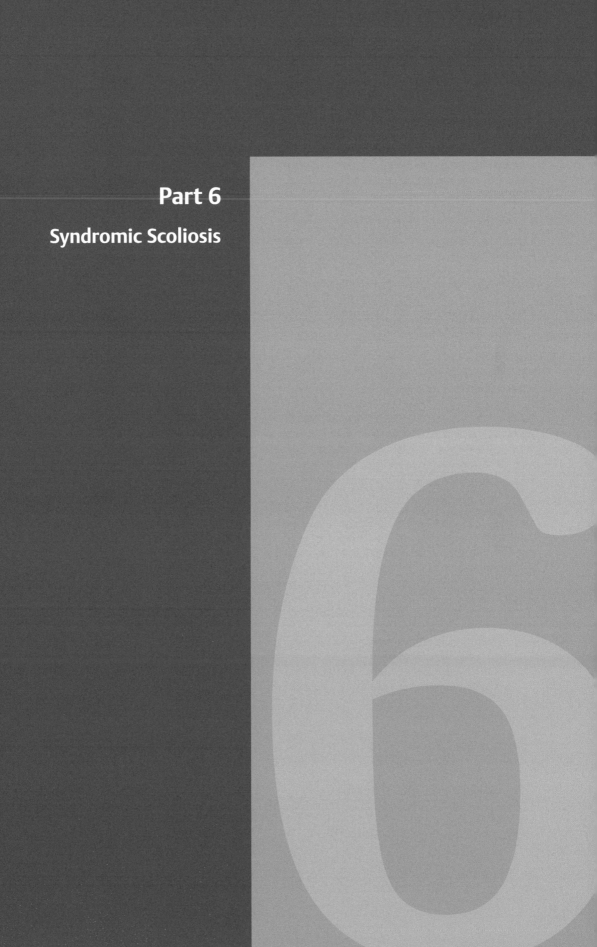

Part 6

Syndromic Scoliosis

20 Medical Intervention and Advances in Medical Management

Anne H. Thomson and Sandeep Jayawant

This chapter considers the medical aspects of neuromuscular and syndromic scoliosis and the interventions that support safe and effective surgery. The causes of scoliosis are myriad; important ones include:

- Syndromic / genetic conditions (e.g., Rett syndrome, neurofibromatosis, VACTERL [vertebral, anal, cardiac, tracheo-esophageal fistula, renal dysplasia, limb defects] association)
- Cerebral palsy: hypoxic ischemic encephalopathy
- Dystonia: genetic, cerebral palsy–associated, metabolic
- Malformations (e.g., Chiari malformation, syringomyelia, spinal dysraphism)
- Following trauma or demyelination (Guillain–Barré syndrome)
- Spinal neoplasia
- Neuromuscular disorders
- Inborn errors of metabolism: mucopolysaccharidoses, mucolipidoses
- Collagen disorders (e.g., Marfan syndrome, Ehlers–Danlos syndrome)

Scoliosis may be evident at birth, such as in children with structural developmental abnormalities of the vertebrae (e.g., hemivertebrae) or bony anomalies in association with other conditions (e.g., VACTERL [vertebral, anal, cardiac, tracheo-esophageal fistula, renal dysplasia, limb defects] disorder or metabolic disorders like the mucopolysaccharidoses). Scoliosis may be a marker of an underlying spinal dysraphism. If profound weakness or neuromuscular transmission defects occur in utero, the child is often born with arthrogryposis, the severity of which is in proportion to the degree of immobility of the fetus in utero. Scoliosis may also be part of general arthrogryposis.

Some of the causes of acquired scoliosis are dealt with elsewhere in the book. Although any muscle disease can cause scoliosis, some of the common neuromuscular disorders that cause scoliosis are:

- Congenital myopathies (e.g., core myopathies, rigid spine syndrome, myotubular myopathy, nemaline myopathy)
- Spinal muscular atrophy
- Muscular dystrophies (e.g., limb girdle muscular dystrophy, Xp21 dystrophies)
- Congenital muscular dystrophies
- Charcot–Marie–Tooth disease
- Spinocerebellar ataxias (e.g., Friedreich ataxia)
- Connective tissue disorders (e.g., Ehlers–Danlos syndrome, Ullrich myopathy)
- Arthrogryposis multiplex congenita

20.1 Neuromuscular Disorders

Congenital myopathies are inherited disorders characterized by a structural developmental abnormality of the muscles. Examples are core myopathies, nemaline myopathy, and centronuclear myopathy. Ultrastructural examination of the muscle often shows the underlying abnormality, such as disorganized Z bands with an altered and ineffective contractile apparatus in nemaline myopathy or an abnormality of oxidative enzymes within the muscle creating the appearance of cores on immunohistochemistry in core myopathy. These are relatively static or slowly progressive disorders. However, scoliosis can occur early in the clinical course of these disorders, and patients need to be carefully monitored from early on. ▶ Fig. 20.1 a shows a muscle biopsy specimen from a patient with core myopathy, and the specimen in ▶ Fig. 20.1 b demonstrates nemaline myopathy.

Muscular dystrophies are progressive destructive conditions; like the myopathies, they are inherited. They may be congenital, with the destructive process beginning in utero; in others, such as Duchenne muscular dystrophy (DMD), the process starts a bit later. Scoliosis may develop early in some cases or often in early teens. Histology reveals a dystrophic process with muscle fibers replaced by fat and connective tissue. ▶ Fig. 20.2 shows the typical histologic features of a dystrophic muscle.

Spinal muscular atrophy is another large category of disorders in which a genetically predetermined progressive degeneration of the anterior horn cells leads to areflexia, profound hypotonia, and weakness. There is an early onset of scoliosis and in some cases early death. Inherited neuropathies and spinocerebellar degeneration account for some of the other cases of neuromuscular scoliosis. Other neuromuscular conditions rarely cause significant scoliosis.

20.1.1 Diagnosis of Neuromuscular Disorders

Huge advances have been made in the genetic diagnosis of some of the conditions causing scoliosis. Chromosomal abnormalities are being more readily identified because of techniques such as array comparative genomic hybridization (CGH) testing. Some centers are performing exome sequencing or whole-genome sequencing, allowing the early genetic diagnosis of these conditions. Specialized DNA laboratories have acquired chips for the DNA diagnosis of conditions like the spinocerebellar ataxias.

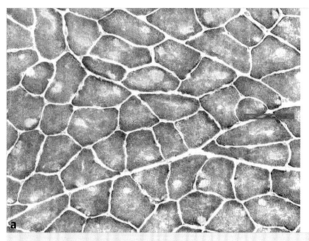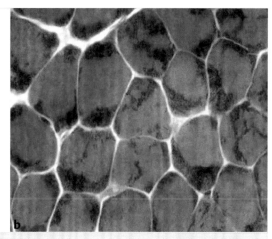

Fig. 20.1 (a) Oxidative stain showing cores in core myopathy. (b) Gomori trichrome stain showing nemaline rods in nemaline myopathy. (Figures used with kind permission from Victor Dubowitz and Caroline Sewry. *Muscle Biopsy: A Practical Approach.* 3rd ed. Philadelphia, Pennsylvania: Elsevier; 2007.)

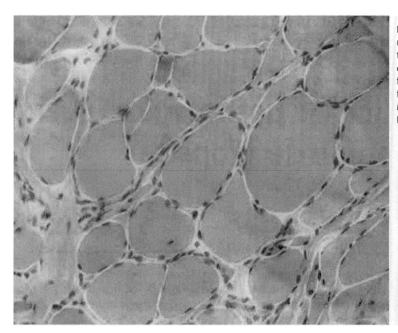

Fig. 20.2 Dystrophic muscle in Duchenne muscular dystrophy showing histologic features of inflammatory change and increased connective tissue with marked variability in fiber size. (Figure used with kind permission from Victor Dubowitz and Caroline Sewry. *Muscle Biopsy: A Practical Approach.* 3rd ed. Philadelphia, Pennsylvania: Elsevier; 2007.)

Muscle biopsy and neurophysiology remain useful in the clinical diagnosis of these conditions.

20.1.2 Medical Management of Neuromuscular Disorders

In keeping with the diagnostic advances, rapid progress has been made in the medical management of these conditions. Genetic engineering to correct or mitigate genetic defects remains the forerunner in the newer treatment strategies. Recent treatment options proposed for the management of some neuromuscular conditions include:

- Genetic advances: trial of antisense oligonucleotides (molecular patch therapy) in Duchenne muscular dystrophy
- Use of drugs to upregulate utrophin in Duchenne muscular dystrophy
- Use of salbutamol in spinal muscular atrophy
- Steroids (prednisolone / deflazacort) in Duchenne muscular dystrophy

Antisense oligonucleotides. The development of effective therapies for neuromuscular disorders such as DMD is hampered by considerable challenges; skeletal muscle is the most abundant tissue in the body, and many neuromuscular disorders are multisystemic conditions. However, despite these barriers, substantial progress has recently been made in the search for novel treatments. In particular, the use of antisense oligonucleotides, which are designed to target RNA and modulate pre-mRNA splicing to restore functional protein isoforms or directly inhibit the toxic effects of pathogenic RNAs, offers great promise, and this approach is now being tested in the clinic.[1]

Utrophin upregulation. Another experimental strategy is the upregulation of alternative muscle proteins, such as utrophin. In the mouse model, these strategies seem to reduce severity significantly. It remains to be seen whether they will be effective in boys with DMD.

Several drugs, such as valproic acid, carnitine, and hydroxyurea, have been tested in spinal muscular atrophy (SMA). They work by different putative mechanisms. Salbutamol seems to increase survival motor neuron transcript levels, thereby slowing the relentless progression of weakness, and it has been shown to be effective in SMA types 2 and 3. Other drugs have been used in other neuromuscular conditions and are primarily directed toward stabilizing or improving cardiac function; examples are idebenone in Friedreich ataxia and combinations of angiotensin-converting inhibitors and β-blockers in DMD. The use of intermittent low-dose steroid regimens seems to prolong ambulation in DMD.

Most of these treatments remain experimental, and studies are ongoing. Until such time as definitive trial data become available, supportive treatments are the only realistic treatment option for most patients. Some of the supportive treatments used in the management of neuromuscular conditions include:

- Physiotherapy: tackling contractures aggressively, chest physiotherapy
- Occupational therapy: seating
- Bracing
- Monitoring of respiratory and cardiac function
- Early intervention in cardiomyopathy
- Prevention and management of early respiratory failure: "therapeutic window" for safe anesthesia
- Surgical spine stabilization
- Use of β-blockers and angiotensin-converting enzyme inhibitors in prevention of cardiomyopathy in Duchenne muscular dystrophy
- Meticulous monitoring of respiratory function in all neuromuscular disorders
- Early initiation of noninvasive ventilation
- Steroids and monitoring for side effects (dual-energy X-ray absorptiometry [DXA])
- Orthopedic intervention

Guidelines have been published in the United Kingdom and elsewhere on standards of care for the management of scoliosis in children with neuromuscular disorders.[2,3,4] Of all the treatment strategies, the intervention that has had the biggest impact in terms of improving quality of

life and survival is the early diagnosis of hypoventilation and the initiation of noninvasive ventilatory support.[5]

20.2 Respiratory Function in Children with Neuromuscular Weakness

Respiratory failure is the predominant mode of death in children with neuromuscular weakness. It is not always easy to predict which children with neuromuscular weakness will have impaired respiratory function. In many disorders, such as DMD and SMA, it is unusual for major respiratory problems to develop while the child retains the ability to walk. However, children with structural myopathies or conditions affecting the chest wall, diaphragm, or intercostal muscles can, even while mobile, have nighttime hypoventilation with carbon dioxide retention and hypoxia.

Scoliosis has the potential to affect lung function by the following mechanisms:
- Impeding the efficient action of respiratory muscles;
- Reducing the thoracic volume;
- Decreasing the compliance of the chest wall.

The effect of scoliosis on lung function is amplified in children with muscle weakness.

20.2.1 Detecting Hypoventilation

All infants who are weak should have an overnight oxygen saturation measurement at a minimum and, if any abnormality is noted, then full respiratory polysomnography. Older children should be assessed for nighttime hypoventilation. Evidence includes a history of the following:
- Disturbed sleep;
- Difficulty waking in the morning;
- Morning headache;
- Morning nausea (Do they eat breakfast?);
- Daytime sleepiness (uncommon in children);
- Difficulty concentrating during the day, manifesting as poor school performance, and evidence of impaired lung function by spirometry (< 60% of predicted vital capacity). Evidence also includes these symptoms:
- Frequent respiratory infections;
- Impaired cough.

The examination should include observation of the respiratory movements (chest and abdomen) with the child in the sitting, standing, and supine positions, and the examiner should witness the power of a voluntary cough.

Where there is any concern, then polysomnography, including carbon dioxide measurement, should be carried out. Some children with neuromuscular weakness also

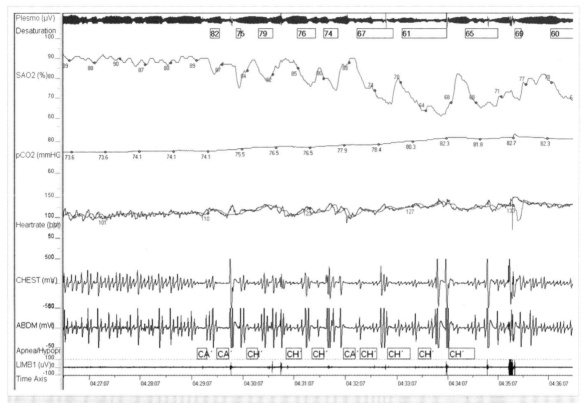

Fig. 20.3 Respiratory polysomnography tracing over a 10-minute period showing evidence of hypoventilation: fall in oxygen saturation and a steady rise in transcutaneous carbon dioxide with decreased respiratory effort during a period of active sleep.

have abnormal respiratory control (e.g., myotonic dystrophy and mitochondrial disease), and this will be detected on polysomnography. A common pattern of abnormality is evidence of hypoventilation, particularly during active (rapid eye movement) sleep (▶ Fig. 20.3).

20.2.2 Respiratory Intervention

The aims of intervention are the following:
- Prevent respiratory infection when possible (e.g., ensure vaccination against pneumococcal pneumonia and influenza);
- Treat early with antibiotics when infection occurs;
- Support the clearance of respiratory secretions with good physiotherapy, including augmented insufflation and assistance with coughing when needed (see later section on cough);
- Improve quality of life and reduce the impact of respiratory infections by preventing nighttime hypoventilation with ventilatory support, usually noninvasive ventilation (see below).

In patients with severe weakness and frank respiratory failure, ventilatory support is needed for survival, but for most children in whom nocturnal hypoventilation develops, the timing of the introduction of ventilatory support

can be difficult. Children with symptoms are most likely to recognize the benefit. If scoliosis surgery is planned, then the preoperative introduction of ventilatory support aids postoperative management.

Noninvasive Ventilation

Noninvasive ventilation is a technique that increases alveolar ventilation without the use of an endotracheal tube or tracheostomy tube. The children who benefit most are those who are able to self-ventilate for periods of time (e.g., those who require support only during sleep). Children with neuromuscular conditions are the largest group using noninvasive ventilation long term. Noninvasive ventilation can be used in the short term to support children after extubation following either an operative procedure or a respiratory illness requiring ventilation with an endotracheal tube. Most commonly, noninvasive ventilation is delivered with a positive pressure ventilator and either a nasal mask or a full face mask as an interface between the child and the ventilator.

Positive Pressure Ventilation

Pressure-cycled ventilators are often referred to as BiPAP (*bi*-level *p*ositive *a*irway *p*ressure) machines. The two levels referred to are a higher supportive pressure during inspiration (a preset inspiratory pressure to support a patient-triggered breathing effort) and a lower supportive pressure during expiration (to maintain functional residual capacity and prevent alveolar collapse and atelectasis). The ventilator delivers air flow to achieve the set pressure (e.g., 18/4 cm H_2O) independently of a small or moderate leak at the mask, and thus the ventilation delivered to the patient is relatively stable, even with a variable leak.

Mask Interfaces

Nasal masks are the most common type of mask, and a large variety of shapes and styles are now available for children (although more limited for infants). The correct size of mask depends on nose size and face shape. It is helpful when possible to permit the child to try several different mask and head piece combinations to see which feels most comfortable.

Face masks cover the nose and mouth. They are particularly useful in some weak children whose mouth hangs open during sleep.

Initiation of Mask Ventilation

It is helpful to take time to familiarize the child and the family with the mask and the ventilator apparatus. The mask should be fit well but not be too tight because a poorly fitting mask can cause skin and eye irritation. The child may try several masks to find the most comfortable fit. The BiPAP machine provides a constant flow of gas to the mask, and any mask system must have a built-in leak. The child should be introduced to the mask and machine gradually, and initially to just the mask without ventilation. At first, a low pressure setting on the ventilator may improve tolerance, and the pressure can then be increased gradually to the target pressure.

20.3 Planning for Scoliosis Surgery in a Child with Medical Problems

It is essential that a multidisciplinary approach be taken to preparing children with medical syndromes or neuromuscular weakness for scoliosis surgery. Predicting which children are at risk for postoperative respiratory failure or other problems is an imprecise science and depends on information gathered from the history, examination, and lung function tests (when the child is capable of performing them).

A detailed history should be taken that encompasses the following areas:

1. Comorbidities. Each diagnosis will have its own co-morbidities. For example, children with VACTERL association, Friedreich ataxia, or Marfan syndrome may have ongoing cardiac conditions. Children with cerebral palsy may be at risk for functional upper airway dysfunction or may have seizures. Concurrent medications should be detailed.

2. A history of the child's previous surgery and response to previous anesthetics is important. There is a known association of malignant hyperthermia–like reactions and rhabdomyolysis with the use of certain inhaled anaesthetics in children who have a number of neuromuscular diseases, including DMD, myotubular myopathy, and myoclonic dystrophy. The child's response and recovery from previous surgery, including the duration of all hospital stays, are important to document along, with any change in the child's medical condition since the last operation.

3. Many children who have a syndromic condition have poor growth and poor nutrition, and these may need to be addressed with supplemental feeding preoperatively, particularly when a device like the vertical expandable prosthetic titanium rib (VEPTR) is to be placed.

4. The cognitive abilities should be documented, in particular along with the ability of the child to understand instructions and respond.

5. Any previous history of chest disease must be elicited. How frequently does the child have "chest infections," and what treatment has been required previously? Have any such episodes required hospital admission or intensive care unit admission with ventilatory support? What was the duration of the illness from start to full recovery?

6. Does the child have a good cough, and can he or she clear secretions? What is the child's current handling of secretions when awake and when asleep; can they be swallowed, or does the child drool? Does the child feed normally? Is any drug being used to aid the handling of secretions, such as oral glycopyrrolate or hyoscine patches?

7. Does the child have any symptoms of nocturnal hypoventilation? (see above). The following should be assessed:
- Strength;
- Chest movements while the child is erect and supine;
- Strength of voluntary cough;
- Cognitive abilities.

20.3.1 Respiratory Function Testing

Vital Capacity

In children with normal cognitive function, repeatable measurement of the vital capacity can generally be achieved from about 6 years of age. Normal values can be predicted from height and age. In children with scoliosis, the height measurement is usually unreliable, and the arm span can be used as a surrogate measure for height. The vital capacity is then measured in the standing or sitting position to allow gravity to assist with diaphragmatic descent. Even in weak children, the vital capacity can be reliably measured by using a slow maneuver in which the child is asked to breathe in as deeply as possible and then to breathe out for as long as possible through a spirometer. In children who are weak and cannot create a tight seal with their lips around a mouthpiece, a face mask held firmly over the mouth and nose can be used.

There is evidence that the vital capacity can be used as an indicator of respiratory morbidity in children undergoing scoliosis surgery. In several retrospective studies, the likelihood of remaining intubated and ventilated for more than 3 days after surgery was higher in children with a lower preoperative vital capacity. In one of these studies, which examined 125 children (57 with neuromuscular disease), a preoperative vital capacity of less than 60% predicted the need for prolonged ventilation (> 3 days) with a sensitivity of 77% and a specificity of 56%.[6] However, there are also good data to indicate that even in children with a low vital capacity, scoliosis surgery can be undertaken successfully with minimal morbidity provided the appropriate support is in place. The routine postoperative use of noninvasive ventilation facilitates successful early extubation in these children.[7,8]

Polysomnography

Children with neuromuscular disease should undergo preoperative polysomnography to assess whether they have nocturnal hypoventilation, and if they do, they should be introduced to noninvasive support preoperatively. Children with upper airway obstruction are also at increased risk postoperatively. Those who have significant obstructive sleep apnea snore every night, with varying patterns of breathing effort and arousal. If there is the possibility of either obstructive sleep apnea or hypoventilation during sleep, an overnight sleep study should be carried out preoperatively. If upper airway obstruction is confirmed, an assessment of whether the child would benefit from adenotonsillectomy should be made. Such surgery should precede scoliosis surgery.

Cough Clearance

Secretions are transported from the peripheral airways to the main airways by ciliary activity, but the removal of airway secretions from the trachea requires a huff or a cough. To cough effectively, the following maneuvers are required:
• A deep inspiration, followed by
• Glottic closure, then
• Contraction of the expiratory muscles (abdominal and intercostal muscles) to generate high pressures and rapid expiratory flow rates.

Postoperatively, pain and sedation can inhibit deep inspiration; in addition, anesthesia can inhibit ciliary clearance, resulting in some retention of airway secretions and atelectasis. Pain and sedation can also decrease the effectiveness of expiratory muscle contraction; a weak cough is therefore further weakened postoperatively, so that cough effectiveness is reduced at a critical time. It is therefore important to obtain a history of the effectiveness of cough clearance preoperatively and, when possible, to measure the cough peak flow rate.

The cough peak flow rate can be measured with a face mask or a mouthpiece connected to a peak flow meter, into which the child makes a maximal cough effort after a deep inspiration. Healthy adults have a cough peak flow rate exceeding 400 L/min, and adults who have a cough peak flow below 160 L/min are not able to clear their airway secretions effectively. A number of studies have shown that in adults, a postoperative cough peak flow rate below 160 L/min substantially decreases the chances of successful extubation.[9] Standard values for cough peak flow rates in normal children aged 4 to 18 years have been published,[10] but there is not yet good evidence to define a cough peak flow rate necessary for effective secretion clearance in children. For children older than 12 years, a cough peak flow rate of less than 160 L/min is likely to be highly suggestive of the need for special care postoperatively with noninvasive ventilation and augmented cough techniques, which can be carried out either manually or with a cough assist device.

In children with poor cognitive function who are unable to perform any respiratory maneuvers, the physician relies on the history or on observation of the effectiveness of cough clearance and secretion handling. A judgment then has to be made as to whether there will be a need for a noninvasive ventilator or other support postoperatively.

20.3.2 Cardiac Assessment

A cardiac assessment is important for children with conditions that affect the cardiac muscle, such as DMD. Cardiac arrhythmias are a well-documented complication of anesthesia in some such children, and a careful choice of anesthetic agents is required.

20.3.3 General Assessment

At the preoperative assessment, the physician will be able to give specific advice as to whether any particular child is at increased risk during the perioperative period. In general, they are those who have the following:
• Vital capacity below 60% predicted;
• Previous history of failed extubation;
• Ineffective cough;
• Symptoms or signs of nocturnal hypoventilation. In addition, those who use noninvasive ventilation at night are at increased risk and need special care.

In this group, preoperative measures can be helpful and may include training the child and the family in the use of airway clearance techniques (see below) and introducing them to the use of noninvasive ventilation preoperatively. In particular, it is very useful to acquaint a child with the kind of mask and the feel of a mask that may be used for noninvasive ventilation postoperatively. It is helpful to ensure that the child's chest is in the best shape possible preoperatively with the use of antibiotics and physiotherapy. If nutrition is poor, a period of nutritional support with oral supplements in the weeks before the operation may be helpful.

20.3.4 Airway Clearance Techniques

An effective cough requires a cough peak flow of 160 L/min. A normal adolescent will produce a cough peak flow of more than 700 L/min. Children with neuromuscular weakness may be unable to generate sufficient flows for the following reasons:
- They are unable to take in a sufficiently large breath.
- They are unable to generate sufficient expiratory force.
- They have glottic weakness.

Children with other medical conditions may similarly be unable to generate sufficient cough flows.

Inspiratory lung volumes can be augmented either manually with a resuscitation bag and mask or mechanically with either a ventilator or a cough assist machine. Expiratory flows during coughing can be improved manually by compressing the upper abdomen or chest wall as the child coughs or with a mechanical cough assist device.

Mechanical Cough-Assist Devices

These devices use a face mask to deliver insufflation at relatively high-pressure ($+25$ to $+40$ cm H_2O) for 2 to 3 seconds followed by exsufflation at similar pressure for 1 to 2 seconds while the child attempts to cough. Airway secretions are then either expelled into the mask or suctioned from the oropharynx. The timing of insufflation or exsufflation can be manual or automated. There are no clinical trials comparing the efficacy of cough assist devices with the manual augmentation of inspiratory volumes with bag and mask, but the machines appear to be a useful addition to secretion clearance techniques.

20.4 Postoperative Care

Postoperatively, the child who is at risk should be extubated onto noninvasive ventilation, and secretion clearance techniques should be used as necessary, including a cough assist machine.

For children who are weak, specific additional precautions are needed:

1. The protocol for extubation postoperatively in a weak child should be similar to that used after a respiratory exacerbation.[9] In particular, the child should be ventilated with positive end expiratory pressure (PEEP) of 3 to 5 cm H_2O to maintain functional residual capacity, and attention should be paid to secretion clearance. Extubation should not be considered until the oxygen saturation is maintained above 94% on air (hypoxemia may be caused by atelectasis, hypoventilation, and retained airway secretions, and supplemental oxygen should be used with caution). Extubation should be to noninvasive ventilation, and any subsequent episodes of desaturation should be treated with a secretion clearance maneuver, such as with a cough assist device. Children who are weak should not be extubated until they are in air and then extubated onto noninvasive ventilation.
2. Children with neuromuscular weakness are at increased risk for respiratory depression associated with opiate analgesics, and epidural analgesia may be a safer and more effective method of pain control.
3. Some children with neuromuscular disease are prone to intestinal immotility, and the use of prokinetic agents and an open gastric tube can be helpful.
4. Some neuromuscular disorders—for example, SMA type 2—can be associated with troublesome acidosis during starvation. Glucose infusion and early nutritional support are helpful.

20.5 Conclusion

The advance preparation for the surgical treatment of scoliosis in a child with a medical condition is complex. However, abundant evidence now indicates that reconstructive spinal surgery in children with severe restrictive lung disease and/or serious medical problems can be conducted safely with minimal perioperative morbidity provided that a multidisciplinary management approach is taken; an example of the chronology of a complex case follows:
- Born preterm (36 weeks)
- VACTERL association
- VSD—repaired in infancy. Tiny residual VSD with high velocity left to right shunt.
- Heart block (postoperative complication in infancy). Transvenous ventricular pacemaker
- Pulmonary hypertension
- Oesophageal atresia and tracheoesophageal fistula—repaired as neonate
- Chronic lung disease. Noninvasive ventilation (NIV) for 2 years in infancy; development of restrictive lung disease. Reestablished nocturnal NIV age 11 years. On overnight NIV/oxygen
- Recurrent chest infections, two High Dependency Unit (HDU) stays in the past year

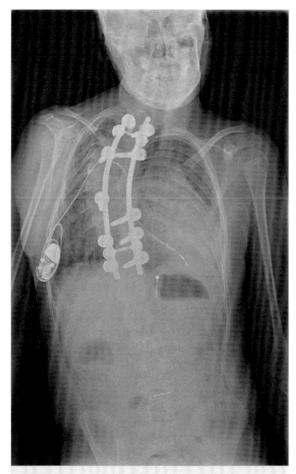

Fig. 20.4 Post-operative radiograph after T3-T11 posterior fusion and instrumentation.

- ACTH and growth hormone deficiency. On daily hydrocortisone
- Kyphoscoliosis
- T3-T11 posterior fusion and instrumentation (▶ Fig. 20.4)

- One night pediatric intensive care unit; two nights HDU noninvasive ventilation
- Day 10—ready for home
- No complications

The multidisciplinary team needs to adopt the Boy Scout motto, "Be Prepared."

References

[1] Cirak S, Arechavala-Gomeza V, Guglieri M et al. Exon skipping and dystrophin restoration in patients with Duchenne muscular dystrophy after systemic phosphorodiamidate morpholino oligomer treatment: an open-label, phase 2, dose-escalation study. Lancet 2011; 378: 595–605

[2] Mullender M, Blom N, De Kleuver M et al. A Dutch guideline for the treatment of scoliosis in neuromuscular disorders. Scoliosis 2008; 3: 14

[3] Muntoni F, Bushby K, Manzur AY. Muscular Dystrophy Campaign Funded Workshop on Management of Scoliosis in Duchenne Muscular Dystrophy 24 January 2005, London, UK. Neuromuscul Disord 2006; 16: 210–219

[4] Sejerson T, Bushby K TREAT-NMD EU Network of Excellence. Standards of care for Duchenne muscular dystrophy: brief TREAT-NMD recommendations. Adv Exp Med Biol 2009; 652: 13–21

[5] Eagle M, Bourke J, Bullock R et al. Managing Duchenne muscular dystrophy—the additive effect of spinal surgery and home nocturnal ventilation in improving survival. Neuromuscul Disord 2007; 17: 470–475

[6] Yuan N, Skaggs DL, Dorey F, Keens TG. Preoperative predictors of prolonged postoperative mechanical ventilation in children following scoliosis repair. Pediatr Pulmonol 2005; 40: 414–419

[7] Chong HS, Moon ES, Park JO et al. Value of preoperative pulmonary function test in flaccid neuromuscular scoliosis surgery. Spine 2011; 36: E1391–E1394

[8] Gill I, Eagle M, Mehta JS, Gibson MJ, Bushby K, Bullock R. Correction of neuromuscular scoliosis in patients with preexisting respiratory failure. Spine 2006; 31: 2478–2483

[9] Bach JR, Gonçalves MR, Hamdani I, Winck JC. Extubation of patients with neuromuscular weakness: a new management paradigm. Chest 2010; 137: 1033–1039

[10] Bianchi C, Baiardi P. Cough peak flows: standard values for children and adolescents. Am J Phys Med Rehabil 2008; 87: 461–467

21 Surgical Treatment of Syndromic Scoliosis

Ahmet Alanay and Ozgur Dede

A multitude of syndromic conditions are associated with the development of spinal deformity in young children. The curve characteristics, soft tissue, and bone structure vary grossly depending on the specific condition; therefore, stacking these quite different conditions in the same section may appear somewhat simplistic. However, because of the rarity of the conditions, similarities in management strategies, and stark differences between syndromic and idiopathic scoliosis, a discussion under a common heading is justified.

21.1 General Considerations

The spine deformities associated with syndromic conditions typically do not respond to conservative measures as much as idiopathic deformities do, and a detailed discussion of nonoperative management is provided in Chapter 22. Casting and bracing are rarely successful. Casting may not be even tolerable or feasible in some patients with multiple comorbidities. Because of the associated abnormalities, the treatment goals in these children also need to be tailored accordingly. As an example, a noticeable residual cosmetic deformity, but a stable spine, is considered a very good result in a patient with syndromic scoliosis if this has been achieved without major complications. Intraoperative problems, such as excessive bleeding and anesthesia-related issues, are more common in this group. Because of the inherent abnormalities of the soft tissues and bone as well as the nervous system, spontaneous correction from the levels that are not included in the fusion mass may not be as dependable as in idiopathic deformity. Junctional deformity is more common in certain conditions, possibly because of the combination of these factors.

For these reasons, a longer fusion, which is attempted to be avoided in idiopathic deformity, may not be undesirable in patients with syndromic scoliosis. Given that the functional demand on the spine will be less in most patients with syndromic scoliosis, a long fusion probably is not as negative as it would be in a patient with idiopathic deformity. Therefore, selective and short fusion should be reserved for the rare patients with good muscle tone, neural control, mental acuity, and bone of good quality. Poor bone quality and a high rate of fixation failure justify longer fusions with the use of more anchors.

In a certain group of patients with syndromic scoliosis, postoperative external supports, most commonly in the form of thoracolumbosacral orthoses (TLSOs), should be considered. Decreased truncal control in some of these children, in addition to poor bone quality, may compromise the internal fixation before bony fusion occurs. There is evidence suggesting that pseudarthrosis and

junctional kyphotic deformities may be more common in patients with syndromic scoliosis following posterior instrumentation procedures. Therefore, it is a safe approach to use external bracing in some cases, especially if the neurologic or cognitive status is compromised.

Because of the multitude of comorbidities typically seen in these patients, a multidisciplinary approach is warranted that begins at the first preoperative visit and continues all through the postoperative course. The surgeon should be familiar with the various syndromes and meticulous about noting the patient's associated medical problems. Consequently, the relevant specialties should be consulted and involved in the preoperative care and preparation. Most commonly, cardiac, pulmonary, gastrointestinal, and neurology / neurosurgery consultations may be necessary. Involving a geneticist may ensure the diagnosis and help with the overall treatment plan. The medical management of patients with syndromic conditions is discussed in Chapter 20.

The surgical plan should include the type of approach and the implant type, size, and material. The bone quality, size and stiffness of the deformity, and desired degree of correction are important factors when an implant is chosen. Smaller implants should be made available because normal-size implants may not fit the dysplastic bones of these children. Preoperative radiographs should be well studied, and a computed tomographic (CT) scan should be acquired if there are any questions about structural anomalies, such as dysplastic or absent pedicles and underdeveloped posterior elements, that may alter the surgical plan. In the presence of positive neural findings or suggestive signs, magnetic resonance (MR) images of the whole neural axis should be acquired. Additionally, in complex deformities and syndromes with connective tissue involvement, MR imaging will prove useful for showing anomalies such as dural ectasia and intraspinal abnormalities that may alter the surgical plan. Specifically, it is wise to avoid canal-occupying implants like hooks, wires, or polyester tape in patients who have conditions associated with dural ectasia (e.g., connective tissue disorders, neurofibromatosis).

Transcranial motor evoked potentials (Tc-MEPs) and somatosensory evoked potentials (SSEPs) are routinely used to monitor all neurologically intact patients during spinal surgeries. Preoperative blood typing and cross-matching are mandatory because a higher rate of bleeding may be encountered, especially in patients with connective tissue disorders. The surgeon must involve the patient's family at every step of the management. It is very important that the family and the child understand the treatment goals and plans. The parents should be well informed about the potential complications and the possible need for revision procedures, as well as the care and rehabilitation that will be required in the postoperative period.

21.2 Specific Syndromes

The complete list of syndromic conditions is exhaustive, and the reader is directed to Chapter 16 for a discussion of the natural history of the spine in some of the various conditions associated with scoliosis. However, this section provides an overview of the authors' approach to the treatment of the most common syndromic conditions associated with early onset scoliosis. The treatment of thoracic insufficiency syndrome is not discussed here because it is covered in Chapter 4.

21.2.1 Marfan Syndrome

Early onset scoliosis that progresses despite bracing is the typical spinal deformity in Marfan syndrome. Dural ectasia is common finding (up to 95% of cases), and preoperative MR imaging of the whole spine should be done before these children undergo surgery. Possible dural tears and the need for repair should be included in the preoperative planning. Pedicle fixation is the preferred method because the laminae are often thin in children with dural ectasia. The pedicles are also affected by dural ectasia and therefore are thinner. The anatomy should be studied on the preoperative MR images or CT scans so that the instrumentation plan can be plotted. Growing rods can be used successfully to delay fusion in children with Marfan syndrome. The rates of junctional kyphosis and implant failure may be high. Current evidence shows that although the curve patterns are similar to those of idiopathic curves, selective fusion results in a high rate of progression in the spared secondary curve. Therefore, when definitive fusion is considered, all curves should be instrumented and fused.

The sagittal plane also requires attention because thoracolumbar kyphosis is not uncommon. Poor bone quality is another consideration; however, pedicle fixation has proved to provide sufficient anchor strength. Intraoperative bleeding is typically greater than in idiopathic deformity, and this must be considered in the preoperative planning.

21.2.2 Ehlers–Danlos Syndrome

One specific type of this connective tissue disorder is especially associated with the severe and early onset of kyphoscoliosis (▶ Fig. 21.1). Because of the ligamentous laxity and low muscle tone, the deformity progresses early and quickly, and surgical treatment is often necessary.

One of the major intraoperative concerns is vascular friability. Anterior surgery should be avoided because of the high risk for injury to the major vessels. All correction can and should be achieved posteriorly. Dural ectasia is another common finding, and the surgeon should be prepared for potential dural tears. As in all collagen disorders, wound healing may be problematic, and the utmost care should be taken for a meticulous and minimally traumatic closure. Postoperatively, patients should be closely monitored for junctional issues because low muscle tone and hyperelasticity may predispose them to junctional deformity above and below the last instrumented level.

Loeys–Dietz syndrome and Beals syndrome are characterized by connective tissue abnormalities in association with early onset scoliosis. The spinal abnormalities and deformities are similar to those of Marfan syndrome. The rate of dural ectasia has been reported to be as high as 67% in patients with Loeys–Dietz syndrome. A surgical approach and precautions similar to those appropriate for Marfan syndrome are also valid for these conditions. The cervical spine requires attention in connective tissue disorders and should be evaluated for instability.

We recommend caution when halo traction is used in patients who have disorders associated with ligamentous laxity because there has been at least one report of the development of iatrogenic cervical kyphosis after halo traction in a patient with Marfan syndrome.

21.2.3 Rett Syndrome

Scoliosis develops in more than 50% of children with Rett syndrome, and most of the curves develop before the age of 8 years. This is a rapidly progressive, c-shaped, long thoracolumbar curve, and it does not respond to bracing. For curves that present early, growing rods or growth guidance systems, such as the Shilla or a trolley-type method, can be used. At later ages, the curves tend to be rigid with significant rib deformity. Pelvic obliquity is common, and in order to control the obliquity, fusion and instrumentation may need to be extended to the pelvis (▶ Fig. 21.2). Pulmonary problems are common after surgery; therefore, an intensive care unit bed should be readily available. These patients may similarly be managed as patients with cerebral palsy.

21.2.4 Osteogenesis Imperfecta

This abnormality of collagen type I presents multiple challenges because of poor bone quality as well as ligamentous laxity. Severe cases (Sillence type III) are more often associated with spinal deformity, which typically is a rigid kyphoscoliosis. Surprisingly, the contemporary literature is very scarce on the management of spinal deformity in osteogenesis imperfecta. However, in our experience, nonsurgical treatment has a very limited role, and early surgical intervention must be contemplated for patients with progressive deformities. The poor quality of bone, deformed vertebrae, and rigidity of the deformity

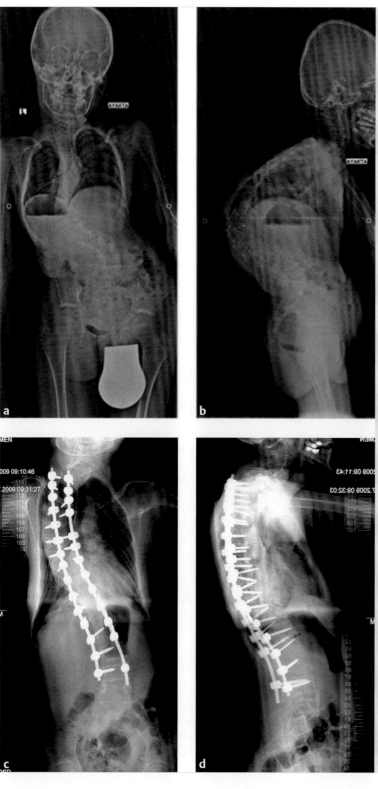

Fig. 21.1 Anteroposterior (**a**) and lateral (**b**) views of a 10-year-old female patient with a diagnosis of Ehlers–Danlos syndrome and severe kyphoscoliosis. Anteroposterior (**c**) and lateral (**d**) views of the patient at 2-year follow-up. Asymptomatic proximal junctional kyphosis was observed.

limit the options for fixation and correction in late-presenting, severe cases.

Cyclic intravenous bisphosphonate treatment has been shown to improve bone quality in children with osteogenesis imperfecta. Preoperative bisphosphonate treatment can be contemplated, months before the scheduled surgery, in order to improve bone quality. The challenge in the operating room starts with positioning.

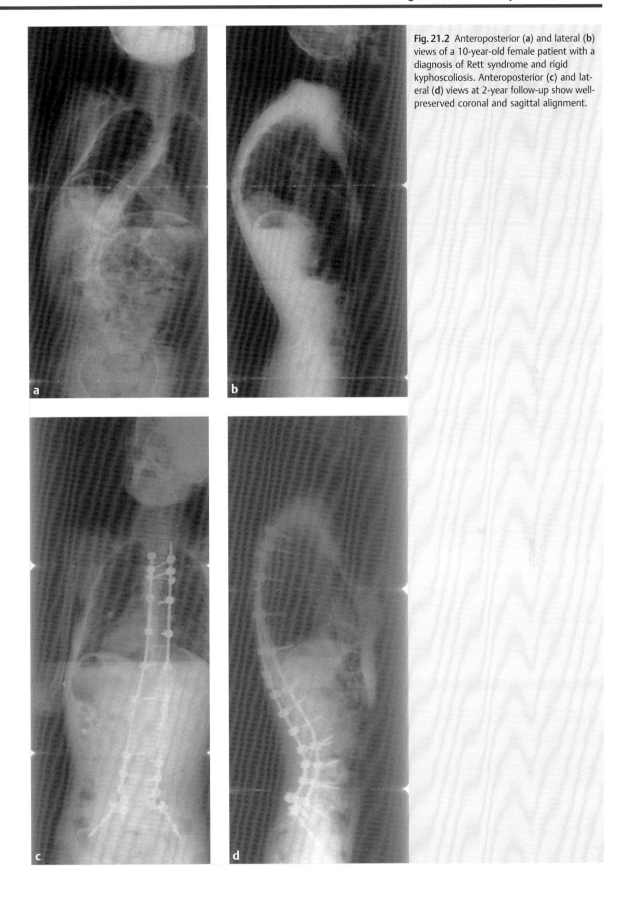

Fig. 21.2 Anteroposterior (**a**) and lateral (**b**) views of a 10-year-old female patient with a diagnosis of Rett syndrome and rigid kyphoscoliosis. Anteroposterior (**c**) and lateral (**d**) views at 2-year follow-up show well-preserved coronal and sagittal alignment.

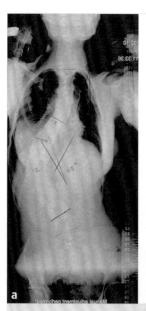
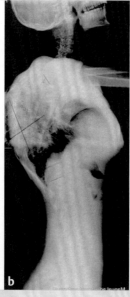
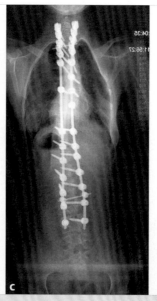
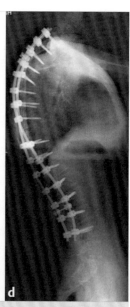

Fig. 21.3 Anteroposterior (**a**) and lateral (**b**) views of a 12-year-old female patient with a diagnosis of arthrogryposis multiplex congenita. The patient had progressive kyphoscoliosis that was unresponsive to brace treatment and underwent a posterior instrumentation and fusion. (**c**) Postoperative anteroposterior and (**d**)lateral radiographs.

All personnel must be very careful while handling the child with *osteogenesis imperfecta* in order to avoid iatrogenic fractures of the long bones and ribs. Variously sized pedicle screws, sublaminar wires, and hooks should be all readily available. Polymethylmethacrylate may be used to augment pedicle screw fixation. In severe disease, a hybrid fixation with wires and screws should be used. The goals of deformity correction should be kept modest because anchor pullout or iatrogenic fractures may ensue. The sagittal plane alignment should be carefully adjusted in an attempt to decrease junctional kyphosis. Stress fractures of the vertebrae may occur at the proximal or distal extent of the fusion and result in junctional kyphosis. There is even a report of a transverse pelvic wing stress fracture after instrumented posterior fusion in a child with osteogenesis imperfecta. There is evidence showing that systemic bisphosphonate treatment enhances screw fixation in long bones; therefore, continuing treatment in the postoperative period appears to be a reasonable choice.

21.2.5 Larsen Syndrome

Larsen syndrome is a genetic condition associated with hyperlaxity. The most commonly reported features of Larsen syndrome are multiple joint dislocations; facial features such as frontal bossing, midface hypoplasia, and ocular hypertelorism; cervical spine instability; tracheomalacia; and a hypermobile airway with related anesthetic concerns. Spinal deformity has been reported only scarcely. The cervical spine is the most commonly involved spinal region, and a high number of patients will have some abnormality of

the cervical spine (e.g., kyphosis, instability, basilar impression, spina bifida). Therefore, the cervical spine of any patient about to undergo surgery should be evaluated, and if necessary, cervical fusion should be accomplished before any other surgical procedure. The scoliosis is typically an early onset deformity, although generally not very severe. Initially, brace treatment may be used in patients with mild curves. There may be associated vertebral anomalies, and the chest wall may be compromised. In such patients, a thoracic expansion procedure, such as the vertical expandable prosthetic titanium rib (VEPTR), can be used. If the chest is not severely affected, a growing rod construct can be used to enhance growth in a patient who does not respond to brace treatment. When satisfactory spinal growth is achieved, a formal posterior fusion should be done. In our experience, the stable vertebra is the lower extent of the fusion in Larsen syndrome. If there is an associated hip dislocation, the spine deformity should be addressed before the hips.

21.2.6 Arthrogryposis

The spinal deformity in arthrogrypotic syndromes can present early or late (▶ Fig. 21.3). The early presenting curves are typically progressive and rigid with a neuromuscular pattern. If the thorax is compromised, a VEPTR-type device can be used to increase the volume on the concave side. Growing rods can also be an option to buy time before definitive fusion. Classic texts recommend anterior and posterior surgery for spinal fusion in arthrogryposis; however, these are from an era when the spinal instrumentation was not as advanced as it is now.

Unfortunately, there is not much evidence on modern posterior-only instrumented fusion in arthrogryposis; however, in our experience, anterior surgery may be obsolete except for very sharp and rigid curves.

Reports on arthrogryposis typically include multiple different diagnoses that present with joint contractures. Multiple pterygium syndrome is one of the arthrogrypotic conditions that is associated with early onset scoliosis. The rate of early developing scoliosis, with numerous congenital vertebral anomalies, is reported to be as high as 81% in multiple pterygium syndrome. These curves can be managed as in thoracic insufficiency syndrome and congenital scoliosis, depending on the curve type.

21.2.7 Neurofibromatosis

The early onset spinal deformity in neurofibromatosis is typically a dystrophic curve and may be associated with kyphosis. These curves tend to progress rapidly despite conservative measures, and early surgical intervention is necessary. For very young children, growing rods and VEPTR can be used as temporizing measures; however, most of these children require definitive fusion at a juvenile age.

Spinal deformity associated with dystrophic neurofibromatosis is one of the few exceptions in which anterior and posterior combined fusion is still the treatment of choice, for two reasons: (1) The rate of pseudarthrosis is high in neurofibromatosis as a result of tissue abnormalities; and (2) because of the young age of these children, the crankshaft phenomenon may ensue as a consequence of continued growth of the anterior vertebral bodies. For severe and rigid kyphoscoliotic deformities, a staged approach can be used in which anterior release is followed by 4 to 6 weeks of halo traction. Then, a posterior instrumented fusion is undertaken. For the correction of very sharp deformities, vertebral column resection is an option; however, given the spinal cord abnormalities in patients with neurofibromatosis, this technique requires a high level of skill and an experienced surgical team. We recommend that this technique be used only by surgeons who are familiar with spinal deformity in neurofibromatosis and very experienced with the technique.

Neurofibromatosis is associated with cervical spine abnormalities, especially kyphotic deformities. The cervical spine of these children should be evaluated, and any abnormality should be addressed before other procedures are contemplated. Dural ectasia is an inherent abnormality in neurofibromatosis and should be expected in all cases. Preoperative MR imaging and CT are necessary and valuable for the operative plan.

21.2.8 Skeletal Dysplasias

The skeletal dysplasias include an extensive number of abnormalities, and a detailed discussion of each condition is beyond the scope of this chapter. However, certain principles apply in the management of skeletal deformity in all these conditions.

In skeletal dysplasia, kyphosis is more common than scoliosis. The deformities are almost always early in onset and can be progressive. Because of the rarity of these conditions, there are multiple unknowns in the management of spinal deformities in patients with skeletal dysplasias. However, once the curves progress to a surgical limit, dual growing rod constructs can be used if the child is young enough. However, given the limited growth potential of the spine, definitive surgery need not be delayed until late. In patients with deformities that deplete the thoracic volume, VEPTR or another thoracic expansion construct can be used to improve the pulmonary capacity. Once the patient's pulmonary function has improved, definitive posterior instrumented fusion can be contemplated. Patients with severe deformities may require osteotomies, and these can all be done posteriorly. Anterior surgery is avoided in these patients in order not to compromise their already limited pulmonary function.

Because of the dysplastic nature of the vertebral elements, fixation may pose a problem. Multiple methods of fixation should be considered in the preoperative plan, and a CT scan should be included in the management of patients with complex deformities. Deficient laminae, fusion defects, pedicle abnormalities, and floating posterior elements (campomelic dysplasia) may be present and should be looked for with the preoperative imaging modalities. Additionally, junctional kyphosis secondary to associated bone dysplasia and hyperlaxity may be seen. Follow-up clinic visits should always include a lateral radiograph in addition to the posteroanterior view.

Spinal stenosis is another common issue and should be addressed with the appropriate amount of decompression during deformity surgery if deemed necessary. Careful evaluation of the preoperative symptomatology and function along with a meticulous neural examination is mostly helpful. In almost all of these children, preoperative MR images are acquired of the whole spine to look for spinal stenosis and intraspinal abnormalities.

Cervical spine abnormalities are common in some skeletal dysplasia syndromes. The cervical spine is recommended to be evaluated in all patients who have skeletal dysplasia with flexion and extension lateral radiographs. If there is associated cervical spine instability, stenosis, or severe kyphosis, this needs to be addressed before any other surgical procedure is undertaken.

21.3 Conclusion

The treatment of early onset scoliosis in the setting of syndromic conditions requires a multidisciplinary approach. Because of medical comorbidities and complications, spine surgery is associated with a higher complication rate in these patients than in those with idiopathic scoliosis. The anesthesiologist should evaluate the patient in advance, and both the surgeon and the anesthesiologist should be knowledgeable about the specific syndrome. Detailed preoperative imaging should be acquired. Multiple different fixation methods and various implants sizes should be readily available in the operating room. The role of halo–gravity traction should not be dismissed, and such traction should be considered in patients with severe deformities. The surgeon should be on the lookout for loss of fixation and junctional deformity during the follow-up. Despite the complexity of these conditions, good results can be achieved by setting realistic goals and executing a well-contemplated plan for surgical and post-surgical care.

Further Reading

Campbell RM Jr. Spine deformities in rare congenital syndromes: clinical issues. Spine 2009; 34: 1815–1827

Crawford AH, Herrera-Soto J. Scoliosis associated with neurofibromatosis. Orthop Clin North Am 2007; 38: 553–562, vii

Demetracopoulos CA, Sponseller PD. Spinal deformities in Marfan syndrome. Orthop Clin North Am 2007; 38: 563–572, vii

Gjolaj JP, Sponseller PD, Shah SA et al. Spinal deformity correction in Marfan syndrome versus adolescent idiopathic scoliosis: learning from the differences. Spine 2012; 37: 1558–1565

Harrison DJ, Webb PJ. Scoliosis in the Rett syndrome: natural history and treatment. Brain Dev 1990; 12: 154–156

Laville JM, Lakermance P, Limouzy F. Larsen's syndrome: review of the literature and analysis of thirty-eight cases. J Pediatr Orthop 1994; 14: 63–73

Lerman JA, Emans JB, Hall JE, Karlin LI. Spinal arthrodesis for scoliosis in Down syndrome. J Pediatr Orthop 2003; 23: 159–161

Sanders JO. Spinal deformity in skeletal dysplasias [published online ahead of print August 27, 2012]. Spine Deformity. In press

Sponseller P, Yang J. Syndromic spinal deformities in the growing child. In: Akbarnia B, Yazici M, Thompson G, eds. The Growing Spine. Berlin, Germany: Springer; 2010:187–196

Tolo VT. Spinal deformity in short-stature syndromes. Instr Course Lect 1990; 39: 399–405

Yingsakmongkol W, Kumar SJ. Scoliosis in arthrogryposis multiplex congenita: results after nonsurgical and surgical treatment. J Pediatr Orthop 2000; 20: 656–661

22 Nonoperative Treatment of Syndromic Scoliosis

Ian W. Nelson

Syndromic scoliosis occurs in a broad group of conditions of varying etiology:

- Neurofibromatosis
- Heritable disorders of connective tissue: osteogenesis imperfecta, Marfan syndrome, Ehlers–Danlos syndrome
- Mucopolysaccharidoses
- Skeletal dysplasias
- Metabolic bone disease: rickets
- Endocrine disorders
- Down syndrome

The options for the nonoperative treatment of spine deformity, from the treating surgeon's perspective, are more limited than the options that patients may find available to them during a brief Internet search:

- Serial casting: Cotrel (elongation, derotation, flexion); Risser
- Bracing
- Traction: halo–gravity, halo–femoral, halo–pelvic
- Exercise

Serial casting is often used to treat early onset scoliosis (developing before the age of 5 years), and general anesthesia is usually required every 3 or 4 months to refit the cast. Although an advantage of casting is that the cast cannot be removed by the patient or family, tolerance is an issue; however, many younger children function well with a cast on.

The efficacy of bracing is widely debated in the more common condition of adolescent or late onset idiopathic scoliosis, and it is therefore not surprising that there is a relative paucity of literature regarding the role of bracing in the treatment of syndromic scoliosis. Patients and their surgeons may, however, seek what are considered to be "less invasive" treatments for their condition in an attempt to avoid or delay surgery. Patient compliance is considered to be an important issue in brace effectiveness. In adolescent idiopathic scoliosis, the use of a brace during the premenarchal growth spurt (peak height velocity) may be of importance, whereas in syndromic scoliosis, patterns of curve progression are not so well defined, and the effects of the condition may extend beyond the usual peak growth periods. Many brace types exist, further complicating the interpretation of data.

Traction, in its various forms, is often used as a preoperative intervention in an attempt to improve the flexibility of a severe scoliosis and thereby the correction obtained.

Exercise therapy has been proposed in the treatment of idiopathic scoliosis, and research continues. At present, there is no evidence for its efficacy in syndromic scoliosis.

22.1 Casting

Mehta[1] reported the outcome of Cotrel (elongation, derotation, flexion) casting in 136 patients with early onset scoliosis. Treatment started before the age of 4 years, and follow-up was for 9 years. The majority of the cases had idiopathic-type curves, but a group of 36 patients had defined or undefined syndromes. Some of the patients in the group had neurologic disorders, but these did not specifically include neurofibromatosis or Marfan syndrome. The results suggest that some cases of syndromic scoliosis have the potential to respond to casting. The main factors affecting response to treatment were age and Cobb angle at presentation. Delays in referral and subsequent rapid Cobb angle progression were felt to militate against a good outcome. Some patients were subsequently managed in a brace.

22.2 Bracing

22.2.1 Neurofibromatosis

Winter et al[2] reviewed the natural history, associated anomalies, and response to nonoperative and operative treatment in 102 patients with scoliosis and neurofibromatosis. Of these, 80 patients had features of dystrophic scoliosis, with rib penciling, vertebral scalloping, and foraminal enlargement. Milwaukee braces were used to treat 10 patients in this group, and in none of them was curve progression arrested. The average curve at the start of brace treatment was 53 degrees, and at the end it was 80 degrees. The curves of the 22 patients without dystrophic features behaved quite differently, and in the four documented cases in the paper treated with a Milwaukee brace for scoliosis or kyphosis, progression to surgery did not occur. The authors concluded that brace treatment was not indicated for dystrophic curves but might be effective for nondystrophic scoliosis.

22.2.2 Marfan Syndrome

Sponseller et al[3] investigated the effectiveness of bracing in Marfan syndrome. The study group included 22 patients with curves of 45 degrees or less and a Risser grade of 2 or lower. Bracing was recommended for 18 hours or more per day, and follow-up continued until maturity or surgery (minimum, 2 years). The average age at the initiation of bracing was 8.7 years (range, 4–12). The initial correction of the curve in the brace was significant, at 45%. Progression was prevented in four patients, but in 20 of 24 patients, treatment was considered a failure. The mean progression was +6 degrees (mean rate of progression, +8

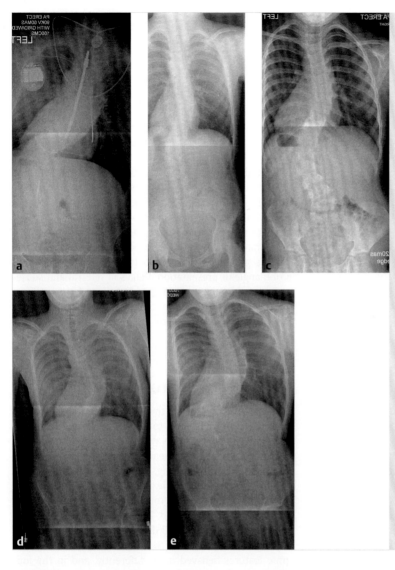

Fig. 22.1 A 45-year-old man with Marfan syndrome had undergone brace treatment for scoliosis, followed by surgery (**a**). He expected that his similarly affected daughters, ages 11 (**b**) and 8 years (**c**), would have brace treatment in the first instance. Not surprisingly, the curves of both progressed (**d, e**) and required surgical correction.

degrees per year), and the average final curve measurement was 49 degrees. Sixteen of the patients underwent or were advised to undergo surgical correction of their scoliosis. The difference between patient age and degree of curvature in the successful group and the unsuccessful group was not statistically significant.

The authors concluded that the majority patients who have Marfan syndrome with a curve of 25 degrees or more and a Risser grade of 2 or lower will continue to have curve progression despite brace treatment, and that consideration of surgical correction is required (▶ Fig. 22.1).

22.2.3 Down Syndrome

Milbrandt and Johnson[4] reported the incidence of scoliosis in 379 patients with Down syndrome to be 8.7% (33 patients). Of the 33 patients, eight (24%) underwent bracing for an average of 26 months. During this period, the average curve progression was 10 degrees (range, 0–44), and three of the eight patients subsequently went on to spinal fusion. A total of seven patients went on to surgical correction of the deformity. The authors concluded that bracing was ineffective for the majority of patients treated.

Bracing has also been recommended in the following:
- Arthrogryposis multiplex congenita in ambulators with curves smaller than 30 degrees[5];
- Spondyloepiphyseal dysplasia, early treatment with a Milwaukee brace[6];
- Successful treatment of kyphosis (not the short angular type) has been reported in osteogenesis imperfecta, Marfan syndrome, mucopolysaccharidosis type IV (Morquio syndrome), spondyloepiphyseal dysplasia tarda, and metatropic dwarfism.

Bracing has been reported *not* to be effective in scoliosis in the following:

- Trisomy 18[7];
- Osteogenesis imperfecta[8,9];
- Ehlers–Danlos syndrome[10];
- Familial dysautonomia or Riley–Day syndrome[11,12];
- Cerebellar gigantism or Sotos syndrome[13];
- Proteus syndrome[14];
- Beals syndrome[15];
- Smith–Magenis syndrome[16];
- Multiple epiphyseal dysplasia.[17]

22.3 Traction

Traction has been reported, primarily as a preoperative procedure for patients with severe scoliosis, in three main forms: halo–femoral, halo–pelvic, and halo–gravity. Most of the reported retrospective series contain a spectrum of diagnoses, including syndromic scoliosis. Of the three techniques, halo–pelvic traction, which was popularized in Hong Kong in the 1970s, was associated with cervical spine complications[18] and cranial nerve palsies, and its use is now rarely reported in the literature. In a series of 83 patients, four patients had neurofibromatosis with only 7% supine correction of the deformity and a 17% incidence of cervical complications.

Mehlman et al[19] reported the use of halo–tibial traction after release and before definitive surgery in 24 patients, four of whom had syndromic scoliosis (two with neurofibromatosis type 1, one with osteogenesis imperfecta, and one with Ehlers–Danlos syndrome). The Cobb angle corrections obtained in these four patients after release and traction and before definitive surgery were 55%, 42%, 53%, and 52%.

In a recent series[20] of 33 patients treated with preoperative halo–gravity traction, 11 of the patients had syndromic scoliosis. Overall, the traction produced coronal Cobb correction of 35% and sagittal Cobb correction of 35%. Improvement in pulmonary function (forced vital capacity [FVC] and forced expiratory volume in 1 second [FEV_1]) of approximately 20% was observed in 19 of 22 patients in whom measurements were made. The overall complication rate was 26%, and there were no long-term neurologic complications.

References

[1] Mehta MH. Growth as a corrective force in the early treatment of progressive infantile scoliosis. J Bone Joint Surg Br 2005; 87: 1237–1247

[2] Winter RB, Moe JH, Bradford DS, Lonstein JE, Pedras CV, Weber AH. Spine deformity in neurofibromatosis. A review of one hundred and two patients. J Bone Joint Surg Am 1979; 61: 677–694

[3] Sponseller PD, Bhimani M, Solacoff D, Dormans JP. Results of brace treatment of scoliosis in Marfan syndrome. Spine 2000; 25: 2350–2354

[4] Milbrandt TA, Johnston CE II. Down syndrome and scoliosis: a review of a 50-year experience at one institution. Spine 2005; 30: 2051–2055

[5] Yingsakmongkol W, Kumar SJ. Scoliosis in arthrogryposis multiplex congenita: results after nonsurgical and surgical treatment. J Pediatr Orthop 2000; 20: 656–661

[6] Bethem D, Winter RB, Lutter L et al. Spinal disorders of dwarfism. Review of the literature and report of eighty cases. J Bone Joint Surg Am 1981; 63: 1412–1425

[7] Ries MD, Ray S, Winter RB, Bowen JR. Scoliosis in trisomy 18. Spine 1990; 15: 1281–1284

[8] Hanscom DA, Winter RB, Lutter L, Lonstein JE, Bloom BA, Bradford DS. Osteogenesis imperfecta. Radiographic classification, natural history, and treatment of spinal deformities. J Bone Joint Surg Am 1992; 74: 598–616

[9] Yong-Hing K, MacEwen GD. Scoliosis associated with osteogenesis imperfecta. J Bone Joint Surg Br 1982; 64: 36–43

[10] McMaster MJ. Spinal deformity in Ehlers-Danlos syndrome. Five patients treated by spinal fusion. J Bone Joint Surg Br 1994; 76: 773–777

[11] Hayek S, Laplaza FJ, Axelrod FB, Burke SW. Spinal deformity in familial dysautonomia. Prevalence, and results of bracing. J Bone Joint Surg Am 2000; 82-A: 1558–1562

[12] Bar-On E, Floman Y, Sagiv S, Katz K, Pollak RD, Maayan C. Orthopaedic manifestations of familial dysautonomia. A review of one hundred and thirty-six patients. J Bone Joint Surg Am 2000; 82-A: 1563–1570

[13] Haga N, Nakamura S, Shimode M, Yanagisako Y, Iwaya T. Scoliosis in cerebral gigantism, Sotos syndrome. A case report. Spine 1996; 21: 1699–1702

[14] Yazar T, Cebesoy O, Basarir K, Karadeniz E. Recalcitrant scoliosis in Proteus syndrome. Acta Orthop Belg 2005; 71: 372–374

[15] Martin AG, Foguet PR, Marks DS, Thompson AG, Child AH. Infantile scoliosis in Beals syndrome: the use of a non-fusion technique for surgical correction. Eur Spine J 2006; 15: 433–439

[16] Tsirikos AI, Baker AD, McClean C. Surgical treatment of scoliosis in Smith-Magenis syndrome: a case report. J Med Case Reports 2010; 4: 26

[17] Herring JA. Rapidly progressive scoliosis in multiple epiphyseal dysplasia. A case report. J Bone Joint Surg Am 1976; 58: 703–704

[18] Dove J, Hsu LC, Yau AC. The cervical spine after halo-pelvic traction. An analysis of the complications of 83 patients. J Bone Joint Surg Br 1980; 62-B: 158–161

[19] Mehlman CT, Al-Sayyad MJ, Crawford AH. Effectiveness of spinal release and halo-femoral traction in the management of severe spinal deformity. J Pediatr Orthop 2004; 24: 667–673

[20] Boginovic L, Lenke LG, Bridwell KH, Luhlman SJ. Preoperative halogravity traction for severe paediatric deformity: complications, radiographic correction, and changes in pulmonary function. Spine Deformity 2013; 1: 33–39

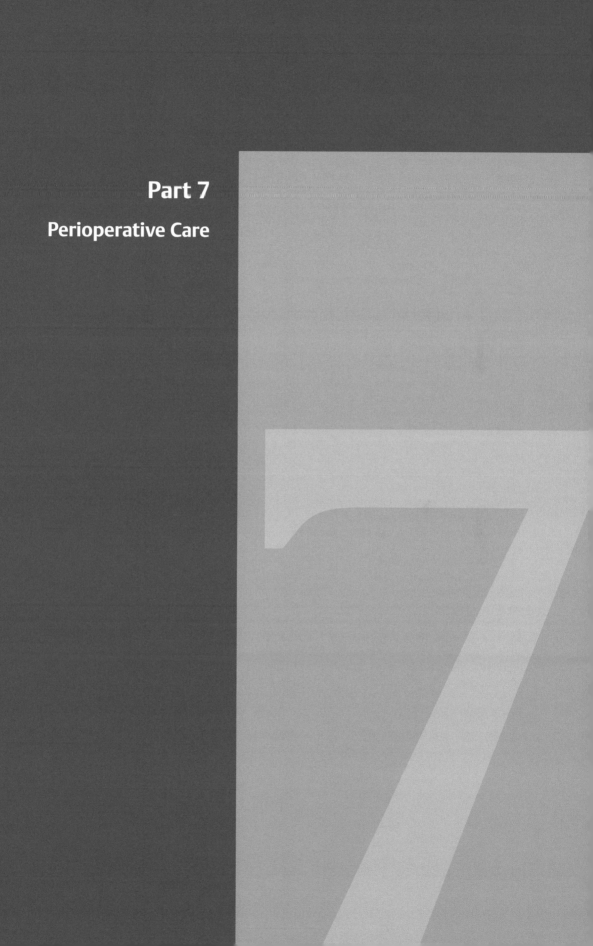

Part 7

Perioperative Care

23 Infection and Bleeding

Evan M. Davies and Andrew Baldock

23.1 Infection

Surgical site infection is a significant cause of postoperative morbidity in patients undergoing scoliosis surgery. Patients with early onset scoliosis and associated co-morbidities are particularly at risk. The effects can be debilitating and life-threatening. Deep surgical infection often requires repeated surgical procedures, delays discharge, and can lead to a poor surgical outcome. Patients with early onset scoliosis and associated medical comorbidities are also at an increased risk for respiratory and line-related sepsis.

As well as the traditional techniques of surgical aseptic techniques, the assessment and prevention of sepsis require a thorough assessment of individual patient risk.

23.1.1 Preoperative Risk Factors for Infection

Comorbidity

Medical comorbidities are associated with an increased risk for superficial and deep infection. As well as the individual comorbidities associated with the specific illness, limited mobility, inability to sit, recurrent respiratory infections, copious secretions, and urinary and bowel incontinence all adversely affect infection rates. Patients with poor social care and community support are also at increased risk for infection. These risk factors are more prevalent in patients with syndromic and neuromuscular scoliosis, who remain at higher risk for infection than those with idiopathic scoliosis, even after preoperative optimization.

Coagulase-negative *Staphylococcus* is the most common colonizing organism overall in pediatric patients undergoing deformity surgery. However, in patients with neuromuscular disease, *Pseudomonas*, *Escherichia coli*, and *Enterococcus* are more prevalent. *Propionibacterium acnes*, a gram-positive rod associated with acne, is increasingly recognized as another infecting organism. *P. acnes* grows slowly, and extended culture (≥ 6 days) is often required.

Poor Nutrition

Patients who are undernourished have a decreased immune capability and are predisposed to infection. A patient's height and weight should be plotted on a growth chart preoperatively. For patients whose weight is in a low centile, pre- and postoperative nutritional support should be considered. Patients with a high body mass index and significant adipose tissue also have an increased risk of infection.

Multiple Surgical Procedures

Multiple surgical procedures, such as are required in patients with growing rods, expose patients to an increase risk for surgical site infection because of sequential exposures, wound healing, and scarring. Techniques that minimize the number of surgical procedures should be associated with a reduced infection rate. Prominent implants, poor soft tissue repair, and inadequate coverage all predispose to infection.

23.1.2 Intraoperative Measures to Prevent Infection

Antibiotics

Perioperative antibiotics reduce the risk for infection. Antibiotics are routinely administered at the induction of anesthesia and continued for 24 hours. In patients with syndromic and early onset scoliosis, microbiological prophylaxis may need to be modified to cover the different organisms encountered. The use of topical antibiotics in the surgical field is becoming more widespread in spine surgery, but currently the evidence of its effectiveness is not clear.

Skin Preparation

Surgical skin preparation and bio-occlusive drapes impregnated with iodine appear to reduce skin site infection. The effectiveness of the use of topical glues to reduce bacterial load at the skin edges remains unproven.

Laminar Flow

Operating theaters with laminar flow and a high rate of air exchange have lower bacterial counts than do conventional theaters. Reducing operating room traffic, staff numbers, and turnover reduces bacterial counts in the airflow.

23.1.3 Postoperative Risk Factors for Infection

Patients who are poorly mobile or are wheelchair ambulators are more likely to have difficulties with wound healing because of additional surgical site trauma and pressure. Patients with impaired postoperative nutrition and ileus at a time of increased metabolic demand are more likely to have infectious complications. Surgical lines, epidural catheters, urinary catheters, and drains can all be sources of infection leading to bacteremia in the postoperative stage. Prompt removal of these devices reduces risk.

Bleeding and Hematoma Formation

Significant bleeding and hematoma formation make the soft tissues susceptible to secondary bacterial infection. Whether suction drainage reduces infection rates by reducing hematoma formation or increases infection rates by acting as a contaminating source of infection of deep spinal metalwork by superficial skin flora is controversial.

23.1.4 Treatment of Infection

Recognition

Larger curves (both preoperatively and postoperatively), greater blood loss, longer procedures, allogeneic transfusions, skin breakdown, and poor healing are all associated with higher infection rates. The differentiation between a superficial and a deep wound infection is important in all aspects of management. Should deep contamination be suspected, then urgent intervention is required. Inflammatory markers are raised in the postoperative period, but persistently raised markers or increasing levels of markers are indicative of infection. Spinal imaging studies, such as ultrasound, may show collections of fluid in the surgical field. Magnetic resonance (MR) imaging and computed tomography (CT) are both affected by implants but again may show collections and abscess formation. CT scans will often identify implant loosening, which can be challenging for MR imaging.

Surgical Débridement with or without Implant Removal

Deep infections in patients with medical comorbidities are unlikely to respond to conservative treatment with antibiotics. Aggressive surgical débridement, wound lavage, and prolonged intravenous antibiotics may salvage the situation or allow control until fusion has occurred and implants can be removed. It is important to culture any organisms present in the surgical field, so antibiotic therapy should be avoided until débridement has been performed.

During surgical débridement, multiple specimens should be taken, with clean instruments used for each specimen to avoid cross-contamination. Samples should be taken first from deep tissues and last from superficial tissues. The location of each specimen should be individually described because organisms can differ between areas.

Previous literature has suggested that 50% of implants in patients with deep infection will require removal. In our own institution, aggressive early surgical débridement and prolonged intravenous therapy has led to implant retention in 90% of cases.

Infection presenting late can be the result of either chronic infection since implant placement or secondary seeding from systemic bacteremia. If stable arthrodesis has occurred in this situation, then implant removal does not necessarily lead to a loss of clinical correction (▶ Fig. 23.1).

23.2 Blood Conservation

Allogeneic blood products are seldom needed for children undergoing the surgical correction of scoliosis if a well-developed blood conservation strategy is in place. However, the use of such products remains commonplace. This is expensive for the hospital and exposes the patient to risks that include the following: metabolic disturbance, infection, hypothermia, incompatibility reactions, transfusion-related lung injury, and immunomodulation. Some patients will not accept blood products for religious or cultural reasons. It is better to avoid blood transfusion whenever it is possible and clinically appropriate to do so. The implementation of optimal blood management starts at the preoperative assessment, continues through surgery into the postoperative period, and involves all members of the multidisciplinary team.

23.2.1 Preoperative Period

Anemia should be identified during the preoperative assessment and treated with oral iron and folate supplementation when appropriate. Recombinant erythropoietin has been used successfully to increase the hematocrit preoperatively but is not used in our institution. Any personal or family history of a bleeding disorder should be identified. These patients require clotting studies and review by a hematologist.

Preoperative autologous donation and acute normovolemic hemodilution are not currently recommended in the United Kingdom. Neither technique has been shown to reduce perioperative exposure to allogeneic blood.

23.2.2 Intraoperative Period

Surgical Technique

Poor surgical technique without soft tissue preservation and careful hemostasis will counteract and render ineffective all other measures aimed at blood conservation. The use of diathermy and a subperiosteal dissection reduces bleeding from muscle layers. Significant bleeding can occur from epidural veins if the spinal canal is opened. Careful exposure, bipolar diathermy, and topical agents may reduce the risk for bleeding. The cannulation of pedicles and osteotomies expose cancellous bone and in young children can cause excessive bleeding, which can be mitigated with the use of topical agents and bone wax. Following surgical procedures, attention to ensure

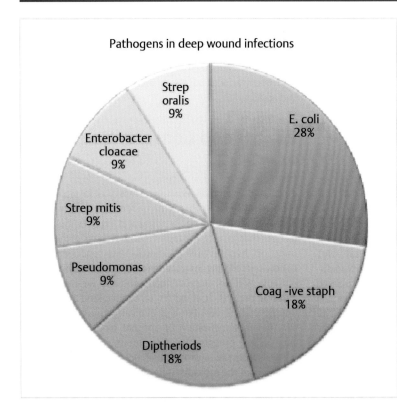

Pathogens in deep wound infections

Fig. 23.1 Pie chart showing pathogen identification in scoliosis infections at University Hospital Southampton, Hampshire, United Kingdom, 2003–2009.

that no surfaces are left bleeding and to prevent hematoma formation is mandatory. The use of ultrasound devices and pressure devices to reduce bleeding in scoliosis has yet to be validated.

Topical Agents

Topical collagens and gelatins can be applied to the surgical field. It is important not to pack these products inside the spinal canal because they may expand and compress the cord. Topical agents that promote hemostasis have become more widely available. Topical thrombin derived from either a bovine or human plasma source can provide local hemostasis. Topical fibrin sealants applied directly or via an aerosol can cover large bleeding surfaces. However, overuse of these products can affect the coagulation cascade directly. Should significant use be necessary, then the bleeding and coagulation cascades should be measured. Direct instillation of these products into vascular channels under pressure can cause lung injury and coagulopathy.

Anesthetic Technique

Controlled hypotension (systolic blood pressure 20–30% lower than the preoperative value, or mean blood pressure of 50–60 mm Hg) has been shown to reduce blood loss in spinal surgery. In our institution, totally intravenous anesthesia with infusions of remifentanil (0.1–0.5 mcg/kg/h) and propofol (3–6 µg/mL) is used to achieve

controlled hypotension. This sympatholytic combination maintains both hemodynamic stability and depth of anesthesia. The agents are also compatible with intraoperative neurophysiologic monitoring, which is mandatory because the combination of hypotension and surgical manipulation is a threat to cord perfusion. Invasive blood pressure monitoring is required.

Patients are carefully positioned to avoid inferior vena cava compression and impaired venous return. Hypothermia impairs coagulation and can be avoided with the use of a warming blanket, a fluid-warming device, and an esophageal temperature probe. Large volumes of crystalloids and colloids cause dilutional coagulopathy and anemia, and they should be avoided.

Antifibrinolytics

Antifibrinolytics have been shown to reduce blood loss significantly in scoliosis surgery. Since aprotinin was withdrawn in 2007, tranexamic acid has been the drug of choice, although the dosing for both loading and ongoing infusion varies enormously (2–100 mg/kg and 0–10 mg/kg/h, respectively). There is little prospective evidence to guide practice. We use 30 mg/kg at induction and do not routinely follow with an infusion.

Cell Salvage

Cell salvage has been shown to decrease the use of allogeneic blood in major surgery. Intraoperatively, blood is

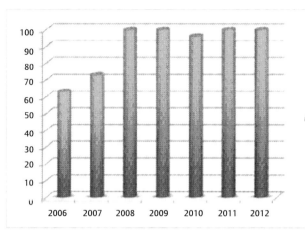

Fig. 23.2 Graph showing the percentage of patients undergoing surgical correction of idiopathic scoliosis at University Hospital Southampton, Hampshire, United Kingdom, without requiring the transfusion of allogeneic blood products. After the implementation of a blood conservation strategy in late 2006, no patients required transfusion in 2008, 2009, 2011, and 2012.

collected directly from the surgical site and by rinsing swabs. It is then anticoagulated, filtered, and centrifuged to separate the noncellular matter from the red blood cells, which are suspended in saline and can be returned to the patient. More than 50% of lost bloods can be salvaged in this way, making it is a crucial part of blood conservation.

23.2.3 Postoperative Period

At the end of surgery, a reinfusion drain is placed, and filtered blood is collected and reinfused at 6 hours. Thromboprophylaxis is achieved with compression stockings (and intraoperative pneumatic boots for older patients). Anticoagulants are avoided. It is also important to avoid large volumes of synthetic fluids in the postoperative period. We use epidurals for pain control, and to reverse hypotension associated with vasodilation, we encourage the use of a peripheral vasopressor, such as phenylephrine (1–5 µg/kg/min), in preference to repeated fluid boluses. Mild to moderate anemia can be treated with iron supplements.

23.2.4 How Important Is Anemia?

This is a contentious question. There is evidence from critically ill patients, both adults and children, that a restrictive strategy of red cell transfusion (hemoglobin < 7 g/dL) is at least as effective as and possibly superior to a liberal transfusion strategy. This practice has been widely adopted. The specific fear in scoliosis surgery is that anemia may contribute to cord injury in some circumstances; however, it has not been identified as an independent risk factor. A lower hematocrit results in lower resistance to flow, but this advantage is offset by a decreased oxygen-carrying capacity. We have agreed on a postoperative transfusion trigger of 6.5 g/dL if the patient is asymptomatic. Whatever the trigger, agreement among the surgical, anesthesiology, and intensive care teams is vital to ensure consistency.

23.2.5 Conclusion

Freedom from the need for the transfusion of allogeneic blood products can be routinely achieved with simple and safe techniques. This is cost-saving and reduces risk to patients (▶ Fig. 23.2).

Further Reading

Bird S, McGill N. Blood conservation and pain control in scoliosis corrective surgery: an online survey of UK practice. Paediatr Anaesth 2011; 21: 50–53

Carless PA, Henry DA, Moxey AJ et al. Cell salvage for minimising perioperative allogeneic blood transfusion. Cochrane Database Syst Rev 2010; 17 (4): CD001888

Grant JA, Howard J, Luntley J, Harder J, Aleissa S, Parsons D. Perioperative blood transfusion requirements in pediatric scoliosis surgery: the efficacy of tranexamic acid. J Pediatr Orthop 2009; 29: 300–304

Hassan N, Halanski M, Wincek J et al. Blood management in pediatric spinal deformity surgery: review of a 2-year experience. Transfusion 2011; 51: 2133–2141

Ho C, Skaggs DL, Weiss JM, Tolo VT. Management of infection after instrumented posterior spine fusion in pediatric scoliosis. Spine 2007; 32: 2739–2744

Joint United Kingdom Blood Transfusion and Tissue Transplantation Services Professional Advisory Committee. Better blood transfusion. www.tranfusionguidelines.org.uk/uk-transfusion-committees/national-blood-transfusion-committee/better-blood-transfusion. Accessed July 14, 2014

Lacroix J, Hébert PC, Hutchison JS et al. TRIPICU Investigators. Canadian Critical Care Trials Group. Pediatric Acute Lung Injury and Sepsis Investigators Network. Transfusion strategies for patients in pediatric intensive care units. N Engl J Med 2007; 356: 1609–1619

Mohamed Ali MH, Koutharawu DN, Miller F et al. Operative and clinical markers of deep wound infection after spine fusion in children with cerebral palsy. J Pediatr Orthop 2010; 30: 851–857

Murphy NA, Firth S, Jorgensen T, Young PC. Spinal surgery in children with idiopathic and neuromuscular scoliosis. What's the difference? J Pediatr Orthop 2006; 26: 216–220

Smith JS, Shaffrey CI, Sansur CA et al. Scoliosis Research Society Morbidity and Mortality Committee. Rates of infection after spine surgery based on 108,419 procedures: a report from the Scoliosis Research Society Morbidity and Mortality Committee. Spine 2011; 36: 556–563

Sponseller PD, LaPorte DM, Hungerford MW, Eck K, Bridwell KH, Lenke LG. Deep wound infections after neuromuscular scoliosis surgery: a multicenter study of risk factors and treatment outcomes. Spine 2000; 25: 2461–2466

24 Perioperative Session: Neurologic Complications

Jorge Mineiro

The concept of early onset scoliosis was introduced by Robert Dickson[1] to define scoliosis starting before the age of 5 years, regardless of the etiology. Over the last two decades, the management of these conditions has changed drastically. Physicians became rather disappointed with the outcomes of treatment with the very conservative approach of serial plaster casts, and they have now adopted a more aggressive attitude, using surgery to reduce the progression of severe deformities. Modern developments in surgical techniques and appliances have brought new hope that rapidly progressive scoliotic curves in these very unfortunate children can be controlled. However, with the introduction of a more sophisticated surgical armamentarium and the treatment of higher-risk patients with scoliosis of different pathogenetic mechanisms, the frequency of perioperative complications has increased.

The complexity and diversity of perioperative complications result from the different conditions diagnosed in association with early onset scoliosis—congenitally abnormal vertebrae, neuromuscular conditions, syndromic spinal deformities, connective tissue disorders, and idiopathic spinal deformities—each carrying its own potential problems. Not only are associated medical problems the cause of complications; in addition, pulmonary function and lung development can be compromised when spine and chest deformities start very early in life.

Procedures that allow the spine and the chest to develop and grow have become popular for the treatment of early onset scoliosis. However, the high rates of complications reported may result from both the need for repeated operations and issues related to the critical health conditions of these children.[2,3]

24.1 The Context

The report of the Scoliosis Research Society on complications in the surgical treatment of pediatric scoliosis (patients younger than 18 years) included the following etiologic groups: idiopathic, congenital, neuromuscular, and others.[4] With an overall rate of 10.2%, the complications did differ significantly among the three main groups.

Regarding neurologic complications, an overall rate of 0.72% was reported in the Scoliosis Research Society series,[4] but the rates of neurologic deficit differed among the three groups; the highest rate was reported in the treatment of congenital scoliosis (2%), followed by neuromuscular (1.1%) and idiopathic (0.8%) scoliosis. An association between the type of instrumentation used and type of procedure performed and the occurrence of new neurologic deficit was also established, with revision surgery having the highest risk.

However, these are overall figures for neurologic complications in the population of patients younger than 18 years of age, and they do not address specifically the group of patients with early onset scoliosis. In order to focus on this particular problem, we must review the principles of treatment and the types of procedures used, assuming that they do include scoliosis with a variety of etiologies.

24.2 The Principles

Because the development of rapidly progressive spinal deformities early in life leads to significant pulmonary compromise in adulthood, more recent treatment options have addressed not only spinal deformity but also chest development to improve the patient's quality of life. A new nomenclature (growth-sparing surgery, also known as fusionless surgical technique) has been created to include a group of different procedures with the same therapeutic objectives of preserving growth of the spine, thorax, and lungs while controlling the deformity. The surgical options are complex, and complications are understandably common if we consider that children with early onset scoliosis are high-risk patients because of their numerous associated comorbidities.

If we focus on the mechanism of treatment of severe spinal deformities in these very young patients, growth-sparing surgical procedures can be divided in three main groups: distraction-based, guided-growth, and tension-based procedures. The first group, distraction-based, includes growing rods and vertical expandable prosthetic titanium rib (VEPTR) techniques; the second group, guided-growth, includes procedures like the Shilla and the Luque trolley; and the third group, tension-based, includes spinal stapling and spinal tether (still experimental). The theoretical benefit of a guided-growth procedure is that it may not require the patient to undergo serial lengthening procedures (but occasionally rod exchange) and therefore may be definitive, although the original operation is more demanding and aggressive.

Because these procedures have been developed to help the young deformed spine to grow, they are not definitive operations per se; rather, they are done in stages: original insertion of the rods or implant, then several interval procedures for rod lengthening and implant exchange (often repeated several times) until the definitive procedure during adolescence.

When we talk about neurologic deficit, we must realize that the type of injury that can arise after one of these procedures is not always the same. On the one hand, types of deficit differ; they may be a cord lesion (total or partial), brachial plexopathy, or radiculopathy; on the other hand, however, it is important to mention that the mechanisms of neurologic injury can also differ; the injury can result from direct trauma, ischemia, or compression of any of the neural structures.

In order to assess the rate of neurologic complications associated with these procedures, we will look into the occurrence of new neurologic deficit in the first two groups of procedures.

24.3 Types of Treatment

24.3.1 Distraction-Based Devices: Growing Rods and the Vertical Expandable Prosthetic Titanium Rib

Sankar et al in 2009[5] reviewed the multicenter data from 252 patients undergoing 782 growing rod procedures, 73% of which were performed with neuromonitoring of the patient. In this series, only one clinical injury was detected on neuromonitoring at implant exchange and attempted screw insertion (1 of 782, 0.1%), and the patient recovered completely by 3 months postoperatively. However, four other neuromonitoring changes were identified, two at implant insertion (2 of 213, 0.9%), one at implant exchange (1 of 116, 0.9%), and one at rod lengthening (1 of 222, 0.5%).

Bess et al[6] also used the Growing Spine Study Group database and in 2010 published an analysis of 140 patients who underwent a total of 897 growing rod procedures. The neurologic complication rate in this series was 2% (three patients); two patients had a postoperative gait change due to leg weakness, and one had changes noted during intraoperative neurologic monitoring. The last complication occurred at the time of growing rod revision; of the other two reported, one occurred at growing rod insertion and one at rod lengthening; neurologic complications were more common in the group of patients in whom dual rods were implanted. Postoperatively, all three patients recovered completely.

Akbarnia and Emans[7] reviewed the literature to describe the complications of fusionless techniques used for the treatment early onset scoliosis. They included not only patients treated with growing rods but also those treated with the VEPTR and concluded that neuromonitoring is indicated for rod insertion and exchange but is controversial for rod lengthening. They also advised that rod lengthening, either at the initial procedure or at subsequent staged procedures, should be done with caution and that excessive distraction should be avoided to reduce the risk for neurologic complications.

The same authors[7] also addressed another type of neurologic deficit, known as brachial plexopathy.[8,9] The brachial plexus is neural structure that is at risk when the VEPTR is used in patients who have congenital deformities associated with major anomalies of the chest wall and shoulder. Brachial plexopathy can be caused by direct trauma or by compression of the plexus from an implant placed too cephalad or laterally in the uppermost chest wall during the initial distraction or an expansion procedure. Brachial plexus palsy may be delayed until compression gradually increases and postoperative swelling ensues. Awareness of the problem and motor and sensory monitoring of the upper limb during the initial, revision, or exchange procedures is recommended to avoid this complication. However, when this implant is used purely as a distraction device without expansion thoracostomy, such injury is less likely to occur because the anchor point on the rib is placed very medially.[10]

Although the single growing rod fell out of use because of an increased complication rate, Miladi et al in 2013[11] reported on 23 patients with progressive early onset scoliosis who failed conservative treatment and underwent fusionless surgery with a single growing rod construct. These patients had 65 staged procedures; two of them were definitive fusions, and three others were in patients who had reached skeletal maturity. There was an overall complication rate of 22% (5 of 23), but no neurologic complication rate has been reported.

24.3.2 Guided-Growth Devices: Shilla Procedure and Luque Trolley

At the 2012 Scoliosis Research Society meeting, McCarthy[12] reported a 5-year follow-up of 40 patients who underwent a Shilla procedure for the treatment of early onset scoliosis. Each patient underwent a mean of 2.7 procedures; six had reached skeletal maturity and underwent the definitive fusion. Although 27 of the 40 patients (67%) experienced complications, most of them were implant-related, and no neurologic changes occurred.

Regarding the Luque trolley, either as a standalone or together with a convex epiphysiodesis, the original results from the Nottingham group[13,14] have not been replicated. Of the 25 patients in the original series of Pratt et al, 10 (40%) experienced complications of different types, but no neurologic complications were reported.

More recently, a new generation of growing rod devices has been developed, including the Phenix rod and the MAGEC (magnetic expansion control) Remote Control Spinal Deformity System (Ellipse Technologies, Irvine, California).[15] These magnetic growing rods are also distraction-based systems that allow spinal growth by remote control. Thus, many of the known complications resulting from repeated surgical procedures for implant exchange, revision, and lengthening are avoided. Although some of these devices are already in clinical trials, long-term results are needed to assess the efficacy and safety of the technology.

24.3.3 Tension-Based Devices

Most of the devices based on this mechanism are experimental, and there is no clinical experience available to validate their efficacy and safety. The one in this group for which the most clinical experience has been acquired is the shape memory alloy, but it is used in older children, not for early onset scoliosis.[16]

24.4 Conclusion

Neurologic complications in the surgical treatment of early onset scoliosis are not frequent. However, if we take into account the various causes and levels of severity of these rapidly progressive curves, we cannot be unaware that we are treating very high-risk patients, and that they are therefore prone to the development of different types of complications, including neurologic complications.

Upon review of the present literature on growth-sparing surgery, we may conclude that the use of neuromonitoring is indicated for rod insertion and exchange but is controversial for rod lengthening.

References

[1] Dickson, RA. Early Onset Idiopathic Scoliosis. New York: Raven; 1994

[2] Akbarnia BA, Emans JB. Complications of growth-sparing surgery in early onset scoliosis. Spine 2010; 35: 2193–2204

[3] Accadbled F, Odent T, Moine A et al. Complications of scoliosis surgery in Prader-Willi syndrome. Spine 2008; 33: 394–401

[4] Reames DL, Smith JS, Fu KM et al. Scoliosis Research Society Morbidity and Mortality Committee. Complications in the surgical treatment of 19,360 cases of pediatric scoliosis: a review of the Scoliosis Research Society Morbidity and Mortality database. Spine 2011; 36: 1484–1491

[5] Sankar WN, Skaggs DL, Emans JB et al. Neurologic risk in growing rod spine surgery in early onset scoliosis: is neuromonitoring necessary for all cases? Spine 2009; 34: 1952–1955

[6] Bess S, Akbarnia BA, Thompson GH et al. Complications of growing-rod treatment for early-onset scoliosis: analysis of one hundred and forty patients. J Bone Joint Surg Am 2010; 92: 2533–2543

[7] Akbarnia BA, Emans JB. Complications of growth-sparing surgery in early onset scoliosis. Spine 2010; 35: 2193–2204

[8] Nassr A, Larson AN, Crane B, Hammerberg KW, Sturm PF, Mardjetko SM. Iatrogenic thoracic outlet syndrome secondary to vertical expandable prosthetic titanium rib expansion thoracoplasty: pathogenesis and strategies for prevention/treatment. J Pediatr Orthop 2009; 29: 31–34

[9] Skaggs DL, Choi PD, Rice C et al. Efficacy of intraoperative neurologic monitoring in surgery involving a vertical expandable prosthetic titanium rib for early-onset spinal deformity. J Bone Joint Surg Am 2009; 91: 1657–1663

[10] Smith JT. The use of growth-sparing instrumentation in pediatric spinal deformity. Orthop Clin North Am 2007; 38: 547–552, vii

[11] Miladi L, Journe A, Mousny M. H3S2 (3 hooks, 2 screws) construct: a simple growing rod technique for early onset scoliosis. Eur Spine J 2013; 22 Suppl 2: S96–S105

[12] McCarthy RE. Five-year follow-up of 40 patients with original Shilla procedure. Presented at: Scoliosis Research Society 47th Annual Meeting and Course; September 5–8, 2012; Chicago, IL

[13] Pratt RK, Webb JK, Burwell RG, Cummings SL. Luque trolley and convex epiphysiodesis in the management of infantile and juvenile idiopathic scoliosis. Spine 1999; 24: 1538–1547

[14] Sengupta D, Freeman B, Grevitt M, Mehdian S, Webb J. Long-term follow-up of Luque trolley growing-rod construct in the surgical treatment of early onset idiopathic scoliosis. Presented at: Scoliosis Research Society 37th Annual Meeting; September 18–21, 2002; Seattle, WA

[15] Tis JE, Karlin LI, Akbarnia BA et al. Growing Spine Committee of the Scoliosis Research Society. Early onset scoliosis: modern treatment and results. J Pediatr Orthop 2012; 32: 647–657

[16] Betz RR, Kim J, D'Andrea LP, Mulcahey MJ, Balsara RK, Clements DH. An innovative technique of vertebral body stapling for the treatment of patients with adolescent idiopathic scoliosis: a feasibility, safety, and utility study. Spine 2003; 28: S255–S265

25 Physiotherapy

Laura Streeton

During the first decade of life, many milestones are reached, many skills are learned and developed, and the environment in which a child lives becomes ever-expanding. Early onset scoliosis can pose a great challenge to development, but with the advances made in treatment options over the last two decades, goals are becoming more achievable.[1]

Developmental milestones are reached through everyday activity, and play has a vital role in enabling children to reach them. In the first few months and years of life, many milestones are related to mobility. If children struggle to turn onto their hands and knees, they will not be able to crawl, and if they also have no sitting balance, they will not bottom shuffle. Both problems hinder independent play because the children are unable to move, and thus, they become reliant on others to give them access to the toys they wish to enjoy.

25.1 Aims of the Chapter

- To outline the role of physiotherapy for children with early onset scoliosis, the importance of family involvement, and the use of play for assessment and treatment;
- To review the physiotherapy program that immediately follows surgical intervention;
- To consider ongoing development through play and activity.

With the vast changes in the surgical options available for treating children with early onset scoliosis that have been made over the last 10 to 20 years have come changes regarding the aims of therapy and the approach to therapy. The framework provided by the International Classification of Functioning Disability and Health (ICF)[2] highlights the importance of activity and participation in a person's life. It describes mobility as "changing location or transferring from one place to another." It is therefore inevitable that the more effective and close to optimal a child's mobility can be, the easier will be the child's execution of activities and the greater will be his or her ability to participate. The ICF has underscored the need for therapists to provide a holistic approach to treatment, focusing not only on exercises, stretches, and what a child is unable to do, but also on the child's abilities. The approach to therapy is functional and questions whether a child can actively participate with his or her current level of function. If not, an assessment must be made of what can be done to achieve participation. Many factors are involved, including the pathology of the child's condition, family input and expectations, the child's environment, the equipment needs, and the ability to access services. This assessment is necessary to establish what is required for each individual.

25.2 Physiotherapy Assessment

A physiotherapy assessment is required for children with early onset scoliosis to enable them to function to their fullest potential within society. Assessments provide a baseline for future interventions and establish goals that are appropriate and achievable for the child and the family within their environment.

An initial assessment may consist of observation of the child at play. This is most appropriately undertaken within the home environment, where the child will be most at ease and will play with his or her own toys. However, this may not always be possible. Play provides many benefits for both child and therapist:
- Creates a happy and fun environment;
- Is achievable;
- Can be done by children with varying levels of mobility;
- Allows an assessment of functional muscle strength, range of movement, and compensatory movements;
- Is active;
- Is interactive;
- Enables development appropriate for the child's age and preexisting abilities;
- Enables the child to participate with peers;
- Is enjoyable.

Play is the most likely way in which rapport will be established between the child and the therapist, but it also provides the opportunity to observe a variety of factors:
- In what position does the child play?
  - Lying on the floor or a bed
    - Supine
    - On the side
    - Prone
  - Sitting on the floor or at a table
    - Propped
    - Unsupported
    - With compensatory fixed postures
  - Standing
    - Freestanding
    - Holding onto an object (e.g., furniture) for support with one hand or two
    - With asymmetries
- Does the child move from one position to another?
  - Does the child remain fairly static throughout play, ignoring toys out of reach?
  - Does the child move to nearby toys, but not those at a greater distance?
  - Does the child move to toys well out of reach?
    - By reaching from within his or her base of support?
    - By moving out of the base of support?

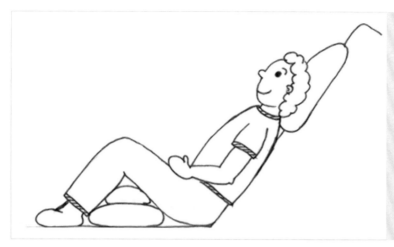

Fig. 25.1 Child sitting up in bed with knees bent and back straight.

- ○ Can the child move from one position to another, or is he or she placed in a position that compromises freedom of movement?
- How does the child move?
  - ○ Does the child remain in a sitting position, crawl from one toy to another, or stand up and walk to toys placed at a greater distance?
- When does the child move?
  - ○ Does the child move regularly throughout the play session or a limited number of times?
  - ○ Does the child move with ease or great effort?
  - ○ With compensatory patterns?
- What motivates the child in his or her play?
  - ○ Finding a task that motivates the child will make the introduction of new concepts easier and increase the child's compliance.
- What kind of toys does the child choose?
  - ○ Static toys, moving toys, noisy toys, functional toys?

The role of the physiotherapist is multifaceted as he or she considers ways to improve the quality of life of each child and family. Law et al studied therapy programs for children with cerebral palsy; however, their concepts of "family-centered functional therapy" are relevant to children with musculoskeletal disorders, such as early onset scoliosis. They discuss how their "therapy programmes included identification of constraints within the person, environment, or activity and [how] therapy intervention aimed to change these constraints and enable function."[3] Thus, it is important within the role of physiotherapist to consider the following:

- The child's abilities, needs, hobbies;
- Needs of the family members and what is important to them;
- Role of the child within the family, especially if the child has siblings;
- The environments inside and outside the home to which the child has access and the child's level of activity and participation.

The physiotherapist serves as a resource for the family members to enable them to have access to and be able to participate in their choice of activities, and also discusses hindrances to activity, function, and participation. An integrated team approach involving the child and family makes it possible to identify appropriate functional goals and work toward them.

25.3 Physiotherapy Program after Insertion of Instrumentation

Children with early onset scoliosis are regularly reviewed by their spinal consultant, and in some cases, the decision is made for them to undergo surgery. The day following the surgery, the physiotherapist assesses the child from a respiratory and orthopedic perspective. Even at this early stage, it is important to keep the child moving so as to facilitate respiration and preventing aching due to lack of movement. Rolling from side to side or onto the back is an ideal way for the child to start gaining movement. The back of the bed can be used to help sit the child up in the early stages (▶ Fig. 25.1). The child must be well positioned in the bed before this is done. The pelvis must be positioned at the fold where the head of the bed rises, with the knees bent over a pillow. The knee bend function of the bed should not be used because this will simply raise the child's feet. With the knees bent, the feet can be flat on the bed or elevated. When the feet are elevated, the heels should remain away from the mattress or pillows to prevent heel pressure sores.

Children often enjoy the control they gain in this position. They are in charge of how much they can raise or lower the back of the bed, and they can also look around from this position. Hospitals can be frightening places, especially environments such as the high dependency unit, where such children often are kept following this type of surgery. The primary condition often determines the child's ability to mobilize, so that the postoperative level of mobility is variable. It is vital at this stage to discuss with the parents the child's usual level of mobility, whether any aids are used, and for how long the child has been walking. Other useful information can include how the child usually gets in and out of bed. Should the usual method not bend or twist the spine, it may be worth considering using this method when getting the child up for the first time (Box 1).

Box 1 Case Study

Example of a child mobilizing from his bed in a way familiar to him that is not the log-rolling technique but does not bend or twist his back

James is 6 years old, has congenital scoliosis, and is autistic. He underwent surgery for his scoliosis with growing rods. James normally gets in and out of bed on all fours. After James was observed mobilizing on the second day following his surgery, it was deemed appropriate that he should continue with this usual way. It was familiar to him, he was independent with this method, and he did not bend or twist his spine. If James been taught only to log roll and sit on the edge of the bed, the method would have been alien to him, he would not have been independent, and if he had tried to do this alone, he would have been at risk of falling from the bed.

A child's normal mobility should be investigated, and although it may not be conventional, it may be safer and more manageable for the child.

For those children who are either occasionally or often carried, advice on lifting or manual handling is essential. The child should not be picked up under the arms because this is likely to tension the instrumentation. The method for lifting and handling the child will be unique to each child and each parent, and thus, the time spent giving advice will be time well spent because the comfort and safety of all parties are ensured.

On either the first or second day following surgery, the aim is to sit the child on the edge of the bed. Some children have their own unique method of getting out of bed that is familiar to them. Provided that they do not bend or twist during this action, the method can be continued. Before any movement is made, lower limb sensation and strength are checked, with particular focus on quadriceps strength, in preparation for standing. Pain medication should be in place before movement.

The lying-to-sitting action is carried out by rolling the child to the favored side; then, with a pendular action, the child's legs are lowered and the trunk raised (▶ Fig. 25.2).

Careful observation of the child is critical during this first sit. When seated in an upright position, the child will often feel dizzy and disoriented. Keeping the eyes open, breathing deeply, and taking a few sips of water and time are often sufficient to alleviate the dizziness.

If pain and dizziness are under control, treatment can be continued:
- Gentle leg swinging;
- Thoracic expansion exercises;
- Moving forward on the bed until the feet reach the floor;
- Foot tapping;
- Standing;
- Stepping on the spot.

The child is usually transferred to the ward on the second day following surgery, and it is at this stage that mobility progresses, with short walks to the end of the bed initially, then functional walks to the toilet or day room. A wheelchair is provided for temporary use to encourage the child and the family to have a change of environment off the ward while the child's sitting tolerance is built up.

Upper limb mobility is assessed from approximately the second day following surgery. If full range from abduction or flexion into elevation cannot be achieved in sitting or standing, range of movement exercises are given in lying. It is explained to the child and parents that the activities of daily living will gradually increase the upper limb range.

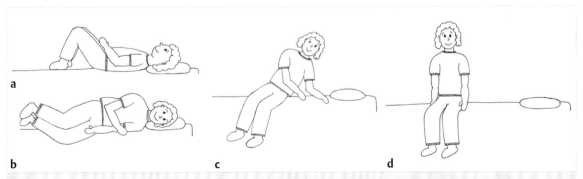

Fig. 25.2 Lying to sitting on the edge of the bed. (**a**) Crook lying. (**b**) Side lying. (**c**) Pendular action. (**d**) Sitting on the edge of the bed.

Some children commence a program of core stability exercises; however, for many children with early onset scoliosis, play is the target exercise. The physiotherapist discusses hobbies with the child, giving advice on which hobbies can be continued and those that need to be discussed with the surgeon at subsequent clinic appointments. It is ideal for a younger child to be seen by the physiotherapist in the ward playroom. The physiotherapist initially observes what the child does and discusses with the parents the child's usual levels of mobility. Advice can then be offered with regard to how the child is currently moving, compared with what is usual.

The surgeon may request that a younger child wear a removable jacket, to protect the surgery, for 3 months. Once the child is wearing the jacket, the physiotherapist should join the child for play while the child is on the floor, sitting at a table, and engaging in activities on his or her feet. The purpose of the jacket is to ensure that the child does not bend or twist the back or engage in acrobatics such as forward rolls. The jacket also protects the instrumentation while the fixation points consolidate. If it is normal for the child to negotiate the stairs, a stair assessment is carried out before discharge.

25.4 Ongoing Development and Activity after Surgical Intervention

On most occasions, children with early onset scoliosis do not require regular physiotherapy because they rapidly resume full mobility and function. Parents always have access to a pediatric physiotherapist should they require further advice or a review of the child. The children are regularly monitored by the orthopedic team, which includes a pediatric physiotherapist. Ongoing exercise for the child largely consists of play activities to whatever level the child can manage, and advice can be given as ability improves. This too can be monitored by the orthopedic team at follow-up clinic visits.

Outcome measures, such as the ASK (Activities Scale for Kids)[4] and the EOSQ (Early Onset Scoliosis Questionnaire),[5] are important in establishing the progress of the child with musculoskeletal limitations, with a focus on relevant aspects of everyday life.[6] These measures are vital for therapists to identify needs of the child and the family, appropriately set goals and monitor treatment, and provide advice regarding hobbies and activities.

Active participation is encouraged through hobbies; this not only provides good exercise but also bring children into regular contact with their peers. Participation in activities brings many other benefits, including friendships and being part of a social group. The case study (Box 2) demonstrates that children can return to their active hobbies, although occasionally adaptations to technique or equipment are necessary. The role of the physiotherapist is extended beyond just providing exercise in ensuring that the child is able to participate in favorite hobbies and sports.

Box 2 Case Study

Example of problem solving in an activity when surgery has altered a child's functional ability

Thomas has returned to playing wheelchair basketball since his initial surgery for the insertion of instrumentation. He explained that he was now unable to bounce the ball beside his wheelchair in the same way as before. With Thomas, his mother, and his older brother (who also plays wheelchair basketball), we discussed the different positions in which he could sit in his chair, different ways of handling the ball, and a potential adaptation to his sports chair. Thomas is now trying out the different options.

25.5 Conclusion

Much can be achieved through everyday activity and function. Children must be given opportunities to extend their boundaries through their own exploration. Play is the most appropriate form of exercise and is vital to all aspects of a child's development. The role of the physiotherapist is to guide the family in encouraging appropriate levels of targeted play. Through play, the child will gain increased ability and confidence. Also, many aspects of play are necessary for optimal function on a day-to-day basis. These include mobility, dexterity, social interaction, and of course laughter and fun. The last two are vital to any physiotherapy program.

References

[1] Gomez JA, Vitale MG. Measuring outcomes in children with early-onset scoliosis Semin Spine Surg 2012; 24: 140–143

[2] International Classification of Functioning, Disability and Health (ICF). Geneva, Switzerland: World Health Organization; 2001

[3] Law M, Darrah J, Pollock N et al. Family-centered functional therapy for children with cerebral palsy: an emerging practice model Phys Occup Ther Pediatr 1998; 18: 83–102

[4] Young NL, Williams JI, Yoshida KK, Wright JG. Measurement properties of the activities scale for kids. J Clin Epidemiol 2000; 53: 125–137

[5] Corona J, Matsumoto H, Roye DP, Vitale MG. Measuring quality of life in children with early onset scoliosis: development and initial validation of the early onset scoliosis questionnaire. J Pediatr Orthop 2011; 31: 180–185

[6] Young NL. Revised activities scale for kids, performance version (ASK-performance). www.activitiesscaleforkids.com Updated 2007. Accessed November 25, 2012

Part 8

International Viewpoints

26 The North American Experience

Jaime A. Gómez, Howard Park, and Michael G. Vitale

The North American approach to early onset scoliosis has been heavily influenced by the recognition that both the natural history of early onset scoliosis and early fusion are associated with poor outcomes. Over the past few decades, physicians who care for children with this potentially devastating disease have faced obstacles in understanding, studying, and disseminating their experiences. Out of these obstacles, study groups based in North America have formed and laid the research infrastructure for future research while bolstering the evidence base for early onset scoliosis.

Notwithstanding the title of this chapter, the European contributions to our understanding of early onset scoliosis have also been invaluable. Foundational work by Dimeglio and Bonnel elucidated spinal and thoracic growth characteristics, which form the basis for comparisons in patients with early onset scoliosis. Early descriptions of the disease by James, novel surgical techniques from Cotrel and Dubousset, and innovative concepts in spinal growth modulation by Roaf and Smith have informed many elements of the North American experience with early onset scoliosis.

26.1 Overcoming Obstacles to the Study of Early Onset Scoliosis

Early onset scoliosis is a rare diagnosis that affects a heterogeneous patient population; in regard to etiology, scoliosis may be related to congenital, neuromuscular, syndromic, or idiopathic conditions. The natural history of this disease spans decades and can lead to devastating pulmonary outcomes. Arguably the most important conceptual development in the field of early onset scoliosis was the description of thoracic insufficiency syndrome. In a milestone paper, Campbell et al in 2003 defined thoracic insufficiency syndrome as the inability of the thorax to support normal respiration or lung growth.[1] This article formalized the concept of spine and thoracic developmental interdependence, and it altered the considerations for the treatment of early onset scoliosis. It led to studies investigating the radiographic evaluation of thoracic and spinal deformity, emphasized the importance of pulmonary outcomes, and contributed to new treatments for early onset scoliosis.

Because of the rarity and heterogeneity of early onset scoliosis, and the nature of its course, there exist significant obstacles to undertaking meaningful research. Furthermore, the treatment methods are evolving simultaneously with the elucidation of disease characteristics, so that another layer of complexity is added to the study of early onset scoliosis.

To overcome these obstacles, two study groups based in North America have been formed to study early onset scoliosis: the Growing Spine Study Group (GSSG) and the Chest Wall and Spine Deformity (CW&SD) Study Group. Founded in 2002 and 2005, respectively, both study groups maintain national registries including data from nearly 50 medical centers serving the population of patients with early onset scoliosis. Patients are prospectively enrolled with the collection of de-identified demographic data, such as age and sex, as well as clinical data, such as radiographs and complications. The patients' courses are tracked over time, and data are entered into the registry for potential inclusion into ongoing prospective or future retrospective studies. As a result of the establishment and maintenance of these two national registries, research efforts by their members have produced significant advances, not the least of which is an identification of the methodologic challenges to producing high-level evidence for early onset scoliosis. These challenges include a lack of the following:
- A disease-specific measure of patient outcome;
- An evaluation of clinical equipoise;
- A classification system that delineates patient subgroups for communication.

To address the need for an outcome measure specific for early onset scoliosis, a quality-of-life assessment was developed with contributions from sites across North America. The need for such an outcome measure was identified through studies that used existing generic assessments to examine the quality of life of patients undergoing surgery for early onset scoliosis.[2] In addition to these studies, literature review and expert opinion yielded elements of an assessment specific for early onset scoliosis that were presented to physicians, patients, and their caregivers. Based on their input, and after multiple iterations, the Early Onset Scoliosis 24-Item Questionnaire (EOSQ-24) was produced. The EOSQ-24 covers 11 domains, including General Health, Pain / Discomfort, Physical Function / Transfer, Pulmonary Function, Daily Living, Fatigue / Energy Level, Emotion, Parental Burden, Financial Burden, Patient Satisfaction, and Parent Satisfaction, which can produce an overall and domain-specific scaled score ranging from 0 to 100. Through validation studies, the EOSQ-24 has been shown to be sensitive to quality-of-life and burden-of-care issues relevant to early onset scoliosis. Currently and in the future, investigators will be able to employ the EOSQ-24 as a robust outcome measure in studies of early onset scoliosis.[3,4]

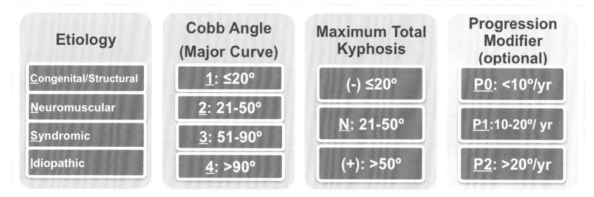

Fig. 26.1 Classification of early onset scoliosis.

To evaluate clinical equipoise, a formal study of members of both the GSSG and the CW&SD Study Group was conducted to identify areas of uncertainty among providers of treatment for early onset scoliosis. Case scenarios were presented in a treatment preference survey to 11 surgeons, who proposed treatment options for each case at two points in time separated by a 6-month interval. Numerous scenarios were identified as areas of equipoise, including the optimal management of patients who have completed their lengthening course, the ideal lengthening intervals, and the comparative advantages of using rib- or spine-based proximal fixation.[5] This study was the basis for a prospective study of rib- vs. spine-based proximal anchors in which the resources of the GSSG and the CW&SD Study Group were used as conduits for research.

To facilitate communication and collaboration among providers of treatment for patients with early onset scoliosis, multiple classification schemes have been developed, including the Classification for Early Onset Scoliosis (C-EOS), the Complication Classification System in Growing Spine Surgery, and a system for classifying the treatments for early onset scoliosis. The C-EOS is a consensus-based classification system that was developed through iterative voting processes by a group of 14 experienced providers of treatment for early onset scoliosis. In its final iteration, it has variables for etiology, Cobb angle, and kyphosis, and an optional progression modifier (▶ Fig. 26.1).[6] Its validity is now being studied through its application to clinically salient scenarios, such as its ability to predict proximal fixation failure in vertical expandable prosthetic titanium rib (VEPTR) surgery and its prognostic potential in patients with 5 years of follow-up. The Complication Classification System in Growing Spine Surgery was developed by group consensus in a method similar to that used for the C-EOS, and studies are currently in development to validate its use. It distinguishes between device- and disease-related complications and categorizes them by levels of severity according to the need for unplanned surgery or an alteration in the treatment course.[7] Furthermore, Skaggs and investigators have developed a system for classifying the treatment methodologies used in this field that divides the approaches to treatment into distraction-based, guided-growth, and compression techniques.[8]

These efforts over the past decade have produced the infrastructure necessary to perform high-level evidence studies. For example, out of the equipoise study, the multicenter prospective study of rib- vs. spine-based proximal anchors was conceived. It uses the EOSQ-24 as an outcome measure, and once the enrollment requirement has been met through the CW&SD Study Group and GSSG registries, it will categorize patients with the C-EOS and report complications with the Complication Classification System in Growing Spine Surgery. This joint effort by the two study groups is the first of many collaborations; the two database registries were merged in 2013.

26.2 Research Contributions by North American Investigators

26.2.1 Non-operative Treatment: Casting and Bracing

Landmark studies by Dr. Min Mehta from England in the 1960s described the derotational serial casting technique, which was virtually abandoned after the subsequent introduction of spinal instrumentation and bracing. However, renewed interest in casting for early onset scoliosis has been prompted by the need for nonoperative interventions for very young children with significant deformity. In a 2009 study of 55 patients, Sanders et al reported positive results in children who underwent casting before 20 months of age.[9] The Shriners Hospital System in the United States paved the way for a resurgence of casting. Many major pediatric orthopedic programs currently use derotational casting for "ideal" patients—namely, those with infantile idiopathic curves that are less than 60 degrees and those with a rib–vertebral angle difference of more than 20 degrees.

The modern use of halo–gravity traction was popularized in 1968 by Stagnara at Rancho Los Amigos Hospital in Downey, California. Like casting, halo–gravity traction declined in use after the introduction of spinal instrumentation for early onset scoliosis. However, interest has been renewed in the use of halo–gravity traction for patients who may benefit from gradual deformity reduction before instrumentation. Generally, patients who benefit from halo–gravity traction are those at risk for neurologic injury during acute reduction, including young children, patients with large and rigid curves, and those with severe upper thoracic kyphosis.[10] In the correction of kyphosis, halo–gravity traction has the added benefit of reducing stress loads on proximal points of fixation, which can contribute to failure. In addition to gradual deformity reduction, this technique may have beneficial effects on pulmonary function and nutrition, and as a result, it may optimize the condition of patients before they undergo growth-friendly surgery.[11]

26.2.2 Early Definitive Fusion and Pulmonary Outcomes in Early Onset Scoliosis

Several studies convincingly showed that untreated scoliosis of the very young led to increased rates of mortality later in life, largely due to pulmonary compromise. To alter the course of early onset scoliosis, early definitive fusion was employed because a short and straight spine was thought to be preferable to the natural history of scoliosis. However, studies of early definitive fusion documented adverse results, including decreased pulmonary function, increased pain, and iatrogenic deformities, such as the crankshaft phenomenon.[12]

Operative Treatment: Growing Constructs

Growing constructs were born out of the notion that sustained growth and correction of scoliosis were necessary to treat the growing spine. In 1962, Harrington introduced the concept of instrumentation without fusion, using a rod on the concavity of the curve and anchoring it with hooks following subperiosteal dissection. Moe later modified this technique by passing rods subcutaneously. In 1977, Dr. Eduardo Luque of Mexico City described the Luque trolley technique, which used sublaminar wires and l-shaped rods. Over time, these techniques fell out of favor because of the risk for spontaneous fusion secondary to subperiosteal dissection, but they were the conceptual basis of modern growth-friendly constructs.

The modern technique using dual growing rods evolved from extensive study. After implantation, patients undergo repeated (at about 4- to 8-month intervals) lengthening procedures at the physician's discretion based on the anticipated velocity and progression of their growth. The GSSG has been instrumental in forming the evidence base for current practice regarding the implementation of growing rods. The GSSG has contributed to comparative therapeutic studies pertaining to the use of single vs. dual rods, frequency of lengthening, and pelvic vs. nonpelvic fixation.[13,14,15] Several retrospective case series have also demonstrated the corrective potential and effect of growing rods on thoracic growth. In North America, growing rods are widely employed, and they represent a significant portion of the operative interventions for early onset scoliosis. Although externally controlled devices for spinal lengthening, which may obviate the need for frequent lengthening procedures, have been available in Europe for several years, such devices have just this year been approved by the FDA in the U.S.

As previously described, the VEPTR was developed by Dr. Campbell to address the unmet needs of patients with thoracic insufficiency syndrome. The VEPTR is approved by the U.S. Food and Drug Administration (FDA) under the Humanitarian Device Exemption for the indication of thoracic insufficiency syndrome in skeletally immature patients with one of the following:

- Absent ribs;
- Constrictive chest wall syndrome;
- Hypoplastic thorax;
- Congenital or neurogenic scoliosis without rib anomaly;
- Progressive scoliosis.

Campbell et al[1] have further characterized four main types of three-dimensional thoracic deformity. These four types of volume depletion deformity represent unique patterns of thoracic / lung volume loss, and a surgical technique is indicated for each type (▶ Table 26.1).

Much of the North American literature pertaining to growing rod and VEPTR surgery reports complications. As a whole, surgery for early onset scoliosis and the repeated lengthening procedures confer a high complication rate. One study that reported the complication rates for growing rods, VEPTR, and hybrid constructs (proximal rib fixation / distal spine fixation) found the number of complications per patient to be 2.30, 2.37, and 0.86, respectively.[16] At the same time, many of these complications are relatively manageable "obstacles" that do not necessarily change outcome or even the course of treatment.

Self-guided techniques such as the Shilla and modern Luque trolley have been developed in order to avoid repetitive lengthening. The Shilla technique fuses the apex of the deformity and uses extraperiosteally implanted pedicle screws that slide along the rods at both

Table 26.1 Characteristics of thoracic volume depletion deformities

Volume depletion deformity type	Thoracic / lung volume deficit	Examples	Suggested surgical techniques
Type I: absent ribs	Unilateral hypoplasia with lung prolapse	VATER association	Opening wedge thoracostomy + flail chest stabilization: rib–rib VEPTR; if scoliosis, rib–spine; if lumbar scoliosis, rib–pelvis
Type II: fused ribs	Unilateral hypoplasia with constricted lung	VATER association	Thoracoplasty after fused rib osteotomies + stabilization with horizontalized ribs (VEPTR as above)
Type IIIA: foreshortened thorax	Bilateral longitudinal lung constriction	Jarcho–Levin syndrome	Staged (concave, 3 months, convex) bilateral opening wedge thoracoplasty ± rib osteotomy
Type IIIB: transverse constriction	Bilateral transverse lung constriction	Jeune dystrophy, windswept scoliosis	Unilateral or bilateral thoracoplasty following intercostal muscle release

Abbreviations: VATER, vertebral defects, anal defects, tracheo-esophageal fistulas, renal defects; VEPTR, vertical expandable prosthetic titanium rib.

ends of the construct. Animal models showed promise at 6-month follow-up, with successful spinal growth.[17] McCarthy et al reported midterm results for 40 patients treated with the Shilla procedure. At 2-year follow-up, scoliosis correction was comparable with that of growing rods and VEPTR. At 5 years, the investigators reported 80% fewer revisions compared with distraction devices, such as growing rods and VEPTR.[18] Recent work done in Canada attempting to modernize the Luque trolley will perhaps provide another option for self-guided techniques.[19]

Although the options for the growth-friendly treatment of early onset scoliosis have rapidly expanded, our knowledge of the comparative effectiveness of treatments has not kept pace. In fact, it has been documented that surgeons vary in the way they approach the treatment of early onset scoliosis, perhaps signifying that the delivery of care is not optimized.[8] Therefore, high-level studies are being planned through the North American study groups and are in progress to compare the efficacy rates of treatments.

Growth Modulation

Growth modulation by tethering has been used in other areas of orthopedics. For the spine, Smith in 1954 reported vertebral body stapling in three patients with variable results. Today, hemiepiphysiodesis of the spine is accomplished with shape memory alloy staples, tethers, and transpedicular growth modulation. Most of these techniques are still under study, with multiple animal models exhibiting promising results.

Anterior spinal tethering in animal models has resulted in decreases in the width of the physis with preservation of the intervertebral disks.[20] In a case report, Crawford and Lenke demonstrated correction of scoliosis with tethering in a patient who had juvenile idiopathic scoliosis, although tethering has not been studied in larger cohorts of patients with early onset scoliosis.[21] Recently, human subject research pertaining to growth modulation has been published in the North American literature. Using nitinol (nickel titanium naval ordnance lab) vertebral staples, Betz et al showed improvement in patients with mild to moderate curves but reported multiple complications, including diaphragmatic hernia rupture, overcorrection in one patient, atelectasis, and superior mesenteric artery syndrome.[22] Anterior spinal tethering and vertebral body stapling may become viable treatment options for skeletally immature children with scoliosis, but further evidence elucidating the indications and long-term outcomes is needed.

26.3 Conclusion

The knowledge base for early onset scoliosis has rapidly evolved in the past five decades. Newer and revisited techniques are currently being studied, and long-term follow-up of more established treatment options is being reported. The North American experience with early onset scoliosis has yielded substantial contributions as groups like the CW&SD Study Group and the GSSG continue their mission to better understand this condition. With the framework established by the efforts of study groups to improve outcome measures and investigate areas of uncertainty, we believe that the evolution of the evidence base will continue its rapid pace, and that the providers of treatment for early onset scoliosis will better understand and treat this disease in the future.

References

[1] Campbell RM Jr Smith MD, Mayes TC et al. The characteristics of thoracic insufficiency syndrome associated with fused ribs and congenital scoliosis. J Bone Joint Surg Am 2003; 85-A: 399–408

[2] Vitale MG, Matsumoto H, Roye DP Jr. et al. Health-related quality of life in children with thoracic insufficiency syndrome. J Pediatr Orthop 2008; 28: 239–243

[3] Corona J, Matsumoto H, Roye DP, Vitale MG. Measuring quality of life in children with early onset scoliosis: development and initial validation of the early onset scoliosis questionnaire. J Pediatr Orthop 2011; 31: 180–185

[4] Matsumoto H, Williams B, McCalla D, et al. The Early-Onset Scoliosis Questionnaire (EOSQ) reflects improvement in quality of life after growth rod surgery. Presented at: Scoliosis Research Society 47th Annual Meeting and Course; September 5–8, 2012; Chicago, IL

[5] Vitale MG, Gomez JA, Matsumoto H, Roye DP Jr. Variability of expertert opinion on treatmetn of early-onset scoliosis. Clin Orthop Relat Res 2011; 469: 1317–1322

[6] Williams B, McCalla D, Matsumoto H, et al. Introducing the early onset scoliosis classification system. Presented at: American Academy of Pediatrics National Conference & Exhibition; October 20–23, 2012; New Orleans, LA and 19th International Meeting on Advanced Spine Techniques; July 18–21, 2012; Istanbul, Turkey

[7] Smith J, Johnston C, Skaggs D, Flynn J, Vitale M. A new classification system to report complications in growing spine surgery. A multicenter consensus study. Presented at: 6th International Congress on Early Onset Scoliosis and Growing Spine (ICEOS); November 15–16, 2012; Dublin, Ireland

[8] Skaggs DB, Flynn J, Myung K, Sponseller P, Vitale M. Classification of treatment of early onset scoliosis. Presented at: 2nd International Congress on Early Onset Scoliosis and Growing Spine (ICEOS); November 7–8, 2008; Montreal, Canada

[9] Sanders JO, D'Astous J, Fitzgerald M, Khoury JG, Kishan S, Sturm PF. Derotational casting for progressive infantile scoliosis. J Pediatr Orthop 2009; 29: 581–587

[10] Caubet JF, Emans JB. Halo-gravity traction versus surgical release before implantation of expandable spinal devices: a comparison of re-

sults and complications in early-onset spinal deformity. J Spinal Disord Tech 2011; 24: 99–104

[11] Emans J, Johnston CI, Smith J. Preliminary halo-gravity traction facilitates insertion of growing rods or VEPTR devices in severe early onset spinal deformity. Presented at: Scoliosis Research Society 42nd Annual Meeting; September 5–8, 2007; Edinburgh, Scotland

[12] Vitale MG, Matsumoto H, Bye MR et al. A retrospective cohort study of pulmonary function, radiographic measures, and quality of life in children with congenital scoliosis: an evaluation of patient outcomes after early spinal fusion. Spine 2008; 33: 1242–1249

[13] Bess S, Akbarnia BA, Thompson GH et al. Complications of growing-rod treatment for early-onset scoliosis: analysis of one hundred and forty patients. J Bone Joint Surg Am 2010; 92: 2533–2543

[14] Akbarnia BA, Breakwell LM, Marks DS et al. Growing Spine Study Group. Dual growing rod technique followed for three to eleven years until final fusion: the effect of frequency of lengthening. Spine 2008; 33: 984–990

[15] Sponseller PD, Yang JS, Thompson GH et al. Pelvic fixation of growing rods: comparison of constructs. Spine 2009; 34: 1706–1710

[16] Sankar WN, Acevedo DC, Skaggs DL. Comparison of complications among growing spinal implants. Spine 2010; 35: 2091–2096

[17] McCarthy RE, Sucato D, Turner JL, Zhang H, Henson MAW, McCarthy K. Shilla growing rods in a caprine animal model: a pilot study. Clin Orthop Relat Res 2010; 468: 705–710

[18] McCarthy R. Basic science of the Shilla procedure. Presented at: American Academy of Orthopaedic Surgeons Annual Meeting; March 19–23, 2013; Chicago, IL

[19] Ouellet J. Surgical technique: modern Luqué trolley, a self-growing rod technique. Clin Orthop Relat Res 2011; 469: 1356–1367

[20] Upasani VV, Farnsworth CL, Chambers RC et al. Intervertebral disc health preservation after six months of spinal growth modulation. J Bone Joint Surg Am 2011; 93: 1408–1416

[21] Crawford CH III Lenke LG. Growth modulation by means of anterior tethering resulting in progressive correction of juvenile idiopathic scoliosis: a case report. J Bone Joint Surg Am 2010; 92: 202–209

[22] Betz RR, Ranade A, Samdani AF et al. Vertebral body stapling: a fusionless treatment option for a growing child with moderate idiopathic scoliosis. Spine 2010; 35: 169–176

27 The French Experience

Jean Dubousset

27.1 Classifying Early Onset Scoliosis

The concept of early onset scoliosis, popularized by Dickson et al,[1] is a good one because on the one hand, it is a paradigm of spinal deformity occurring at a young age (yet to be correctly defined) in a child with a large potential for growth. On the other hand, it is not entirely adequate because conditions with many different etiologies are included within the one term (attractive and popular), even though they have very little in common except for the young age of the patients. We cannot compare localized hemivertebra pathology, in which only one or two vertebrae are involved; paralytic scoliosis in spinal muscular atrophy (SMA), for example, in which the entire spine is involved; and idiopathic infantile scoliosis, in which the entire thoracic spine may be involved. So, if the concept of early onset scoliosis is to be retained, we must add the etiologic subgroups when we describe this condition. There are clearly two large groups of patients, and it is essential not to mix them. It is also clear, unfortunately, when one listens to presentations or reads articles for the evaluation of methods of treatment or the evaluation of instrumentation, that no clear distinction is being made, and I, for one, find this hard to accept.

The danger of relying on this "all-encompassing" denomination of early onset scoliosis is that many surgeons rush to embrace a "new surgical treatment" under the auspices of a "miracle cure" and gradually lose the expertise to provide nonoperative care with proper casting and bracing (care that is time-consuming, not well paid, often ignored, and often unrewarding). They don't realize that by rushing into surgery they "put their fingers in gear," after which the only escape is repeated surgeries with an exponentially increasing risk for infections and complications as time goes by. So in my view, and generally in France, it is clear that we must categorize cases of early onset scoliosis based on the following:

27.1.1 Age of the Patient

In my experience, the real patients with early onset scoliosis are those in whom the pathology is recognized and treated between birth and 6 years of age (at entry into elementary school). However, we can also create a "prepuberty" group from 6 to 9 years of age and a "late early" group at the beginning of puberty for diagnosis and treatment, and finally a "post-puberty" group. This scheme may be useful because the treatment strategy is different for each group.

27.1.2 Etiology

Here, we can allocate patients to one of five groups: (1) idiopathic, (2) paralytic and neuromuscular, (3) congenitally malformed, (4). dystrophic, and (5) iatrogenic. It is also necessary to recognize that inside each group there are multiple subdivisions (e.g., postpolio syndrome is different from SMA and from congenital muscular dystrophy, post-laminectomy scoliosis is different from post-thoracotomy scoliosis, etc.). So finally, each patient should be considered as an individual and unique case. This chapter will concentrate on the first age group:– patients with "real early onset scoliosis" (developing between birth and 6 years of age). However, a permanently uniform thought process must be maintained across all ages and etiologies in the mind of the orthopedic surgeon.

27.2 Complete Clinical Examination and Imaging Are Mandatory as the First Step

After general information about the pregnancy, birth, and family has been obtained and the classic orthopedic inquiries and measurements have been made, the assessment continues with the most complete neurologic examination possible, which includes an examination of the cranial nerves and abdominal skin reflexes. The quality of the soft tissues, skin, joint laxity, and so forth must be assessed. Imaging, including regular radiography, computed tomography (CT), and magnetic resonance (MR) imaging, is frequently useful, if not mandatory, not only for a proper diagnosis (e.g., association of a syrinx with supposedly infantile scoliosis) but also for treatment (e.g., when asymptomatic instability is discovered in a congenital malformation of the craniocervical junction in a patient with chondrodystrophic scoliosis). A three-dimensional reconstruction, especially with a view from the top, serves as a very reliable prognostic indicator for distinguishing among the three types of idiopathic scoliosis: the spontaneously regressive type; the progressive "benign" type of Min Mehta, which we are able to correct completely with cast and brace only; and the progressive malignant type, which is not correctable with nonoperative techniques (▶ Fig. 27.1). This important information was presented at the Scoliosis Research Society meeting in Chicago, Illinois, in 1980 but was unfortunately overlooked, as was its publication in the French literature[2] a few years later. This clinical and imaging investigational phase leads to a more precise approach for determining

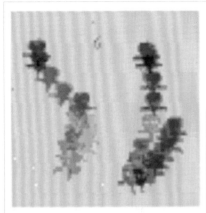

Spontaneously resolving

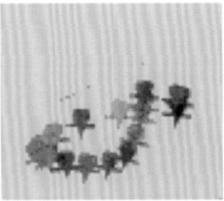

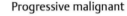

Progressive malignant

Progressive "benign"

Fig. 27.1 The three types of idiopathic early onset scoliosis.

the etiology of the deformity rather than applying a generic label of "early onset scoliosis."

27.3 General Philosophy about Concerns and Priorities to Address in Patients with Early Onset Scoliosis

1. The first priority is to identify significant problems affecting the lungs and respiratory function, which is linked to cardiac function, and subsequently thoracic cage development. Thoracic insufficiency syndrome has been well described by Campbell. We now know that alveolar multiplication stops at about 7 to 8 years of age. This syndrome therefore requires early detection and early therapeutic decision making. There is also a need for the early detection, as soon as possible after birth, of any instability of the spine, from the craniocervical junction to the sacrum, that could lead to an irreversible paralytic disorder after even minor trauma.

2. The second priority is the evaluation of normal or abnormal growth of the skeleton, especially the spine,[3,4] which affects the shape of the spinal canal at any level and can compromise the spinal cord, as well as the evaluation of progressive deformities of the entire trunk (scoliosis, lordosis, or kyphosis) and their subsequent effects on vital organ and locomotor function, balance, and cosmesis.

3. The third priority is the evaluation of the development of the nervous and muscular systems, which are linked to the ability to maintain erect posture when standing or sitting and to locomotion.

4. The synthesis of all these evaluation techniques must always be in the mind of the orthopedic surgeon. Does the deformity modify the shape of the spinal canal and risk damage to the dural sac or the spinal cord? Particularly in kyphoscoliosis, the inner part of the canal may be regular or may have a step-off. Do the vertebral bodies create a kind of "billot"? Is there any cartilaginous protrusion of the disks? Is there any immediate or potential instability? How is the alignment of the pedicles? of the facets? Is the deformity rigid or flexible? The clinical examination is crucial, particularly the neurologic examination, as well as imaging, including traction, bending, and "billot" films. It is therefore mandatory to perform CT and MR imaging, sometimes with three-dimensional reconstruction, for the initial assessment to determine the etiology. For example, infantile scoliosis can be considered idiopathic until MR imaging demonstrates a syringomyelia, which then changes the diagnosis to neurologic scoliosis.

Another question is, What is the influence of the spinal deformity on the adjacent vital structures? Are they normal or abnormal? Are the malformations cardiac, pulmonary (dysplasia, agenesis), thoracic (rib synostosis or agenesis), muscular (aplasia of the thoracic or abdominal walls, of the diaphragm), or visceral (kidneys or bowels)? What are the effects of all these different surrounding pathologies on the normal life and development of the child? All this must be meticulously assessed before any decision for treatment is made.

27.4 Most Important Principles of Treatment

27.4.1 Nonoperative Procedures

The basic requirements for such treatment in a growing young child are the following[4]: cause no thoracic compression, correct or prevent spinal collapse, attempt to produce a derotation of the deformity without too much constraint on the body structures, and allow the most normal life for the child (playing, walking, running) so as to produce the fewest possible psychological adverse effects.

Casting

Casting (► Fig. 27.2) is by far the technique of choice, to be started as soon as the deformity is noticeable, in some cases soon after birth. It is always done while general anesthesia is administered via a nasotracheal tube because traction to the head– pelvis unit (always mild) is required (the patient's teeth will crush the tube if intubation is done through the mouth). Mild traction on the casting frame makes the procedure easier for the patient, technician, and surgeon. It also reduces the rate of respiratory and digestive complications. The child's body is meticulously draped with two or three cotton jerseys, and particular care is taken to avoid creating folds in contact with the skin.

When the deformity is relatively flexible, the EDF (elongation, derotation, and flexion) technique, with the use of linen straps and hand moulding, is our preferred method. During the preparation, we place pieces of felt and padding around the thorax, particularly below the clavicle area, to be removed when the cast is dry, giving room for thoracic expansion and preventing excessive vertical orientation of the ribs. The pressure on the ribs is applied to the convex side below the apex in a posterolateral direction. Windows are created in the cast to allow pressure and counterpressure, produce the desired derotation effect, and minimally restrict the vital capacity.

When the deformity is large and stiff, immediate traction and derotation bands alone will not work. It is necessary to reduce the curve progressively by using the elongation cast of Donaldson and Stagnara. The principle of this cast is to apply progressive distraction between the head and the pelvis through two turnbuckles fitted between the two parts of the cast and turned twice a day by half a turn, causing no more than 4 to 5 mm of elongation each day. This technique is similar to that previously described, with four precise points to be located:

1. A meticulous and precise moulding by hand of the pelvic girdle.
2. The same careful moulding of the occipitomandibular fitting.
3. The addition of sufficient layers of felt and padding all around the thoracic cage, which are removed after the cast dries to allow the skin to be free of pressure and the rib cage to have plenty of room for motion.
4. Minimum of traction to the head–pelvis unit when the patient is on the cast frame.

For patients with very stiff curves, we recommend adding a halo ring to the skull and proceeding to elongation with the child in a lying position and 3 to 4 kg of traction on the halo, which is generally kept on during the night. The

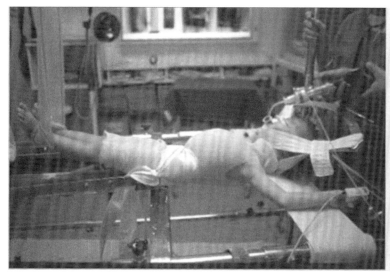

Fig. 27.2 Casting of the patient on the frame. General anesthesia is administered via nasal intubation.

halo is not linked to the cast in order to allow rotation of the head so as to prevent degenerative changes of the posterior facets of the cervical spine. This technique addresses the viscoelasticity of all the soft tissues surrounding the spine skeleton (ligaments, joints capsule, tendons, and muscles). It is used in conjunction with respiratory positive pressure ventilation machines and is continued until improvement in the respiratory measurement graphics reaches a plateau. Treatment should be continued with localized surgery, as in the case of a congenital dystrophic anomaly, or if there is no surgical indication, we change the cast to a new one made according to the EDF principles. The cast is changed as many times as necessary (generally every 3 months) until brace treatment is started. Local hygiene of the skin under the cast is essentially maintained by a regular change (every 15 days) of the thin cotton jersey in contact with the skin.

Bracing

Braces for young children must fulfill many requirements:

1. They must be easy to fit by only one person (generally the mother).
2. There must be no constriction of the thoracic cage in order to prevent respiratory compromise.
3. Bracing is better done after primary casting.
4. If possible, the braces must be adjustable in height, width, and body thickness to follow growth for a minimum of 1 year.
5. Their action must be passive or active, or both, according to the etiology.

The Garchois brace (▶ Fig. 27.3) with or without a chin piece is my favorite for all types of early onset scoliosis, especially when the patient has poor-quality muscles. Monovalve braces or thoracolumbosacral (TLSO) types are difficult to use and often harmful for the thorax. The Milwaukee brace is good for patients with normal muscles but requires a very good and trained physiotherapist. For an underarm brace when muscles are normal, the three-dimensional carbon brace with its derotational and kyphogenic effects is recommended in cases of significant lordoscoliosis. All braces are custom-made, and the expertise of the orthotist is crucial.

Respiratory assistance with machines and physiotherapy is also an important part of the treatment of early onset scoliosis and is better done under the guidance of a pediatric respiratory physician.

Family Implications

The family is of major importance in the treatment of these children because it is mandatory that they understand the goals of treatment. The family members must also appreciate the difficult path they will have to navigate during this period of rapid growth, and that in some cases surgical action will be required. Complete transparency and mutual trust among the participants —the surgeon, members of the surgeon's team (nurses, physiotherapist, orthotist, secretary, social services), parents, and patient—are essential.

27.4.2 Operative Procedures

It is clear that we have three main groups of patients, whatever the etiology of the scoliosis.

Patients with a Localized Lesion Requiring Surgery during Early Childhood

In the case of a patient with a progressive congenital malformation, such as a hemivertebra giving rise to truncal imbalance, kyphosis, or lordosis, a resection fusion with

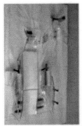
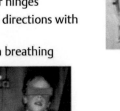
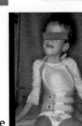

-Completely rigid

+/-Head support

-Pelvic girdle opens like a book due to 2 posterior hinges

- Adjustable in all directions with growth

-No restriction on breathing

Bad brace

Good "Garchois" brace

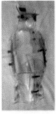

Fig. 27.3 Comparison of a good Garchois brace and a bad brace. The Garchois brace is easy to use and can be adapted to the growth of the child.

or without instrumentation on one or two levels allows a complete correction without disturbing the final growth characteristics. The situation is similar in patients with dystrophic conditions, such as neurofibromatosis type 1 and chondrodystrophy, in whom a localized rotatory dystrophic dislocation may create an irreversible spinal cord disorder. A localized anterior and posterior fusion with or without instrumentation solves the acute problem. The argument is the same for infectious or malignant / benign pathologies (deformity following laminectomy, for example).

In some patients with congenital malformations or dystrophic conditions, the use of epiphysiodesis purely anteriorly to control lordosis or purely posteriorly to control kyphosis, or the use of simultaneous convex anterior and posterior fusion to control scoliosis, has regularly yielded very acceptable results. These good results are achieved when decisions are based on the three-dimensional location of the epiphysiodesis levels and the age of the patient.

In all these cases, it is imperative that the patient's spine be observed and controlled until the end of growth. This principle should be followed even if some of the patients require complementary bracing during the growth period and others require extensive spinal surgery by the end of growth.

Patients with Pathology Involving the Entire Spine and Often the Entire Body

This is the case in patients with various paralytic pathologies resulting from upper or lower motor neuron syndromes, most frequently SMA, cerebral palsy, and spina bifida but also soft tissues diseases, such as Ehlers–Danlos syndrome, Marfan syndrome, muscular dystrophy, and congenital myopathy.

The nonoperative treatment is generally started first, with some excellent results obtained when patient and family compliance is good and the choice and strategy of the orthopedic surgeon are adequate. In most cases, when growth is almost completed, definitive fusion and instrumentation are performed, with the goals of stabilizing the spine and doing away with the brace. In some cases, the definitive fusion is done before the end of growth,[5] for technical or psychological reasons. These patients subsequently require the addition of an anterior fusion to prevent the crankshaft phenomenon,[6] even if in some of them with very little residual torsion crankshaft may be avoided with the bilateral placement of pedicular screw instrumentation at every level.

Occasionally, however, the severity of the deformities and very poor status of the patients have pushed surgeons into undertaking temporary surgical "fusionless treatment" to "help the brace." This is done as a delaying tactic until the definitive fusion when sufficient growth of the trunk has been achieved, usually after a failure of nonoperative treatment in older patients about 7 to 10 years of age. Various techniques have developed; they all have a purely mechanical basis in which elongation forces are applied to implants located on the spinal or thoracic skeleton in the form of hooks, rings, or pedicular screws constructs, linked by rods or bars of various sizes. Variations in the technique relate mainly to the methods used to elongate or compress the spine, which can be divided into three categories.[7]

1. *Purely mechanical surgical action.* Direct distraction can be applied manually with instrumentation that allows elongation of 2, 5, or 8 mm. It is then locked and the wound closed. The maneuver is repeated every 4 or 6 months. The drawbacks of this method are the following:
   a) Necessity for repeated anesthesia and surgical procedures with the subsequent risk for infection, even when a minimally invasive approach is used;
   b) Sudden elongation (amount not exactly controlled) with the subsequent risk for neurologic complications;
   c) Need for hospitalization and its subsequent cost.

In almost 40% of the cases in which this method was used, in addition to the complications mentioned, we observed that at final fusion, there were multiple spontaneously fused levels that had not been broached during the previous mini-surgeries. It has been our experience that this spontaneous fusion is even more pronounced when the *dual rod technique* is used, as we tried this many years ago with pediatric Cotrel–Dubousset rods. I have no experience of the vertical expandable prosthetic titanium rib (VEPTR) designed by my friend Bob Campbell.

1. *An electrically powered system* first developed in 1997, based on the expandable prosthesis mechanism developed in 1993 after tumor resection and replacement. A preloaded spring is embedded in a plastic tube. The spring is released after local heating of the plastic tube by a wire activated through the skin by an induced electrical current. This was an improvement on the previous method for the following reasons:
   a) Elongation is performed in the outpatient clinic without anesthesia.
   b) The treatment is controlled by the patient and the surgeon.
   c) Elongation is still sudden, however. This method was used for some years and lowered the rate of infections due to previous repeated surgeries despite some rod breakages. This allowed a delay until the placement of definitive fusion instrumentation, with better control of curves than in the past.
2. *Magnetically powered systems* (started experimentally in 2003 in our department) are the latest generation of distraction or compression rods for the spine. The principle underlying the first generation was implantation of a small magnet linked to a mechanical reciprocation

system, which itself was linked to a technologically advanced small threaded rod activated by a bigger external magnet. This allowed elongation or compression according to the direction of rotation of the external magnet. Improvements to the system were made with direct action of the magnet on the threaded rod. This powered compartment may vary in size according to the total anticipated elongation (4–8 cm). It must remain straight for obvious biomechanical considerations. So, it must be linked with a "domino" to the rod, which is attached to the spine or ribs. This rod can be bent as required by the anatomy and the surgeon and is inserted through a minimally invasive approach. The advantages are the following:

a) Insertion through a minimally invasive subcutaneous approach;
b) Progressive elongation (varying from 1/10 to 1/2 mm by turn);
c) Lack of pain;
d) No requirement for anesthesia;
e) Can be done at home by the parents.

The preliminary results of this last technique are very encouraging but too early to be widely distributed, and the procedure was limited to a very few centers where the effects had been meticulously studied, but unfortunately stopped because of the end of production by the industry.

We must add to this group some congenital malformations or syndromic lesions involving the whole spine (e. g., Jarcho–Levin syndrome). These deformities are so large and respiratory compromise is so significant that Bob Campbell has described them with the term *thoracic insufficiency syndrome*. When, for example, the defect of segmentation involves the entire thorax on one side or when multiple-rib synostosis is associated with extended bars, hemivertebrae, or asymmetric vertebral fusions, surgical treatment should be attempted because nonoperative treatment in these cases will not work. The VEPTR may be used as a rib distractor, but it can be bulky and sometimes too large for a very young child. It is why I used the baby Cotrel–Dubousset rod, on the ribs or on the spine, or the hybrid construct (spine and rib). The main drawback is that repeated surgeries are needed to expand the device every 6 months. The risk for infection from these repeated surgeries and the rate of distraction is rapid enough not to be physiologic. Furthermore, we have observed that preexisting kyphosis is a relative contraindication and a source of mechanical complications (cutout of the upper fixation, whether it be rings, hooks, pedicular screws, or tape.)

We also have experience with the Luque trolley,[8] especially in some very difficult cases, such as patients who have myelomeningocele with severe scoliosis and pelvic obliquity or severe, acute thoracolumbar kyphosis requiring kyphectomy before the age of 4 years, along with

stabilization and growth of the remaining spine. This technique, when done without too much stripping of the periosteum during passage of the wires, prevents early fusion and allows significant growth of the instrumented segment afterward. This technique was also used in some patients with SMA and similar pathology, with the advantage that postoperative bracing is not required thanks to good pelvic fixation of the rods.

Finally, for those patients with a poor prognosis, these techniques help to surmount some difficult problems, even though it has been noted that the constructs do not control the axial plane of deformity at the end of growth. Thus, in many of the patients who survive, a significant rib hump is still noticeable at the end of growth.

To avoid some of these complications, new technologies have been developed, such as magnetic expansion devices (still in clinical evaluation), which can be distracted noninvasively through the skin without anesthesia, without surgery, and without pain, often at home by the parents, with smaller increments of distraction closer to physiologic growth, as already mentioned.

Patients with Involvement of the Spine That Is Only Partial but Sufficiently Extensive to Affect, for Example, the Entire Thoracic Area

This is the case in patients with so-called infantile or young juvenile idiopathic scoliosis. The proper treatment of this group of patients is clearly nonoperative, with a succession of casts, braces, and casts again; in some cases, it is even possible for a patient to reach the end of growth with a spine that is normal in regard to cosmesis, function, and mobility. On the other hand, some patients will undergo surgery with fusions / instrumentation as soon they reach the peak of growth at adolescence. Because these children are very active, with normal musculature that allows them to run and jump as expected for their age, it is tempting to offer fusionless treatment with growing surgical devices, with the aim of avoiding casts and braces during childhood. Although they allow the most normal growth, casting and bracing are associated with physical and cosmetic restraints.

Many devices have been used all over the world, inserted through either anterior or posterior routes. Anterior vertebral body stapling has been used only in children before onset of adolescence to create a temporary epiphysiodesis, and in our experience the technique is limited. Among the posterior techniques, the mechanical fusionless method of inserting one concave distraction rod attached to a "domino" is the simplest. This provides good longitudinal control to prevent vertical collapse but less control in the sagittal plane and virtually nothing in the axial plane. This is why a severe rib hump may remain at the end of puberty and sometimes require a thoracoplasty for cosmesis, with the subsequent risk for pain and impairment of pulmonary *function.*

In addition to these mechanical techniques, an approach that is very simple, less aggressive, and less expensive than the modern-day advanced technological implants, such as the magnetic devices and the VEPTR, was developed in 2005 by Lofti Miladi, one of my pupils at St. Vincent de Paul Hospital in Paris. However, it does require a meticulous technique. A single concave titanium rod, called the H3S2 construct, is implanted through a minimally invasive technique in which two supralaminar hooks and one pedicular hook (H3) are placed at the top of the construct and two monoaxial pedicular screws (S2) are used for anchorage at the bottom of the construct. Exposure is extraperiosteal. The rod is prebent to restore thoracic kyphosis and lumbar lordosis. It is then inserted transmuscularly in a caudal to cephalic direction (▶ Fig. 27.3). The principle is to have a rod perfectly aligned with the patient's vertical axis on the concavity of the curve. This will determine the anchorage points after longitudinal traction radiographs have been obtained. Preservation of the surrounding soft tissues and bone decreases the risk for concave fibrosis and spontaneous fusion. Preoperative traction is used for curves greater than 50 degrees. Surgery is performed with external traction and spinal cord monitoring. After surgery, the patient is left free of any external supports either when standing or walking. Rod lengthening is done at the lower end every 8 to 12 months according to the specifications of Dr. Miladi. When the Cobb angle after the preoperative correction of scoliosis by traction is more than 70 degrees, surgical correction is supplemented with a simultaneous apical anterior release and fusion. The results for 23 patients reported at 3.5-year follow-up were encouraging, with Cobb angle correction maintained at 57%. The complication rate was 22% (four cases of rod breakage and two of infections, no neurologic complications). The preoperative correction of severe or rigid scoliosis, the absence of a rod connector, which is a weak point in the growing construct, and the distal location of lengthening reserved for future lengthening may explain the low complication rate. It must be understood that this technique can be used for early onset scoliosis of any etiology.

In contrast, in a discussion of technical philosophy, the Shilla method designed and popularized by McCarthy and McCullough[9] is an attractive one because of the very limited circumferential apical fusion and instrumentation without fusion above and below, so that normal growth is maintained, at least theoretically. The results appear encouraging, but I have no personal experience with this technique.

Note: The previously described alternative methods of electrically powered and magnetically powered systems[10] are used with the same philosophy and technique already described.

During my personal experience with fusionless instrumentation for spinal deformities, I have always supplemented internal fixation with a light brace in order to protect the anchorage of the systems from the multiple and undetermined stresses occurring in young children. However, I am encouraged by the experience with the H3S2 construct without postoperative bracing for children in the preadolescent phase, who are even more "uncontrolled" than very young children!

The final issue for this third category of patients was whether just to remove the hardware of the temporary device (so as to remove all sources of possible imaging artifacts during adult life) or also to perform a definitive fusion after removal. More often, it was necessary to perform a definitive instrumentation and fusion (with or without thoracoplasty) in order to obtain the best results for the future.

For all these operative procedures, whatever the type, age of the patient, and duration, the surgeon's paramount concern must be the quality of the respiratory environment and subsequent physiotherapy with or without the help of mechanical respiratory devices.

27.5 Indications for Treatment

The indications for treatment are based on the results of the numerous cases that we have observed during my professional life.

27.5.1 Major Statement

Apart from the odd case, most of the time we must start with nonoperative treatment. We must remember that any surgery anywhere in the body traumatizes the tissues involved, and healing always produces a scar. The fibrous tissues from scarring increase substantially if the surgical wound becomes infected, especially if foreign material is implanted in the surgical field. It must also be noted that repeated surgeries in the same area increase the amount of fibrous scar tissue, and thus increase the risk for infection in the surgical field.

This explains why we must favor the nonoperative treatment of early onset scoliosis as long as possible and decide upon surgery in childhood only when the indications are such that surgery is mandatory. When the surgery is localized and can address the problem in one or two attempts, there should be no restrictions for surgery at any age. However, when the surgery involves a large amount of the spine, such as most of the thoracic area, we must remember that once we embark on surgery, if complications occur, the only remedy is repeated surgery until the child is old enough for definitive surgery. It is why I favor the principle of "semi-delayed" surgery with a minimally invasive approach, such as with the H3S2 construct. This allows more time for new and promising technology like the magnetic expansion devices to demonstrate their efficacy.

27.5.2 Indications According to the Most Frequent Etiologies

Idiopathic Scoliosis

My preference is to use nonoperative treatment as much as possible. Rarely is it preferable or acceptable to terminate growth with a final fusion when growth can be preserved without surgery. Only in very infrequent cases of the malignant type, after repeated failures of well-executed serial casting and brace treatment, should we turn to a surgical solution, and the least invasive technique possible should be used. It is in reality a kind of "delayed" early surgical treatment, such as is done with the H3S2 system. Care should be taken to ensure that surgery involves only a localized part of the spine. The fusionless techniques, when attempted, must treat only the structural part of the spine and avoid excessively long instrumentation, which can restrict the ability of the spine to compensate for any imbalance. In the malignant type,

when only three apical vertebrae are the most axially rotated, the Shilla procedure may play a role. However, we still advocate caution because of the number of complications associated with the fusionless techniques. In our experience, the best outcomes have been obtained with serial casting and bracing until the beginning of the growth spurt, when a final fusion (with or without anterior and posterior instrumentation) can be done (▶ Fig. 27.4).

Congenital Malformations

In the case of congenital malformations, it is easier to understand the great differences between patients who have conditions with the same etiology. A very localized treatment, such as resection of a thoracolumbar, lumbosacral, or cervicothoracic hemivertebra with a subsequent short fusion, solves the problem quickly and definitively. The deformity must be treated as soon as it is confirmed to be progressive. An asymmetric defect of segmentation involving the entire thoracic area, with or without concave multiple-rib synostosis, cannot be treated with early convex fusion because the result is a short, small, and

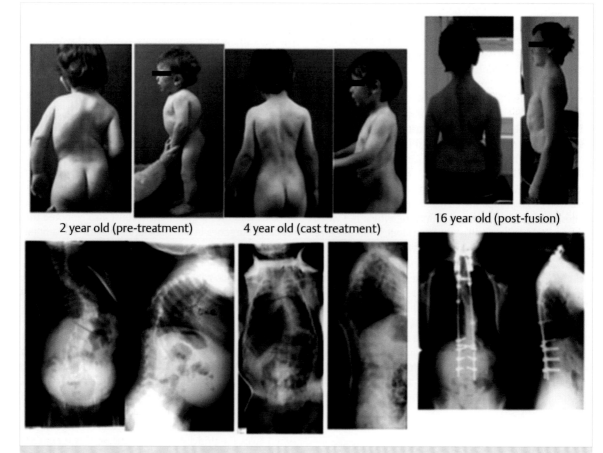

2 year old (pre-treatment)   4 year old (cast treatment)   16 year old (post-fusion)

Fig. 27.4 Photographs and corresponding radiographs of a child undergoing treatment for malignant idiopathic early onset scoliosis (80-degree Cobb angle).

rigid thoracic cage. Experience has demonstrated that the consequences to the respiratory mechanism are disastrous because growth of the spinal column of the thoracic cage is limited, creating highly restrictive conditions. In such cases, it is mandatory to use distraction devices, which carry the least amount of risk during insertion and require the fewest repeated procedures for expansion. Distraction should be done ideally before the age of 8 years to allow room in the thoracic cage for lung development. This process is facilitated by supplementary therapy with positive pressure ventilation, administered as early as possible.

The adaptation and combination of these two basic concepts for congenital scoliosis depend on the individual variations in anatomy, remaining growth potential, balance, and associated anomalies.

Neuromuscular Pathologies

In my view, it would be a mistake to say that nonoperative treatment is not effective in neuromuscular etiologies. We have the data to refute this view, particularly when the Garchois brace is used as a preventive treatment in patients with flaccid pathologies, such as severe SMA. The brace is used as soon as the patient can assume a sitting posture. For those who already have a significant deformity, active treatment starts with a cast and then the Garchois brace with or without a chin piece until the end of growth, when a posterior fusion with instrumentation is carried out. In some cases, a light brace may be useful postoperatively to control and support head alignment in patients with cerebral palsy. If the preventive treatment is started before the onset of significant deformity, and if the patient and family are compliant, it is often sufficient to last until puberty, when a definitive fusion may or may not be performed. Failing this, we are likely to get into a cycle of repeated surgeries with a multitude of expandable devices. It should be understood that there is poor tolerance on the part of parents for this type of treatment, during which some kind of therapy is required every minute. This explains the high failure rates.

The treatment of patients with dystrophic disease, such as neurofibromatosis type 1 or chondrodystrophy, is also long and arduous because of the fact that the apical dystrophic part often requires an early anterior and posterior localized fusion while the rest of the spine requires nonoperative treatment with casting and/or bracing until end of growth with or without final fusion / instrumentation. Patients with soft tissue dystrophy are generally treated in the same way as patients with paralytic neuromuscular disease. Syndromic lesions often comprise a mixture of lesions, and different treatments on a case-by-case basis are required.

27.6 Conclusion

Patients with early onset scoliosis are a specific group with a basic common philosophy of care. The techniques and goals of treatment must be readily adapted individually according to each etiology, each patient, and the prognostic factors.

References

[1] Dickson RA, Lawton JO, Archer IA, Butt WP. The pathogenesis of idiopathic scoliosis. Biplanar spinal asymmetry. J Bone Joint Surg Br 1984; 66: 8–15

[2] Graf H, Hecquet J, Dubousset J. Approche tridimensionnelle des déformations rachidiennes. Application à l'étude du pronostic des scolioses infantiles. Rev Chir Orthop 1983; 69: 407–416

[3] Mehta MH. Growth as a corrective force in the early treatment of progressive infantile scoliosis. J Bone Joint Surg Br 2005; 87: 1237–1247

[4] Dubousset J, Zeller R, Miladi L, Wicart P, Mascard E. Le traitement orthopédique dans la pathologie vertébrale du petit enfant Rev de Chirurgie Orthopédique et Traumatologique 2006; 92: 73–82

[5] Sanders JO, Herring JA, Browne RH. Posterior arthrodesis and instrumentation in the immature (Risser-grade-0) spine in idiopathic scoliosis. J Bone Joint Surg Am 1995; 77: 39–45

[6] Dubousset J, Herring JA, Shufflebarger H. The crankshaft phenomenon. J Pediatr Orthop 1989; 9: 541–550

[7] Moe JH, Kharrat K, Winter RB, Cummine JL. Harrington instrumentation without fusion plus external orthotic support for the treatment of difficult curvature problems in young children. Clin Orthop Relat Res 1984: 35–45

[8] Luque ER. Treatment of scoliosis without arthrodesis or external support, a preliminary report Orthop Trans 1977; 1: 37–38

[9] McCarthy RE, McCullough FL. Growing instrumentation for scoliosis. Presented at: Scoliosis Research Society 28th Annual Meeting; September 18–23, 1993; Dublin, Ireland

[10] Dubousset J, Miladi L, Soubeiran A. Noninvasive expandable spinal rods with magnet: spinal deformity on the cutting edge. Presented at: International Society for the Study of the Lumbar Spine Annual Meeting; May 2009; Miami, FL

28 The Asian Experience

Harwant Singh

Asia is the world's largest and most populous continent, located in the eastern and northern hemispheres of the planet. It covers 30% of the planet's land area and is home to approximately 4.3 billion people, or 60% of the world's current human population. Because of its size and diversity, Asia is a "cultural concept," incorporating diverse regions and heterogeneous peoples, cultures, and environments.

Asian economic growth in the past 30 years has been centered in the nations of the Pacific Rim, most of which have now achieved the status of developed countries; some have the highest numbers for gross domestic product per capita in Asia. East Asia also has the highest overall human development index (HDI), which has doubled over the past 40 years, whereas areas like Afghanistan are rated low. As such, there cannot be a uniform "Asian experience." Certain geographic regions of Asia—for example, Japan, Hong Kong, Korea, Taiwan, Singapore, and major cities in India, Malaysia, Thailand, and the Philippines—have scoliosis treatment facilities comparable with those in Europe and North America.

Definition of early onset scoliosis. Early onset scoliosis is best described as a coronal spinal deformity larger than 10 degrees that starts to develop before the age of 10 years. One cannot exclude the combination of a coronal (scoliotic) deformity and a sagittal (kyphotic) component —kyphoscoliosis—because the two problems frequently occur together. The study of early onset scoliosis is still an expanding area in which new knowledge is added continuously, and presently, the level of evidence worldwide does not allow a standard "best protocol / guideline" of treatment to be implemented across the board. However, most Asian centers rely on their past clinical experience and results from other world centers as guides to treatment.

28.1 Prevalence and Magnitude of the Problem

No study has reported the exact prevalence of early onset scoliosis in Asia, and data can only be inferred from the available published literature on idiopathic scoliosis, which has been well studied. The prevalence of idiopathic scoliosis has been consistently estimated at about 2 to 3% in screened schoolchildren at the peripubertal age of 12 years.[1] In a study conducted in Singapore, the prevalence rates of idiopathic scoliosis among 9-, 10-, 11-, 12-, and 13-year-old female students were 0.27%, 0.64%, 1.58%, 2.22%, and 2.49%, respectively.[2] Another Singapore study demonstrated a prevalence of 0.12% in the 6- and 7-year-old school population. A Korean school screening program in 2000–2008 reported a prevalence of 3.26%, with the highest prevalence seen in the 10- to 12-year-old age group. A Taiwanese study group reported prevalence rates of 6.58% (curve of 5 degrees) and 2.4% (curve of 10 degrees). A large Hong Kong school screening study group demonstrated a 2.8% referral rate for radiography. This study also demonstrated school screening to be predictive and highly sensitive, with low referral rates for radiography, and remains a strong validation for school screening programs. Interestingly, a study in Patiala, India, of a school screening program reported an incidence of scoliosis of 0.13%, and the majority of cases (43.7%) were paralytic curves due to poliomyelitis. A study from Ahwaz, Iran, reported a prevalence of 42.9% in a screened school population of 12-year-olds in 2004.

28.2 Screening for Early Onset Scoliosis: Is It Possible? A Case for Asia

Screening for scoliosis is conducted solely to identify children who are at risk for curve progression and may require referral to a specialist center for treatment.[3] Although some public health authorities consider screening programs not to be cost-effective, there are some very effective programs in Asia. Examples of excellent screening programs for adolescent girls and boys are those in the city state of Singapore[4] and in Hong Kong. These school programs are well placed to detect affected children 10 years of age and older. The programs do not identify early onset scoliosis in those younger than 10 years of age who may already have progressive curves and the attendant pulmonary problems that ensue. Although it is well understood that the prevalence of idiopathic scoliosis is much lower in children younger than 10 years old, the failure to identify a developing curve (of any etiology) may prevent a child from receiving treatment with simple measures, such as bracing. A higher proportion of patients in this group have spinal deformities with congenital, syndromic, or infective causes, which may require early attention. The only way to capture children younger than 10 is to identify them during "grassroots" evaluations conducted by child health care programs when childhood vaccination and nutritional programs are being implemented, usually between the ages of 4 and 5 years. In most nationwide implemented child health programs, anthropometric data are routinely collected to assess nutrition and growth. The Village Health Promoter Programmes implemented in the Borneo States of Malaysia are an example.[5] The simple incorporation of a back examination, neurologic examination, or Adam forward bend test as part of each child's health record is sufficient at least to identify those who are at risk and require referral to a treatment center.

28.3 Public Resource Allocation and Accessibility of the Referral System

The allocation of public resources is a major issue for nations already suffering from overburdened and limited resources. Scoliosis treatment and screening programs may even be considered a luxury in these nations because infectious and communicable diseases still cause high rates of morbidity and mortality in children younger than 5 years of age.[6] Poverty and conflict, although not major concerns in East Asia and South Asia, remain major concerns in West Asia.[7] Integrated "grassroots" public health programs (with the ability to identify children who need assessment) providing direct referral to regional scoliosis treatment centers are best suited to tackle this issue. Such programs are already working in most, if not all, regions in Asia.[5]

28.4 Cultural Attitudes and Compliance

The "acceptability" of treatment can be an issue. It is a challenge to educate the parents and guardians of children who need treatment. Barriers must be overcome, such as views that Western / allopathic medicine is unacceptable and reliance on traditional or shaman treatment methods. Even now, there are parents who distrust the efficacy of modern treatment methods, such as bracing and surgery, and prefer to rely on alternative or complementary methods of massage, osteopathy, and manual manipulation.

Even in regions where excellent public health systems are integrated with regional scoliosis centers, there are children whose parents and guardians choose not to have them undergo treatment. In an audit of the public hospital scoliosis service in Kuala Lumpur, Malaysia, between 1985 and 2000, of the 89 patients who presented with a primary curve larger than 50 degrees and who were advised to have surgery, only 45% underwent surgery; 3.5% elected for brace treatment instead, and 51.5% decided against surgery or any treatment, preferring to be observed.[8] In the same study, of the 75 children who presented with a curve between 30 and 50 degrees, 73.4% declined brace treatment, whereas 17.3% complied with bracing. The rate of acceptance of bracing and surgery, when these are indicated, is less than 50%.[8] Interestingly, those families who were likely to agree to surgical treatment were from urban, middle class backgrounds. The

availability of excellent treatment facilities does not mean that treatment will be accepted. Only public and parental education policy can remedy this attitude.

28.5 Population Differences

Are the physical data similar in different population groups? To answer this question, pedigree population groups should be compared. The populations of Malaysia and Singapore, which historically are diverse, comprising three major Asian ethnic groups (Han Chinese, South Indian, and Malay), present a unique opportunity to make such a comparison.

28.5.1 Menarche

Age at menarche is an important prognostic factor in idiopathic scoliosis. A later mean age at menarche is associated with a higher prevalence of idiopathic scoliosis. This finding is attributed to the longer period during which the spine can undergo rapid growth.[9] The mean age at menarche was 12.35 years in Malay, 12.43 years in Chinese, and 13.00 years in Indian patients who presented at the scoliosis service in Malaysia.[3] Although these differences were not significant, the prevalence of scoliosis was seen to be marginally higher in the Chinese populations of Malaysia and Singapore.

28.5.2 Progression of Untreated Curves

In the cohort of patients with untreated idiopathic scoliosis, the mean premenarchal progression rate was 5.66 degrees per year, and the mean postmenarchal progression rate was 2.94 degrees per year. No significant difference was found between the ethnic groups.[3] When the data were analyzed with respect to curve size at presentation, curves larger than 50 degrees progressed fastest in Chinese patients, at a rate of 14.7 degrees per year, and most slowly in Malay patients, at 8.4 degrees per year. Rates of progression for curves of 30 to 50 degrees at presentation were the same for all groups, as were the rates for curves of less than 30 degrees at presentation.[8,10]

28.5.3 Ethnic Differences in Quality of Life in Adolescents

A very interesting study from Singapore has demonstrated significant differences in adolescent quality of life among Chinese, Malays, and Indians. These differences were independent of socioeconomic and health status, suggesting important cultural differences. Such cultural differences may be important in efforts to develop quality-of-life assessments for patients who have early onset scoliosis.[11]

28.6 Etiology of Curves at Presentation to the Scoliosis Service

In Malaysia, idiopathic scoliosis was the most common type, accounting for 68.1% of all cases; neuromuscular scoliosis accounted for 10.4% of cases, and congenital scoliosis for 14.8%. In the remaining 6.7%, scoliosis was due to neurofibromatosis, Marfan syndrome, infection, and other miscellaneous causes.[8] Data from a Saudi scoliosis service reported that 59% of curves were idiopathic, 17% were congenital, and 7% were due to poliomyelitis.[12]

28.6.1 Curves at Presentation

In the Malaysian study, irrespective of the diagnostic group, the curve size at presentation for treatment was consistently between 37 and 42 degrees.[8] This is probably the size at which curves become clinically apparent to family members. When age at presentation was considered, patients with idiopathic scoliosis were seen at a mean age of 16.3 years, those with neuromuscular scoliosis at a mean age of 13.3 years, and those with congenital scoliosis at a mean age of 9 years.[8] The Saudi study reported that although the curves were first detected at a mean age of 12.5 years, the patients presented to the scoliosis service at a mean age of 16 years.[12] In both study populations, most patients at presentation were past the optimal stage for successful treatment, despite the availability of excellent public health surveillance and scoliosis services.

28.7 Diagnostic Groups

28.7.1 Idiopathic Curves

Goal of Treatment

The goal of treatment in idiopathic early onset scoliosis is to achieve a spine with normal coronal and sagittal alignment at skeletal maturity. The earlier a curve begins, the more likely it is to progress, and the more likely it is that surgical treatment will be required. The chance that curves of more than 30 degrees during the premenarchal period will progress is 100%, with the need for surgery. Evaluation of the patient requires magnetic resonance imaging of the whole spine because the incidence of neuroaxial anomalies in idiopathic scoliosis has been reported to be between 5.9% and 16% in two Indian studies and 3.8% in a Japanese study. The other major factor that is deemed important is that the treatment must be acceptable culturally and socially, so that the utilization of treatment will be maximized.

Observation

Although observation as a method of surveillance / treatment is reserved for curves of less than 30 degrees that present in the postmenarchal period, observation is sometimes used for patients with larger curves who present before 10 years of age and do not want bracing or surgery. This is suboptimal, but at least intervention can be offered when necessary. The risk for the progression of juvenile curves of more than 30 degrees is 100%,[13] and surgery can be offered whenever the patient or parents opt for it.

Rib Hump

Observation is also used to monitor rib humps. The cause of rib humps is still not well understood. They are seen in patients with idiopathic, neuromuscular, and syndromic curves. It is not uncommon to see a significant rib hump in a patient with a "smallish" curve of 20 degrees (▶ Fig. 28.1, ▶ Fig. 28.2, ▶ Fig. 28.3) and, conversely, to see a patient with a large curve and no or a minimal rib hump. Rib humps are integrally related to vertebral rotation and pulmonary function, although no large study has evaluated the exact relationship between rib humps and pulmonary outcome.

Derotation Casting and Bracing

Derotation casting and bracing are usually recommended for early progressive curves of 30 to 50 degrees, and even for smaller curves if they are clinically apparent, in premenarchal patients. Serial casting has been shown to delay the need for definitive surgery[14] and preserves thoracic growth and pulmonary function in early onset scoliosis.[15] Casts are not well tolerated in humid tropical regions; however, no long-term reports on their use in Asia are available in the literature. Bracing has been evaluated. A Hong Kong study has shown that the satisfaction of patients treated with a rigid brace did not improve after brace wear, suggesting that there is little adaptation over a period of time in comparison with observation.[16]

One major issue has been the "usability" of braces in societies that require dexterity in normal social activities, such as sports and religious activities (▶ Fig. 28.4). A "flexible" brace may address this issue. In addition, in humid, tropical regions of Asia, a rigid brace usually causes sweating and fatigue, which are undoubtedly factors in the limited acceptance of this form of treatment (▶ Fig. 28.5). There are conflicting data on the efficacy of flexible braces; a Hong Kong study reported a higher failure rate for the flexible brace (SpineCor; The Spine Corporation, Chesterfield, United Kingdom) compared with the rigid brace for "moderate adolescent curves." Interestingly, the acceptance of the flexible brace was comparable with that of the rigid brace.[17] A Malaysian study, however, reports that the flexible brace (SpineCor) has been

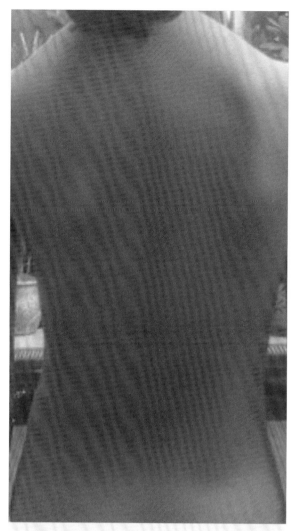

Fig. 28.1 An 8-year-old with an early curve (idiopathic type). Clinically, minimal back deformity is seen. Note the presence of shoulder asymmetry and scapula prominence on the right side.

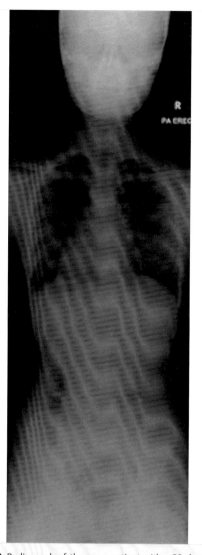

Fig. 28.2 Radiograph of the same patient with a 23-degree curve (T8-L1). The patient is currently at Risser stage 0, with significant growth remaining. Can we guarantee that this curve and the rib hump will not progress?

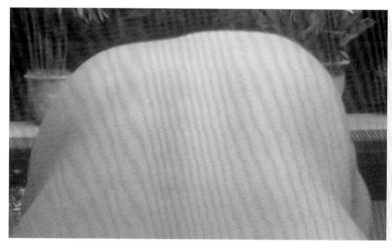

Fig. 28.3 The rib hump in the same 8-year-old at Risser stage 0. There is a 22-degree rib hump in a curve with a Cobb angle of 23 degrees. Should treatment be started?

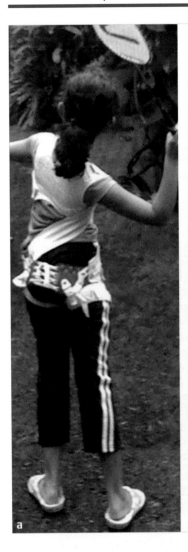
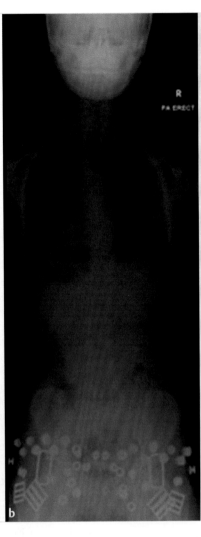

Fig. 28.4 (a) Flexible brace allowing dexterity in sports. This type of brace is well tolerated in humid environments. (b) Flexible brace in the same patient correcting the 23-degree curve to 15 degrees. Note the absence of rigid restraints in the upper torso.

effective for patients with curves presenting before 10 years of age (premenarchal) and smaller than 50 degrees.[18] Recommending brace treatment for young patients with small curves may lead to the overtreatment of curves that would otherwise have reduced spontaneously. What type of early curves will reduce spontaneously? This question can be answered only by a large scale study; however, would it be ethical to withhold simple flexible brace treatment for a patient 5 to 7 years old (during the window of opportunity for treatment) with a curve of 20 degrees in whom we cannot promise or guarantee a spontaneous reduction?

Surgery

Standard teaching recommends that in idiopathic scoliosis, instrumented posterior surgical fusion can be used for fast-progressing curves larger than 50 degrees, and that a combination of an anterior release (with or without instrumentation) with instrumented posterior fusion can be used for curves approaching 70 degrees. The two

surgical procedures can be done at the same time or staged a few days apart. The Risser stage 0 patient who undergoes a posterior fusion before or during peak growth velocity theoretically is at risk for development of the crankshaft phenomenon,[19] in which the posterior fusion acts as a tether for the still-growing anterior vertebral body end plates. It is for this reason that an anterior procedure may be considered at the same time, to include vertebral growth plate fusions at the apical region, so that a balanced spine can be achieved at maturity. However, a long-term study of posterior fusion in Risser stage 0 patients in Hong Kong who were followed to maturity at a mean of 7.8 years after fusion did not report a significant issue with the crankshaft phenomenon. The authors did not recommend routine anterior surgery to prevent crankshaft.[20]

The same group also reported that although early posterior fusion did shorten the thoracic trunk, the final height of the subjects at maturity did not differ much from the height of the subjects in the nonsurgical group because the surgical subjects compensated with longer

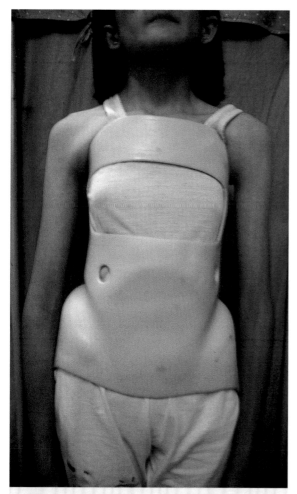

Fig. 28.5 Boston brace made with rigid material. Compliance with this type of brace in the humid tropics is poor, and treatment frequently fails.

lower limb lengths. Perhaps the most prudent management strategy has been outlined in a Korean review, in which the authors recommend initial observation and supervised bracing (for a hypothetical idiopathic curve of 35 to 50 degrees in a patient at Risser stage 0–2 with significant growth potential left). The rationale is to prevent unnecessary surgery, as they report that more than 50% of patients could be well controlled with this strategy.

Outcome Studies

A long-term review (21–41 years) from Japan has reported no pain or adverse mental health effects of surgery and no increased rates of back pain; however, the patients' scores for self-image and function were significantly lower than those of controls. The standard surgical techniques used for idiopathic scoliosis have demonstrated satisfactory or good early and midterm results in Malaysia, India, Hong Kong, Thailand, Pakistan, and Iran. Posterior segmental pedicle screw fixation has been shown to be as effective as anterior surgery, and thoracoscopic instrumentation has been shown to be as effective as posterior surgery in Singapore. Although magnetically controlled growth rods are still considered experimental, early results of the Hong Kong experience show that they are safe and effective, with minimal surgical scarring and psychological distress; in addition, they improve quality of life and are more cost-effective than traditional growth rods. A mainland Chinese study group has reported superior early results with a dual growing rod technique compared with a single growing rod in the correction of early onset scoliosis.

Lung Function

A study in Hong Kong of patients aged 11 to 18 years with idiopathic scoliosis and curves between 40 and 98 degrees has shown associated lung dysfunction to be predominantly restrictive in nature. Thoracotomy in patients younger than 10 years of age has fallen out of favor in recent times because of the risk for pulmonary disturbances, and it may interfere with pulmonary development if the lungs have not yet fully matured. However, in specific situations—for example, a 5-year-old with a progressive idiopathic curve of 70 degrees—most surgeons would offer surgery. The longest follow-up available in Asia for anterior surgery has reported that despite a small percentage reduction in the FEV (forced expiratory volume) and FVC (forced vital capacity), there were no pulmonary symptoms after a mean follow-up of 15.2 years.

Patient Satisfaction

The difficulty in assessing outcome measures in early onset scoliosis has been discussed extensively, and to date no comprehensive, reliable pro forma protocol has been developed. One factor is that the very young children being evaluated may not be able to express their feelings and thoughts as well as adolescents. In a Malaysian study of adolescent idiopathic scoliosis, patients reported being satisfied with the results of the surgery. This was independent of the magnitude of the curve before surgery.

28.7.2 Congenital Curves

Congenital curves account for 15 to 17% of the patient load at scoliosis services in Asia.[8,12] The goal of treatment is to maintain spinal balance. Because these deformities are present from birth, they may be clinically apparent at the first growth spurt of the spine. Also, because the curves are due to anatomical defects (type 1, failure of formation; type 2, failure of segmentation; or type 3, a combination of both), they are usually treated by surgery if they progress. Untreated kyphotic curves due to type 1 or type 3 vertebral defects may be associated with paraplegia, and a thoracic apex kyphotic deformity is associated with respiratory dysfunction. An Indian study demonstrated anatomical anomalies in 44% of cases, with 15% occult intraspinal anomalies (most frequently diastematomyelia), 15% cardiovascular anomalies, and 6% genitourinary anomalies.

Lung Function

In a Hong Kong series of patients with congenital vertebral anomalies, the pulmonary vital capacity was significantly reduced in surgically treated patients (68% of predicted value), especially those with multiple thoracic anomalies. The authors' recommendation was to treat with surgery early, before deformity progression.

Surgery

A recent report from China has described encouraging 2-year results for the dual growing rod technique, combined with an osteotomy of the apical vertebra in severe rigid deformity as well as a short segment fusion. The authors report an average of 4.2 lengthening procedures per patient, with a high rate of patient satisfaction and low complication rates.

28.7.3 Neuromuscular Curves, Including Syndromic Types

These curves account for 6 to 7% of the patient load at scoliosis services in Asia.[8,12] They are difficult to treat, and the goal of treatment is to achieve a functional, balanced spine in an ambulant patient or a balanced pelvis for stable seating in a nonambulant patient. Bracing is not effective except to delay the timing of surgery. Surgery is often the only way to treat these curves. Patients with neuromuscular conditions require a great deal of medical

and psychosocial support, which must continue throughout life. Their life expectancy is usually reduced because of pulmonary complications that develop as a consequence of decreasing muscle power after the adolescent period.

Surgery

Surgery for these curves usually involves instrumentation to the pelvis to maintain pelvic balance, which is important for standing and sitting. A Singapore review reports

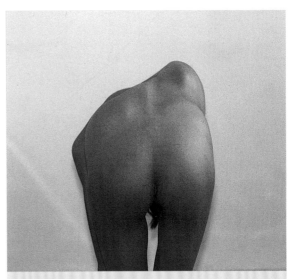

Fig. 28.6 Severe rib hump (razor back) in Marfan syndrome in a 12-year-old. This rib hump was not correctable at the time of surgery for the curve. Could an early flexible brace have "controlled" the rib hump so that a thoracoplasty would have been useful?

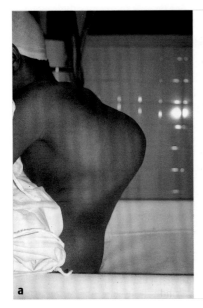
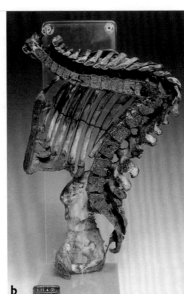

Fig. 28.7 (a) Kyphoscoliosis in a 12-year-old with spinal tuberculosis. This side view demonstrates the sagittal curve, with the apex at the T8 vertebral body. (b) Museum specimen of an adult skeleton showing a pure kyphosis in spinal tuberculosis with the apex at T9-T10. Note that there is a fusion at the apical vertebrae. (Reproduced with kind permission of the President and Fellows of the Royal College of Surgeons of Edinburgh.)

a

b

safe and effective outcomes; however, increases were noted in intensive care unit stays and in the rates of deep and superficial infections, pseudarthrosis, and implant breakage, all of which were treatable. However, pulmonary capacity did not improve after curve correction. Another review by the same group reported that the pulmonary function of patients who had surgery for scoliosis associated with spinal muscular atrophy continued to worsen after surgery. A Chinese study reported good outcomes in curves associated with Marfan syndrome after posterior-only surgery.

Rib Hump

A "razor back" rib hump (▶ Fig. 28.6) in early onset scoliosis is usually seen with syndromic or "infantile" curves. This rib deformity is resistant to bracing. Surgical treatment (thoracoplasty) in patients younger than 5 years may affect pulmonary development. Pulmonary function in older patients undergoing convex thoracoplasty and rib resection decreases 3 to 6 months after surgery and returns to baseline 12 to 24 months after surgery.

28.8 Tuberculosis

Osteoarticular tuberculosis is a unique, paucibacillary, slow-growing disease that is often diagnosed after it produces significant destruction. This is usually seen as a kyphoscoliotic spinal deformity rather than as a purely coronal spinal deformity (▶ Fig. 28.7). The routine availability of magnetic resonance imaging of the spine has made the early diagnosis of spinal tuberculosis easier (▶ Fig. 28.8), as percutaneous biopsy for tissue diagnosis is difficult and controversial. Another unresolved issue is the duration of chemotherapy because it is still not possible to determine when the conversion of bacteriologic positivity to bacteriologic negativity occurs. Multidrug-resistant tuberculosis is likely to develop in the near future, and success in dealing with this issue depends on the early identification of resistant strains.

In children, the spinal deformity often continues to progress, even after the infection has healed, because the normal vertebral growth plates are still maturing. The spine "at risk" should be identified and observed. Surgery to control the developing deformity should be offered once it is determined that the deformity is unstable.

The best series that reviewed the long-term (30-year follow-up) outcomes of children with spinal tuberculosis is from Korea. Of 124 children aged between 2 and 15 years, 73% were treated conservatively with chemotherapy, and the remaining 27% were treated with surgery (focal débridement, posterior interspinous wiring, or posterior instrumentation with rods and segmental wiring). Paraplegia was seen in 15% of patients, all of whom recovered after treatment.

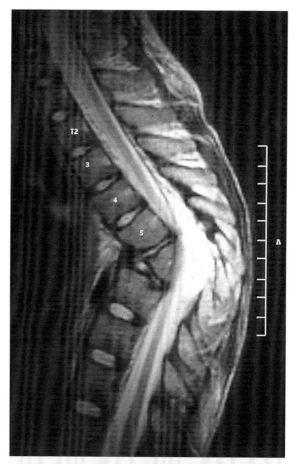

Fig. 28.8 Sagittal magnetic resonance imaging section of a patient with spinal tuberculosis showing apical compression of the neural elements. Note the "mismatch" between the vertebral bodies and spinous processes at the apical area. This indicates resorption of the affected vertebral bodies in long-standing spinal tuberculosis, in which the apices are very often rigid and require an osteotomy.

28.8.1 Surgery

Surgery for tuberculosis of the spine has evolved rapidly over the past 30 years. The goal is to maintain a good sagittal balance. Good results have been achieved with posterior fusion after tubercular kyphosis in a series of patients younger than 8 years. Severe kyphosis in healed tuberculosis has been successfully managed by a combination of anterior release, decompression, deformity correction, and instrumented fusion, followed by posterior osteotomy, deformity correction, and pedicle screw instrumentation.

28.8.2 Lessons Learned from Tuberculosis of the Spine

It has been shown that leg length is increased at maturity in patients who have undergone fusion of the immature thoracic spine for idiopathic scoliosis, possibly as the result of a compensatory mechanism that may be neurally or hormonally mediated. Although patients with spinal deformity due to tuberculosis have shortened standing and spinal heights, they have longer lower limbs compared with normal subjects. This suggests that the same compensatory mechanism may be at work.

28.9 Conclusion

There is no uniform experience in Asia in the management of early onset scoliosis, largely because of vast differences in the availability of resources within the region and possibly different disease patterns, determined by local factors such as culture. Centers in Japan, Korea, and Hong Kong (and China) have led and still do lead in the development of new treatments for this problem. At the other end, there are some regions in Asia that still lack the resources to provide effective treatment, which remains the main challenge of the 21st century.

References

[1] Plaszewski M, Nowobilski R, Kowalski P, Cieslinski M. Screening for scoliosis: different countries' perspectives and evidence-based health care. Int J Rehabil Res 2012; 35: 13–19

[2] Yong F, Wong HK, Chow KY. Prevalence of adolescent idiopathic scoliosis among female school children in Singapore. Ann Acad Med Singapore 2009; 38: 1056–1063

[3] Oh KS, Chuah SL, Harwant S. The need for scoliosis screening in Malaysia. Med J Malaysia 2001; 56 Suppl C: 26–30

[4] Wong HK, Hui JH, Rajan U, Chia HP. Idiopathic scoliosis in Singapore schoolchildren: a prevalence study 15 years into the screening program. Spine 2005; 30: 1188–1196

[5] Mohamed A. Thirty years of Village Health Promoter Programme in Sarawak: promoting health in the community. Int J Pub Health Res Special Issue 2011 (Symposium):21–22

[6] The State of the World's Children 2005. New York, NY: UNICEF; 2004

[7] Collier P, Elliott VL, Hegre H, et al. Breaking the conflict trap: civil war and development policy. A World Bank Policy Research Report. Washington, DC: The World Bank and Oxford University Press; 2003:23–24

[8] Chuah SL, Kareem BA, Selvakumar K, Oh KS, Borhan Tan A, Harwant S. An audit of the Scoliosis Service at Hospital Kuala Lumpur. Med J Malaysia 2001; 56 Suppl C: 31–36

[9] Grivas TB, Vasiliadis E, Mouzakis V, Mihas C, Koufopoulos G. Association between adolescent idiopathic scoliosis prevalence and age at menarche in different geographic latitudes. Scoliosis 2006; 1: 9

[10] Singh H, Soo-lin C,, Kareem BA, Selvakumar K, Kim-Soon O, Abdullah MBT. Does race influence the progression of adolescent idiopathic scoliosis? J Bone Joint Surg Br 2003; 85-B Suppl I III: 189

[11] Ng TP, Lim LC, Jin A, Shinfuku N. Ethnic differences in quality of life in adolescents among Chinese, Malay and Indians in Singapore. Qual Life Res 2005; 14: 1755–1768

[12] Al-Arjani AM, Al-Sebai MW, Al-Khawashki HM, Saadeddin MF. Epidemiological patterns of scoliosis in a spinal center in Saudi Arabia. Saudi Med J 2000; 21: 554–557

[13] Charles YP, Daures JP, de Rosa V, Diméglio A. Progression risk of idiopathic juvenile scoliosis during pubertal growth. Spine 2006; 31: 1933–1942

[14] Fletcher ND, McClung A, Rathjen KE, Denning JR, Browne R, Johnston CE III. Serial casting as a delay tactic in the treatment of moderate-to-severe early-onset scoliosis. J Pediatr Orthop 2012; 32: 664–671

[15] Baulesh DM, Huh J, Judkins T, Garg S, Miller NH, Erickson MA. The role of serial casting in early-onset scoliosis (EOS). J Pediatr Orthop 2012; 32: 658–663

[16] Cheung KM, Cheng EY, Chan SC, Yeung KW, Luk KD. Outcome assessment of bracing in adolescent idiopathic scoliosis by the use of the SRS-22 questionnaire. Int Orthop 2007; 31: 507–511

[17] Wong MS, Cheng JC, Lam TP et al. The effect of rigid versus flexible spinal orthosis on the clinical efficacy and acceptance of the patients with adolescent idiopathic scoliosis. Spine 2008; 33: 1360–1365

[18] Tan YH, Teoh LL, Abader A, Robertson M, Du Plessis J, Singh H. Curve correction in adolescent idiopathic scoliosis (AIS) treated by dynamic bracing (SpineCor): a midterm review. Presented at: MSS-SRS International Spine Congress 2011; December 8–10, 2011; Kuala Lumpur, Malaysia

[19] Sanders JO, Little DG, Richards BS. Prediction of the crankshaft phenomenon by peak height velocity. Spine 1997; 22: 1352–1356, discussion 1356–1357

[20] Mullaji AB, Upadhyay SS, Luk KD, Leong JC. Vertebral growth after posterior spinal fusion for idiopathic scoliosis in skeletally immature adolescents. The effect of growth on spinal deformity. J Bone Joint Surg Br 1994; 76: 870–876

Further Reading

Akazawa T, Minami S, Kotani T, Nemoto T, Koshi T, Takahashi K. Long-term clinical outcomes of surgery for adolescent idiopathic scoliosis 21 to 41 years later. Spine 2012; 37: 402–405

Ameri E, Behtash H, Mobini B, Omidi-Kashani F, Momeni B. Radiographic outcome of surgical treatment of adolescent idiopathic scoliosis in males versus females. Scoliosis 2008; 3: 12

Bowring P. What Is Asia? Far Eastern Economic Review. Feb 12, 1987 (v. 135 n. 7)

Chan CY, Kwan MK, Saw LB et al. Post-operative health related quality of life assessment in scoliosis patients. Med J Malaysia 2008; 63: 137–139

Cheung KM, Cheung JP, Samartzis D et al. Magnetically controlled growing rods for severe spinal curvature in young children: a prospective case series. Lancet 2012; 379: 1967–1974

Chng SY, Wong YQ, Hui JH, Wong HK, Ong HT, Goh DY. Pulmonary function and scoliosis in children with spinal muscular atrophy types II and III. J Paediatr Child Health 2003; 39: 673–676

Chu WC, Li AM, Ng BK et al. Dynamic magnetic resonance imaging in assessing lung volumes, chest wall, and diaphragm motions in adolescent idiopathic scoliosis versus normal controls. Spine 2006; 3119: 2243–2249

Chunguang Z, Limin L, Rigao C et al. Surgical treatment of kyphosis in children in healed stages of spinal tuberculosis. J Pediatr Orthop 2010; 30: 271–276

Corona J, Matsumoto H, Roye DP, Vitale MG. Measuring quality of life in children with early onset scoliosis: development and initial validation of the early onset scoliosis questionnaire. J Pediatr Orthop 2011; 31: 180–185

Daruwalla JS, Balasubramaniam P, Chay SO, Rajan U, Lee HP. Idiopathic scoliosis. Prevalence and ethnic distribution in Singapore schoolchildren. J Bone Joint Surg Br 1985; 67: 182–184

Day GA, Upadhyay SS, Ho EK, Leong JC, Ip M. Pulmonary functions in congenital scoliosis. Spine 1994; 19: 1027–1031

Deshpande SS, Mehta R, Yagnik M. Short term analysis of healed post-tubercular kyphosis in younger children based on principles of congenital kyphosis. Indian J Orthop 2012; 46: 179–185

Fazal A, Lakdawala RH. Fourth-generation spinal instrumentation: experience with adolescent idiopathic scoliosis at a tertiary care hospital in Pakistan. Int J Gen Med 2012; 5: 151–155

Fletcher ND, Larson AN, Richards BS, Johnston CE. Current treatment preferences for early onset scoliosis: a survey of POSNA members. J Pediatr Orthop 2011; 31: 326–330

Hee HT, Yu ZR, Wong HK. Comparison of segmental pedicle screw instrumentation versus anterior instrumentation in adolescent idiopathic thoracolumbar and lumbar scoliosis. Spine 2007; 32: 1533–1542

Hsu LC, Upadhyay SS. Effect of spinal fusion on growth of the spine and lower limbs in girls with adolescent idiopathic scoliosis: a longitudinal study. J Pediatr Orthop 1994; 14: 564–568

Human Development Report 2010. New York, NY: United Nations Development Programme; 2010

Jain AK, Rajasekaran S. Tuberculosis of the spine. Indian J Orthop 2012; 46: 127–129

Krishna M, Upadhyay SS. Increased limb lengths in patients with shortened spines due to tuberculosis in early childhood. Spine 1996; 21: 1045–1047

Leung JP, Lam TP, Ng BK, Cheng JC. Posterior ISOLA segmental spinal system in the treatment of scoliosis. J Pediatr Orthop 2002; 22: 296–301

Li ZC, Liu ZD, Dai LY. Surgical treatment of scoliosis associated with Marfan syndrome by using posterior-only instrumentation. J Pediatr Orthop B 2011; 20: 63–66

Luk KD, Lee CF, Cheung KM et al. Clinical effectiveness of school screening for adolescent idiopathic scoliosis: a large population-based retrospective cohort study. Spine 2010; 35: 1607–1614

McMaster MJ, Ohtsuka K. The natural history of congenital scoliosis. A study of two hundred and fifty-one patients. J Bone Joint Surg Am 1982; 64: 1128–1147

McMaster MJ, Singh H. Natural history of congenital kyphosis and kyphoscoliosis. A study of one hundred and twelve patients. J Bone Joint Surg Am 1999; 81: 1367–1383

McMaster MJ, Glasby MA, Singh H, Cunningham S. Lung function in congenital kyphosis and kyphoscoliosis. J Spinal Disord Tech 2007; 20: 203–208

Mittal RL, Aggerwal R, Sarwal AK. The evaluation of a scoliometer. Int Orthop 1987; 11: 335–338

Mohanty S, Kumar N. Patterns of presentation of congenital scoliosis. J Orthop Surg (Hong Kong) 2000; 8: 33–37

Moon MS, Kim SS, Lee BJ, Moon JL. Spinal tuberculosis in children: retrospective analysis of 124 patients. Indian J Orthop 2012; 46: 150–158

Nakahara D, Yonezawa I, Kobanawa K et al. Magnetic resonance imaging evaluation of patients with idiopathic scoliosis: a prospective study of four hundred seventy-two outpatients. Spine 2011; 36: E482–E485

Pin LH, Mo LY, Lin L et al. Early diagnosis of scoliosis based on school-screening. J Bone Joint Surg Am 1985; 67: 1202–1205

Rajasekaran S, Kamath V, Kiran R, Shetty AP. Intraspinal anomalies in scoliosis: an MRI analysis of 177 consecutive scoliosis patients. Indian J Orthop 2010; 44: 57–63

Safikhani Z, Fakor M, Soori H, Hejazian L. Prevalence of scoliosis in female students 11–15 years of age in Ahwaz, Iran. Neurosciences (Riyadh) 2006; 11: 97–98

Sudo H, Ito M, Kaneda K, Shono Y, Takahata M, Abumi K. Long-term outcomes of anterior sppinal fusion for treating thoracic adolescent idiopathic scoliosis curves: average 15-year follow-up analysis. Spine 201 3; 38: 819–826

Suh SW, Modi HN, Yang JH, Hong JY. Idiopathic scoliosis in Korean schoolchildren: a prospective screening study of over 1 million children. Eur Spine J 2011; 20: 1087–1094

Telang SS, Suh SW, Song HR, Vaidya SV. A large adolescent idiopathic scoliosis curve in a skeletally immature patient: is early surgery the correct approach? Overview of available evidence. J Spinal Disord Tech 2006; 19: 534–540

Thacker M, Hui JH, Wong HK, Chatterjee A, Lee EH. Spinal fusion and instrumentation for paediatric neuromuscular scoliosis: retrospective review. J Orthop Surg (Hong Kong) 2002; 10: 144–151

Unnikrishnan R, Renjitkumar J, Menon VK. Adolescent idiopathic scoliosis: retrospective analysis of 235 surgically treated cases. Indian J Orthop 2010; 44: 35–41

Vitale MG, Gomez JA, Matsumoto H, Roye DP Jr. Chest Wall and Spine Deformity Study Group. Variability of expert opinion in treatment of early-onset scoliosis. Clin Orthop Relat Res 2011; 469: 1317–1322

Wajanavisit W, Laohacharoensombat W. Treatment of adolescent idiopathic scoliosis using Cotrel-Dubousset spinal instrumentation. J Med Assoc Thai 2000; 83: 146–150

Wang S, Zhang J, Qiu G et al. Dual growing rods technique for congenital scoliosis: more than 2 years outcome: the preliminary results of a single centre. Spine 2012; 37: 1639–1644

Wong HK, Hee HT, Yu Z, Wong D. Results of thoracoscopic instrumented fusion versus conventional posterior instrumented fusion in adolescent idiopathic scoliosis undergoing selective thoracic fusion. Spine 2004; 29: 2031–2038, discussion 2039

Zhao Y, Qiu GX, Wang YP et al. Comparison of initial efficacy between single and dual growing rods in treatment of early onset scoliosis. Chin Med J (Engl) 2012; 125: 2862–2866

Zhou C, Liu L, Song Y et al. Pulmonary function changes after operation in patients with severe scoliosis [in Chinese] Zhongguo Xiu Fu Chong Jian Wai Ke Za Zhi 2010; 24: 23–26

29 The North African Experience

Hazem Elsebaie

Egypt, a developing country with a population of 90 million, is deeply rooted in Africa and the Middle East, and the Egyptian experience with spinal surgery, especially in pediatric cases of spinal deformity, is representative of that of the entire North African region. This chapter discusses the ways in which surgeons in developing countries can acquire new techniques and technology and tailor them to match their limited resources; it also explains how local innovations in the field can be designed to fulfill the requirements of the population being served.

The treatment of progressive spinal deformities in childhood has always been challenging. The younger a person's age when a deformity arises, the more detrimental effects the deformity has. Spinal deformity affects children physically, psychologically, and socially; additionally, it can be life-threatening, especially in those with large and progressive curves, which can decrease pulmonary function and in the most severe cases lead to heart failure. In the growing spine, we need not only to correct the deformity but also, even more importantly, to maintain spinal growth and so enable normal development of the heart and lungs. Spinal implants in young children can be risky, and we may not know their long-term effects on growth. Nonoperative treatment for early onset scoliosis is in many cases unsuccessful, and surgical treatment with instrumented spinal fusion and correction prevents further spinal and trunk growth, with numerous detrimental effects. Attempts to correct the spine while preserving its growth potential has always been the goal. This has been achieved to a great extent by using spinal instrumentation without fusion.

The first trials of instrumentation without fusion in Egypt were started in the early 1990s in very small numbers of patients. The Luque trolley was used; however, this limited experience proved very disappointing because of the high rate of complications and failures, including minimal spinal growth, spontaneous fusion, failed implants, loss of correction, metalwork prominence, and infections. This technique was soon abandoned, and the cases were never presented or published.

29.1 Traditional Growing Rods

The techniques of three-dimensional correction and instrumentation for spinal deformities were introduced in Egypt in the late 1990s. A few years later, at Cairo University, surgeons started to learn and gain experience in instrumentation without fusion for the treatment of early onset scoliosis; most of this experience was acquired directly during training in the United Kingdom and from American spinal surgeons visiting spinal centers in Egypt. Experience remained limited to a handful of surgeons,

and it took a while to convince the community of spinal physicians of the importance of growing rods as a valid safe and effective surgical treatment option for patients with early onset scoliosis.

The concept of the single submuscular rod was acquired from Hilali Noordeen, FRCS UK, and modified. The first construct used in Egypt had a proximal foundation consisting of an intrasegmental claw (proximal downward-facing transverse process hook and distal upward-facing facet hook) and a stainless steel sublaminar wire to increase stability and decrease the incidence of pullout failure; the distal foundation consisted of a single pedicle screw. The two rods, attached proximally and distally to the foundations, were connected via a longitudinal connector (tandem) with proximal and distal locking screws (▶ Fig. 29.1). The second version of the single growing rod was acquired from David Marks, FRCS UK; the proximal foundation consisted of a double claw construct (claw in a claw) with double transverse process and double facet hooks, and the distal foundation consisted of adjacent pedicle screws (▶ Fig. 29.2).

The results of the first series of patients who had early onset scoliosis treated with the single growing rod technique were published in 2005 in the *Pan Arab Journal of Orthopaedics and Trauma*.[1] This was one of the first documented case series in the region on the use of growing instrumentation in early onset scoliosis. The study reviewed 12 patients with juvenile and infantile idiopathic early onset scoliosis, whose average age was 6 years and 2 months at the index surgery. The patients underwent surgery between 2001 and 2003; the average follow-up was 1 year and 10 months, and the average number of distractions per patient was 3.5. The wake-up test was routinely used. Three proximal hook pullouts and two rod fractures occurred.

This study was the basis for the first national recommendation and approval for centers and surgeons to start offering growing spine surgical treatment with serial distraction. The study concluded that growing rods could be a valid alternative for children with early onset scoliosis, who had very limited treatment options; however, the surgeons had to accept the high rate of complications and be able to deal with them. The study also recommended that an adequate orthotic capability be available, that surgeons be certain that the families of patients were willing to have their children undergo multiple procedures with anesthesia, and that the families be informed beforehand that at any stage the surgeon might have to discontinue the distraction procedure and proceed to a definitive instrumented fusion.

In subsequent studies, the single growing rod was used in different pathologic conditions, including congenital,

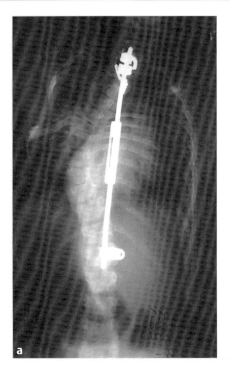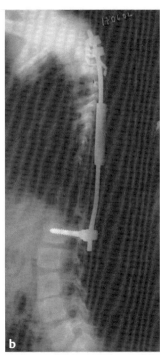

Fig. 29.1 Anteroposterior (**a**) and lateral (**b**) views of a single rod with a single claw, wire, and pedicle screw.

syndromic, and neuromuscular scoliosis and neurofibromatosis; many studies done in Egypt were presented at various international meetings, including the 2005 International Meeting on Advanced Spine Techniques (IMAST) in Canada, the 2006 Scoliosis Research Society European and Middle East Meeting in Turkey, and the 2007 International Congress on Early Onset Scoliosis (ICEOS) in Spain. This international exposure enriched the experience of Egyptian surgeons and led to improvements in their techniques and results. The single rod construct remained the only option in Egypt for the surgical treatment of children with early onset scoliosis until a few years later, when Dr. Behrooz Akbarnia of the United States introduced the double rod construct, with its possible advantages. Since then, double rod constructs have become the standard of care for these children (▶ Fig. 29.3).

Research done on the patients in Egypt treated with growing rods yielded three important original findings in the field of early onset scoliosis; the concepts were discussed for the first time worldwide and have clear implications for the management of these children. The first study looked at the growth of unsegmented bars in patients with congenital scoliosis treated with serial growing rod distraction. Unilateral bars have been identified as having absolutely no growth potential, and it has always been assumed that the concave side of a congenital curve does not grow. In this study, the unilateral bars appeared to grow during concave vertebral distraction with growing rods; their growth was much slower (about 25%) than that of the normal vertebrae in the same circumstances, and the growth appeared to be directly related to the number of distraction procedures (an increase in the bar of 3 to 4% per distraction). The coronal Cobb angle of the unsegmented bars also improved significantly in patients treated with concave growing rods; therefore, it may be possible to correct scoliosis due to unilateral bars with periodic distraction. In addition, the growth of unilateral bars during distraction may help in managing the pulmonary effects of congenital thoracic scoliosis.[2]

The second study was planned to assess the controversial complication of pedicle screw migration; this was the first case series ever to document, quantify, and classify the change of position of distal pedicle screws in relation to the vertebral bodies in children with spinal implants. The change in position of the distal pedicle screws of growing rods in relation to the vertebral bodies was described as "pedicle screw migration, shift or drift?" Pedicle screws in growing rods are subjected to serial distractive forces that push them down during every distraction, in addition to the continuous growth and remodeling of the vertebral bodies during the treatment period; these two factors can affect their position within a vertebra. Two types of migration were identified in this study: one within the pedicle, with pedicle elongation, and the second through and distal to the pedicle. Apart from implant prominence, none of the patients experienced adverse clinical consequences related to this change (▶ Fig. 29.4). The study concluded that a change in distal pedicle screw position with time is a frequent occurrence in single growing rods.[3]

The third study was the first case series to use computed tomography (CT) to evaluate noninstrumented, nonfused segments of the spine in growing rod graduates with early onset scoliosis. The behavior of the growing

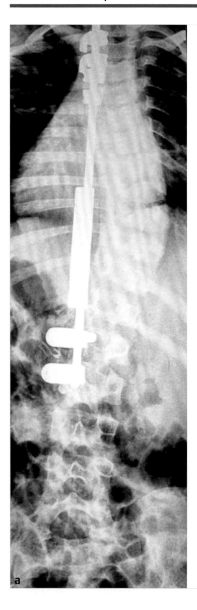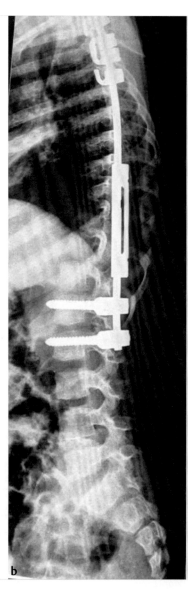

Fig. 29.2 Anteroposterior (**a**) and sagittal (**b**) views of a single rod with double claw and two pedicle screws.

spine after many years of distraction in regard to stiffness and spontaneous fusion, as well as the possibility of curve progression after maturity, remain controversial issues. This area of research is of great importance to understand not only the response of the vertebrae to long periods of serial distractions but also the need for final fusion at the end of the distraction program. In five patients younger than 9 years of age who had idiopathic early onset scoliosis, treatment was started with a single submuscular growing rod. They were evaluated more than 6 years after the index surgery, a minimum of six distractions, and a minimum of 2 years of follow-up after the last distraction with plain anteroposterior and lateral standing radiographs and with CT and sagittal, coronal, and axial reconstructions. The CT scans showed complete fusion of the facet joints at the levels studied; however, they showed severe degeneration and narrowing of the disk spaces

without complete fusion. Also noted were a disproportionate ratio of vertebral body to disk height, irregular end plates, and the overall appearance of an arthritic spine (▶ Fig. 29.5). The CT findings showed a stiff, nonmobile, fixed spine with probably little or no potential for curve progression. We concluded that after a reasonable follow-up period, growing rod graduates with satisfactory results could be treated by removing the growing rods, without the need for final fusion surgery.[4]

In 2006, the Egyptian patients who had early onset scoliosis treated with growing rods were reviewed and included in the data of the Growing Spine Study Group (GSSG), based in the United States. At present, Cairo is still the only center representing Africa and the Middle East that is included in the GSSG, which is supported by the Growing Spine Foundation. The GSSG furthers medical education and scientific research with the purpose of

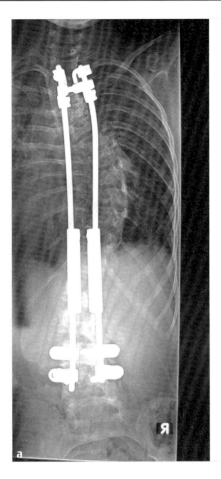
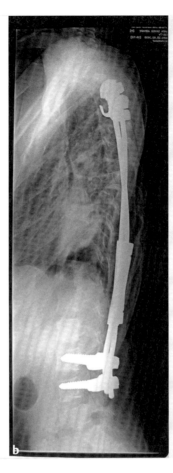

Fig. 29.3 Anteroposterior (a) and sagittal (b) views of a double rod construct.

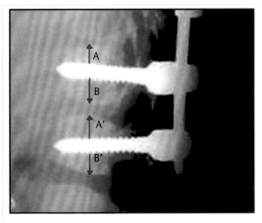

A/B=0.77
A'/B'=1.1

A/B=2
A'/B'=1.5

a

b

Fig. 29.4 Before (a) and after (b) pedicle migration.

optimizing outcomes in patients who have early onset scoliosis. This specialized study group is currently taking the lead worldwide in documenting and exploring the best strategies for the management of early onset scoliosis and is the main driving force behind most of the current research in pediatric spinal deformity.

Two landmark papers published by the GSSG looked at patients with early onset scoliosis; some of these cases

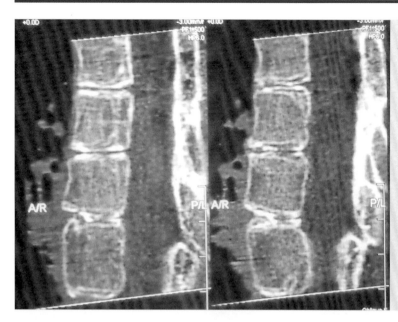

Fig. 29.5 Computed tomographic scans of a growing rod graduate.

were done in Egypt and the papers were co-authored by an Egyptian investigator. One was the first multicenter case series to evaluate the use of growing rods in congenital scoliosis. It reviewed 19 patients from the international multicenter GSSG database with progressive congenital spinal deformities who underwent growing rod surgery and had a minimum of 2 years of follow-up. The mean age at surgery was 6.9 years, the mean number of affected vertebrae per patient was 5.2, and the mean number of lengthening procedures per patient was 4.2. Spinal deformity, spinal growth, and space available for lung all improved. Complications occurred in 8 patients (42%), and there were 14 complications in 100 procedures (14%), with no neurologic complications. The study concluded that growing rods with serial distractions could reliably improve deformity correction in congenital scoliosis, enhance spinal growth (T1–S1 length), and increase space available for lung without any significant increase in the complication rate owing to the congenital nature of the deformities.[5]

Another study was the first dedicated multicenter study to evaluate the clinical and radiographic complications associated with growing rod treatment. Previous reports have indicated high rates of complications after nonfusion surgery in patients with early onset scoliosis. Between 1987 and 2005, 140 patients met the inclusion criteria and underwent a total of 897 growing rod procedures. The mean age at the initial surgery was 6 years, and the mean duration of follow-up was 5 years. Of the 140 patients, 81 (58%) had at least one complication. The authors concluded that regardless of treatment modality, the management of early onset scoliosis is prolonged; therefore, complications are frequent and should be expected. Complications can be reduced by delaying the initial implantation of growing rods if possible, using dual rods, and limiting the number of lengthening procedures. Submuscular placement reduces the complications of wounds and implant prominence and reduces the number of unplanned operations.[6]

29.2 Magnetically Controlled Growing Rods

The concept of distracting growing rods via remote control without the need for multiple surgeries has been realized with the development of the MAGEC (magnetic expansion control) Remote Control Spinal Deformity System (Ellipse Technologies, Irvine, California). MAGEC is a novel, minimally invasive implant used for the treatment of severe spinal deformities. The implant is fixed to the spine proximally and distally, and an external remote controller is used to distract the implant noninvasively. Critically, after the MAGEC rod is surgically implanted, the device is distracted with the external remote controller, so that the additional surgeries required with traditional growing rods are eliminated. Cairo was the second center worldwide to implant this novel distraction-based spinal correction device (▶ Fig. 29.6 and ▶ Fig. 29.7).

The first worldwide multicentric study to use magnetic remotely controlled growth rods, which included the patients treated in Egypt, was subsequently published in the *Journal of Spine*.[7] This was a prospective, nonrandomized study of 14 patients with a mean age of 8 years, 10 months and a mean follow-up of 10 months. The Cobb angle decreased from 60 to 34 degrees after initial surgery and was 31 degrees at latest follow-up. Complications included one superficial infection, one prominent implant, minimal loss of initial distraction in three single rods after index surgery, and partial loss of distraction in

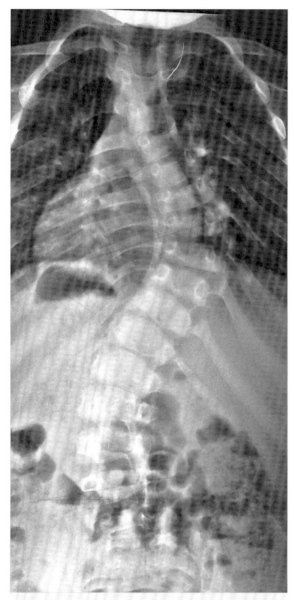

Fig. 29.6 Anteroposterior radiographs before surgery and after distraction with the MAGEC System.

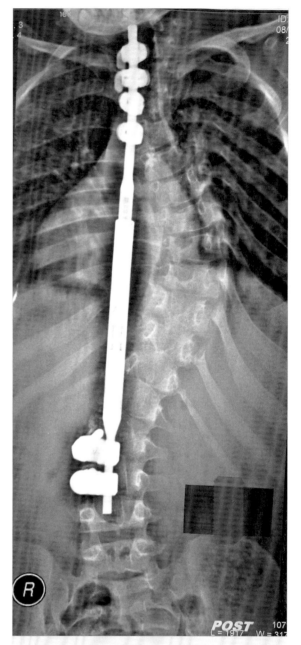

Fig. 29.7 Anteroposterior radiographs before surgery and after distraction with the MAGEC System.

14 of the 68 distractions. The authors concluded that the preliminary results indicate that the magnetically controlled growth rod is safe and provides adequate distraction similar to that of the standard growing rod.[7]

29.3 Growth-Directed Growing Rods with Apical Control

Although Egypt was one of the first countries actively involved in the development of magnetically controlled growing rods, which are now in common use in Europe and are awaiting U.S. Food and Drug Administration approval in the United States, MAGEC is not yet readily available in Egypt except for clinical trials. The difficulty of bringing this latest, relatively expensive technology to Egypt and making it available to Egyptian children with early onset scoliosis led spinal surgeons to think of alternative ideas that could avoid the need for multiple surgeries during rod distraction; the basic answer was growth-directed implants, which can be affordable and have the features required for the management of these children.

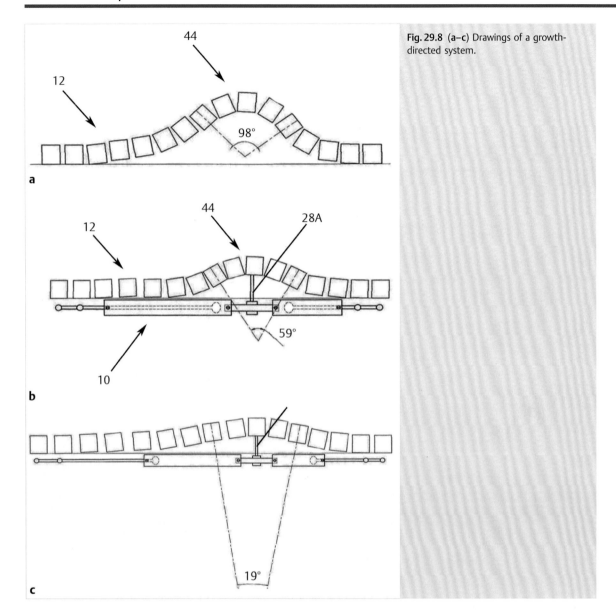

Fig. 29.8 (a–c) Drawings of a growth-directed system.

Growth-directed systems appear to be a valid alternative to remotely controlled growing rods. Multiple surgical interventions for serial rod distractions are not required with these systems because they are designed to allow spinal growth while maintaining correction. A clear advantage of these types of systems, especially in developing countries, is the reduced cost of the implants compared with the cost of more sophisticated technologies. Also avoided are the costs of the multiple surgeries and hospital admissions associated with traditional growing rods. The older versions of growth-directed systems, including the Luque trolley, were far from satisfactory because of the high rate of complications and failures associated with the technique, including minimal spinal growth, spontaneous fusion, failed implants, loss of correction, inability to control rotation, and infections. The

more recent growth-directed implants use multiple segmental pedicle screws, which allow the rod–screw contact points to slide. However, these recent systems still have many potential problems, including the following: possible autofusion after segmental exposure to insert the pedicle screws; jamming of the screw–rod junctions; limited ability to contour the rod to allow sliding; and the increased operative risk, operative time, and exposure to radiation that accompany multiple pedicle screw insertions in this very young age group. In addition, the amount of growth permitted remains questionable in comparison with traditional growth rods. In Egypt, a system was designed and developed to avoid the disadvantages of current growth-directed systems. It controls the apex of the deformity and corrects the deformity during insertion, but in addition, for the first time, it has been

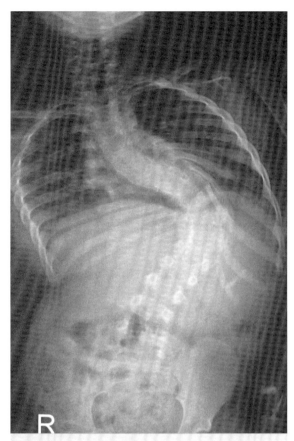

Fig. 29.9 Growth-directed system. Preoperative anteroposterior radiographs.

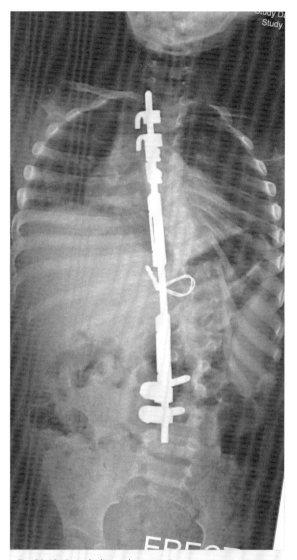

Fig. 29.10 Growth-directed system. Postoperative anteroposterior radiograph.

designed to make use of the forces of growth for distraction, thus ensuring continuous correction of the deformity as long as the child is growing and the system is applied, without the need for any further intervention (▶ Fig. 29.8).

The main idea was to design a growth-directed system that has the fewest possible points of fixation and the ability specifically to control, correct, and derotate the apex of the deformity while allowing the corrected spine to grow. In 2009, an application for a patent for this invention was submitted to the Egyptian patent office, and an Egyptian patent was granted in 2012.[8] Subsequently, a U.S. patent was granted on the 9th of September 2014.[9]

Apical control should be strong and reliable to counteract the main deforming forces at the apex and prevent its rotation and angulation. The main correction of the curve occurs when the system is inserted; then, with time and growth, the system allows longitudinal growth of the spine with additional correction of the curve. Because the distance between the rod and the apex of the deformity is fixed, any increase in the distance between the proximal and distal fixation points of the system results in a proportional decrease in the angle of the scoliosis.

The first trial in human patients started in Egypt in 2012 with promising preliminary results; this new concept is a significant step toward improving the management of children with early onset scoliosis. The system continues to correct the spine dynamically during growth and at the same time controls the apex and retains some mobility of the spine during the years of growth (▶ Fig. 29.9 and ▶ Fig. 29.10).

References

[1] Hazem B, El-Sebaie P. Instrumentation without fusion for progressive pediatric spinal deformities. J Orthop Trauma 200 5; 9: 11–17

[2] Elsebaie H, Skaggs D. Unsegmented unilateral bars: do they grow with distraction? Presented at: 14th International Meeting on Advanced Spine Techniques (IMAST); July 11–14, 2007; Paradise Island, Bahamas

[3] El-Sebaie H, Noordeen H, Akbarnia BA. Incidence, magnitude, and classification of pedicle screw migration. Presented at: Scoliosis Research Society 47th Annual Meeting and Course; September 5–8, 2012; Chicago, IL

[4] Elsebaie H, Akbarnia B. Do all growing rod graduates need final fusion? A CT study of the unfused segments. Presented at: 7th International Congress on Early Onset Scoliosis; November 21–22, 2013; San Diego, California

[5] Elsebaie HB, Yazici M, Thompson GH et al. Safety and efficacy of growing rod technique for pediatric congenital spinal deformities. J Pediatr Orthop 2011; 31: 1–5

[6] Bess S, Akbarnia BA, Thompson GH, Sponseller PD, Shah SA, Elsebaie H. Complications of growing-rod treatment for early-onset scoliosis: analysis of one hundred and forty patients. J Bone Joint Surg Am 2010; 92: 2533–2543

[7] Akbarnia BA, Cheung K, Noordeen H et al. Next generation of growth-sparing techniques: preliminary clinical results of a magnetically controlled growing rod in 14 patients with early-onset scoliosis. Spine 2013; 38: 665–670

[8] Elsebaie H, Akbarnia B, inventors. Self-expandable vertebral instrumentation system with apical deformity control. Egyptian patent EG 25692 A. Publication date: May 20, 2012

[9] Elsebaie H, Akbarnia B, inventors. Growth-directed vertebral fixation system with distractible connector(s) and apical control. United States: Publication No. US8828058 B2. Application No. US 12/873,582. Publication (Grant) date: Sep 9, 2014

30 The Oxford Experience

Jeremy C.T. Fairbank and Arvindera Ghag

Spinal deformity frequently arises in growing children with neuromuscular conditions, such as cerebral palsy, myelodysplasia, spinal muscular atrophy, Friedreich ataxia, Duchenne muscular dystrophy, traumatic paralysis, and, in the past, poliomyelitis. The incidence of deformity varies directly with the severity of neuromuscular disease and ranges from 25% in children with diplegic cerebral palsy to 100% in those with thoracic myelodysplasia or traumatic paralysis who are younger than 10 years of age. Children classified under the Gross Motor Function Classification System (GMFCS) as level 4 or 5—those who require wheeled mobility or lack head and trunk control—are most frequently found to have spinal deformity. In a 2011 review of the pediatric and young adult spinal deformity service of Scotland's National Health Service, it was estimated that 44 patients with neuromuscular scoliosis would require corrective surgery yearly, extrapolated to an annual incidence of 0.07% of the pediatric population undergoing scoliosis correction.[1] A national database study from the United States reported an incidence of neuromuscular spinal deformity of 2.5% in a cohort of nearly 18,000 patients admitted for scoliosis surgery.[2]

Deformity is often characterized by kyphosis and pelvic obliquity, rapid progression at a young age because of the early onset of the conditions, subsequent curve rigidity, and limited patient mobility. There is a pattern of long, *c*-shaped thoracolumbar curves related to the early onset of deformity or of lumbar curves related to a later onset. The risk for progression of deformity is extremely high because of neuromuscular imbalance and is modified by growth. Natural history studies have reported ranges of curve progression from 7 to 40 degrees.[3,4,5] A Japanese study of the natural history of untreated scoliosis in patients with spastic cerebral palsy found that risk factors for progression included a curve with a magnitude of 40 degrees before the age of 15 years, total-body-involvement cerebral palsy, bedridden status, and a thoracolumbar curve.[6] Other factors related to curve progression include early onset and evolution of neuromuscular disease, skeletal immaturity, and severe weakness. Peak skeletal growth is associated with the greatest progression of deformity, as in idiopathic scoliosis. Unlike the deformity in idiopathic scoliosis, however, a neuromuscular deformity is likely to progress after skeletal maturity.

30.1 Management and Complications

Nonoperative management of neuromuscular spinal deformity is indicated as soon as deformity is detected in an attempt to prevent progression. Braces may be used to slow curve progression and improve sitting posture in skeletally immature patients with flexible curves.[7,8] When a brace is chosen, it is imperative to consider the neuromuscular patient's poor motor control, skin sensation, respiratory function, and nutritional status. Because these patients are often mobilized in manually operated or power-assisted chairs, moulded or modular seating within the chair is indicated. The seat and chair are frequently reassessed for modification as the spinal deformity progresses.

Although the traditional indication for operative management in neuromuscular scoliosis is deformity greater than 50 degrees with rapid progression, it is much more important to consider how the patient's overall function, or lack thereof, is affected by progressive deformity. Indeed, Cobb angles become increasingly difficult to measure in weight-bearing films as the magnitude of deformity increases and some curves collapse. It is critical to consider factors such as comfortable sitting with independence and balance, positioning for upper extremity use, and cardiopulmonary compromise. Pain and discomfort secondary to spinal deformity are also factors that persuade families to proceed to surgery. For some, cosmesis is an issue that encourages surgical correction of deformity.

The means to achieve spinal fusion in neuromuscular deformity have evolved over recent decades. Segmental spinal instrumentation with pedicle screws from the upper thoracic spine to the pelvis appears to be the currently accepted method of fixation and has replaced traditional alternatives, such as Harrington rods, Luque–Galveston instrumentation, and Unit rod instrumentation. The outcomes of these fusion techniques are discussed below, with an emphasis on complications rather than the benefits of specific instrumentation systems.

Lonstein and Akbarnia reported on a series of 107 patients who had neuromuscular deformities treated either with cast correction and posterior fusion followed by prolonged supine immobilization, posterior fusion, and Harrington instrumentation, or with combined anterior and posterior fusion and instrumentation followed by short supine immobilization.[9] Functional outcome was worse in one patient, unchanged in 82 patients, and improved in 24 patients. The complication rate was exceedingly high, at 81%; the most frequent complications included pressure sores, wounds, and instrumentation problems. The pseudarthrosis rate was 17%, and the infection rate was 5%. There were three deaths, and one patient was rendered paraplegic. Despite these outcomes, the authors concluded that surgery was still of benefit in these patients.

Comstock et al. reported the results of a series of 79 patients with total-body-involvement spastic cerebral palsy who underwent posterior Luque instrumentation, anterior spinal fusion, or both.[10] Late progression of deformity, pelvic obliquity, or decompensation occurred in more than 30% of the patients, and 21% of these patients required revision procedures to address the progression. Most of the patients were skeletally immature at the time of surgery and underwent posterior fusion only, whereas those without progression underwent combined anterior and posterior fusion. The results of questionnaires administered to caregivers and parents revealed that 85% were satisfied with results of surgery, including improvements in sitting ability, physical appearance, ease of care, and comfort.

Tsirikos et al retrospectively reviewed 241 patients with cerebral palsy who underwent posterior or combined anterior and posterior fusion with Unit rod instrumentation at a single institution performed by one of two surgeons.[11] Satisfactory corrections of coronal deformity and pelvic obliquity were achieved. In posterior-only procedures, the average blood loss was 2.8 L, the intensive care unit (ICU) stay was 4.9 days, and the hospital stay was 19.6 days. In combined procedures, the average blood loss was 3.4 L, the ICU stay was 6.7 days, and the hospital stay was 24.5 days. Major complications included three perioperative deaths and 18 deep wound infections (7.5%). A survey of caretakers reported a 96% satisfaction rate.

Lonstein et al reported an early complication rate of 58% in a series of 93 patients with cerebral palsy who underwent spinal fusion for neuromuscular deformity with Luque–Galveston instrumentation.[12] The infection rate was 1.1%, and the pseudarthrosis rate was 7.5%. The length of stay was statistically significantly increased, from 7 to 9 days, in patients who experienced one complication.

A review of the Scoliosis Research Society morbidity and mortality database by Reames et al revealed 1,971 complications in 19,360 patients with pediatric scoliosis of all etiologies.[13] The complication rate for the correction of neuromuscular scoliosis was significantly higher, at 17.9%, than the complication rate for the correction of scoliosis of all other etiologies. The rate of neurologic deficit in this population was 1.1%, and mortality was 0.3%.

Piazzolla et al reported the results of Cotrel–Dubousset instrumentation and posterior spinal fusion in 24 consecutive patients with neuromuscular scoliosis.[14] Satisfactory corrections of coronal deformity, sagittal imbalance, and pelvic obliquity were achieved. The mean intraoperative blood loss was 2.1 L, major complications affected 8.3% of patients, and one postoperative death occurred.

Modi et al reported the results of all pedicle screw construct posterior spinal fusion procedures in a series of 18 patients with paralytic neuromuscular scoliosis and poor pulmonary function, defined as preoperative forced vital capacity (FVC) of less than 30%.[15] Satisfactory corrections of coronal scoliosis and pelvic obliquity were achieved. There was a subtle decrease in the FVC at 6 weeks postoperatively and a significant decrease at the mean final follow-up of 32 months (from 25.2% preoperatively to 20.6% at follow-up). The forced expiratory volume in 1 second (FEV_1) also significantly decreased in a similar manner. The perioperative complication rate was 44.4%, including five pulmonary complications and one intraoperative death. Granata et al reported similar results in a series of 30 patients with Duchenne muscular dystrophy.[16] Head control was lost in 14 patients who developed severe extension contractures of the neck. There was one death due to cardiac arrest. The mean preoperative FVC was 57%, and this decreased to 34% at 4-year follow-up. Still, more than 90% of parents reported that they would again give their consent for operative intervention.

30.2 Intraoperative Blood Loss

Evidence on the application of blood-sparing techniques in spine surgery has historically been derived from the field of cardiac surgery, with the bulk of the literature considering hemodynamic methods, such as hypotensive anesthesia and planned autologous donation.[17] However, the efficacy of these methods has been reported rarely in spinal surgery, and not at all in pediatric spinal deformity surgery. An extensive review of the literature on blood loss in pediatric spine surgery revealed significantly higher rates of blood loss in neuromuscular scoliosis correction than in adolescent idiopathic scoliosis correction.[18] Mean ranges of blood loss were 1,300 to 2,200 mL in patients with cerebral palsy treated with posterior approaches, 2,500 to 4,000 mL in patients with Duchenne muscular dystrophy, and 2,000 to 3,500 mL in studies that pooled data for all patients with neuromuscular disorders. Blood loss was also shown to be progressively greater in patients having larger numbers of vertebral levels incorporated into the fusion, having posterior fusions vs. anterior fusions, and having both anterior and posterior fusions.

Modern blood-sparing techniques in spinal surgery have been increasingly applied to pediatric spinal deformity surgery. The use of antifibrinolytics was recently reported in 12% of 1,547 neuromuscular scoliosis correction procedures over nearly 4 years at 37 U.S. children's hospitals.[19] However, the median hospital-specific rate of red cell transfusions was 43%, and antifibrinolytic use was not associated with a decrease in the odds of a red cell transfusion requirement. Nevertheless, a matched-cohort therapeutic comparative study reported by Dhawale et al demonstrated significantly less intraoperative blood loss in a group of patients with scoliosis secondary to cerebral palsy who received antifibrinolytics and consequently less cell salvage transfusion.[20] Although no significant differences were found in total transfusion requirements, a trend toward decreased hospital stay was found in the group that received antifibrinolytics.

As demonstrated above, a high complication rate for neuromuscular scoliosis correction has been reported; the range in rates is likely attributable to how *complication* is defined in each study. Nevertheless, the rates of infection, pseudarthrosis, late progression of deformity, intraoperative blood loss, and perioperative mortality are far higher than what is considered acceptable for an intervention that is meant to improve quality of life. Furthermore, the finding of further compromise in respiratory function postoperatively is interesting and contradictory to the classic indication of deformity correction to preserve cardiopulmonary function. Although the reported rate of satisfaction with scoliosis correction among caregivers and parents is high, presumably an inverse relationship between satisfaction rate and complication rate exists.

30.3 Patient Comorbidity

The typical patient with spastic cerebral palsy has a host of comorbidities involving multiple organ systems.[21] Neurologic conditions often include epilepsy, visual and hearing impairments, cognitive dysfunction, and sleeping and pain disorders. Patients often have gastrointestinal motility dysfunction leading to gastroesophageal reflux, delayed gastric emptying, and constipation. Oropharyngeal dysphagia makes oral feeding difficult, and impaired swallowing is associated with a risk for aspiration, so that many children are fed via an endoscopically placed percutaneous gastrostomy tube. Nutrition and growth are impaired by decreased caloric intake and must be monitored by a medical practitioner or nutritionist. Chronic pulmonary conditions include recurrent pneumonia, atelectasis, bronchiectasis, and restrictive lung disease. Frequent urologic conditions include voiding dysfunction, retention, incontinence, and urinary tract infection. These multiple medical comorbidities have obvious effects on life expectancy and must be appropriately addressed preoperatively in the patient with neuromuscular scoliosis. The studies summarized below have explored these issues in greater detail.

Tsirikos et al studied the life expectancy of 288 patients with severe spastic cerebral palsy after neuromuscular scoliosis correction and found the mean predicted survival after surgery to be 11 years.[22] Factors negatively affecting the survival rate were a high number of days in intensive care postoperatively and thoracic hyperkyphosis. Factors that did not affect survival included sex, age at surgery, level of ambulation, cognitive ability, degree of coronal plane spinal deformity, amount of intraoperative blood loss, surgical time, and number of days in the hospital. Cardiopulmonary function and postoperative complications apparently were not studied as risk factors.

Erickson and Baulesh conducted a literature review on the topic of preoperative optimization by identifying relevant comorbidities and placing patients with neuromuscular scoliosis on appropriate care pathways.[23] Risk factors associated with perioperative and postoperative complications included the following: seizure disorders, decreased cognitive ability, poor pulmonary status, restrictive lung disease, history of frequent pneumonias, sleep apnea, malnutrition, cardiac disease, immunocompromise, low social status, poor ambulatory status, and a complex procedure. Along the same theme, Miller et al analyzed a treatment protocol emphasizing perioperative work-up to compare surgical outcomes before and after its implementation.[24] Significant reductions in the overall length of stay, ICU length of stay, and perioperative complication rate were observed in the patient group managed according to the protocol.

Almenrader and Patel conducted a study to determine risk factors for postoperative ventilation in patients with nonidiopathic scoliosis.[25] The rate of postoperative ventilation was 23.8%, with postoperative ventilation having been planned preoperatively for half of the patients, and 40% of the patients with Duchenne muscular dystrophy required postoperative ventilation. An increased tendency for children with Duchenne muscular dystrophy and those with a preoperative FVC below 30% to require postoperative ventilation was observed. Abu-Kishk et al performed a similar study to determine possible associations with prolonged mechanical ventilation postoperatively and found an odds ratio of 31.25 when postoperative mechanical ventilation was correlated with neuromuscular scoliosis correction.[26]

It is critical to discuss the factors mentioned here with patients' families during the preoperative assessment because the perioperative expectations must be guided realistically. Multidisciplinary team involvement is accepted as the standard of care for these complex patients in order to anticipate potential complications and ensure that the patient is in an optimal physiologic state before undergoing surgery.

30.4 Outcomes Measurement

The assessment of surgical outcomes in patients with neuromuscular scoliosis has traditionally been dominated by radiographic measures of curve correction and pelvic obliquity, or the documentation of postoperative complications. Recently, interest has been shown in studying the effect of deformity correction on quality of life; however, no accepted, reliable, and validated outcomes instrument is available to capture this entity. A systematic review of measures of activities of daily living for children with cerebral palsy revealed the Pediatric Evaluation of Disability Inventory (PEDI) to have the strongest psychometric properties, and the Assessment of Motor and Process Skills (AMPS) to be the most comprehensive evaluation of underlying motor and cognitive abilities.[27] However, these tools have not been used to assess outcomes of neuromuscular deformity correction, perhaps in part because further research is required to determine their reliability and stability in this particular patient population. Bagó et al published a literature review of health-related quality of life and disease-specific instruments used to assess scoliosis surgery.[28] The SF-36 (Short Form [36] Health Survey) and the EuroQol EQ-5D have been used to assess generic health-related quality of life, and the SRS-22 (Scoliosis Research Society-22) Patient Questionnaire and QLPSD (Quality of Life Profile for Spinal Deformities) have been used as disease-specific instruments. These have been complemented more recently with the use of instruments to assess a single aspect of spinal deformity, such as perception of trunk deformity and body image or effects of brace use. However, these tools have been used and partially validated only in patients with adolescent idiopathic scoliosis, and none has been sufficiently validated and analyzed in the population of patients with nonidiopathic scoliosis.

Ersberg and Gerdhem used EQ-5D and SRS-22r outcome instruments to report the effect of spinal fusion for neuromuscular scoliosis in 32 patients.[29] At 2-year follow-up, both tools demonstrated statistically significant improvements (EQ-5D score increased 0.15 points, SRS-22r score increased 0.5 points) in quality of life for the cohort. To our knowledge, this is the only published paper that has used these robust measures for quality of life in this patient population. However, it is imperative to note that both the EQ-5D and SRS-22-r indices have not been validated in patients with neuromuscular scoliosis.

Watanabe et al conducted a retrospective study to assess the satisfaction of patients with spastic cerebral palsy and their parents with the results of spinal fusion.[30] Questionnaires were designed to assess expectations, cosmesis, function, patient care, quality of life, pulmonary function, pain, health status, self-image, and satisfaction. Responses were obtained from 84 patients and families with an average follow-up of just over 6 years. The overall satisfaction rate was 92%, and a similar proportion of respondents reported improved sitting balance and cosmesis, whereas 71% reported improved quality of life. Functional improvements were relatively limited, but 8 to 40% still perceived the surgical results as improvement. When the respondents were divided into "satisfied" and "less satisfied" groups, the less satisfied group was observed to have a higher rate of late complications, less major curve correction, and hyperlordosis of the lumbar spine postoperatively. Lumbar hyperlordosis is known to be associated with severe back pain, superior mesenteric artery syndrome, malnourishment, loss of bowel and bladder control, and difficulty with sitting balance. One of the chief reasons for satisfaction was the achievement of expectations; in this case, expectations most commonly were to "prevent progression of deformity" and "prevent cardiopulmonary problems." This finding is in contrast to those of previous studies, which reported improved appearance and improved sitting balance as common expectations.

Obid et al performed a similar retrospective questionnaire study of 32 patients with an average of 3 years of follow-up.[31] Patients and/or their caregivers strongly agreed with statements that quality of life was improved, they were satisfied with surgery, and that expectations were fulfilled. Cassidy et al used a health care worker questionnaire to assess the impact of spinal fusion on patients with severe cerebral palsy with regard to comfort, function, health, and ease of nursing care.[32] When 17 patients who had scoliosis of 35 degrees and underwent fusion were compared with 20 patients who had scoliosis of 76 degrees and did not undergo fusion, no differences were found in any of the parameters except for comfort; the majority of health care workers believed that the patients with fusion were more comfortable. These findings must be tempered by the lack of reported studies on the correlation of caregiver perceptions of discomfort with patients' actual perceptions of pain.

Tsirikos et al compared 190 parents' and 122 professional caretakers' perceptions of functional outcome after spinal fusion in patients with spastic cerebral palsy.[33] Both groups reported a positive impact of surgery on patients' overall function, quality of life, and ease of care. Parents appreciated improvement in appearance, whereas educators and therapists acknowledged improvement in gross and oral motor function. Most parents (95.8%) and caretakers (84.3%) said they would recommend spine surgery.

The majority of reports of caregiver satisfaction after spinal fusion for neuromuscular scoliosis have been retrospective in nature, hence introducing bias. Jones et al reported the results of POSNA (Pediatric Orthopaedic Society of North America) outcomes questionnaires prospectively administered to 20 parents preoperatively, 6 months, and 1 year after spinal fusion.[34] No significant changes were found between preoperative and postoperative assessments of physical function, school absence, co-morbidities, and parental health. Patient pain and frequency of feeling sick and tired decreased, patient happiness increased, and parental satisfaction improved significantly by 1 year postoperatively. The presence of complications did not significantly affect results. The authors concluded that subjective gains noted in previous retrospective studies were substantiated by these prospective results.

A standardized, reliable, and validated outcomes instrument for patients with neuromuscular scoliosis would enhance our understanding of the effect of spinal deformity correction. Ideally, such a tool would encompass surgical outcomes and effects on patient quality of life simultaneously, allowing data to be communicated and extrapolated on an international scale.

30.5 Economic Considerations

Modern health care systems are burdened by increasing costs of care, so that clinicians are pressured to choose more cost-effective methods of care provision whenever possible. A review of a U.S. nationwide inpatient database revealed that surgery for neuromuscular scoliosis was associated with increased hospital length of stay (10.3 vs. 7.7 days) and increased hospitalization expenditures ($80,251 vs. $62,154) in comparison with surgery for idiopathic scoliosis.[2] A retrospective review to assess the hospital and operating room costs of 74 patients with neuromuscular scoliosis who mostly underwent posterior pedicle screw instrumentation and spinal fusion revealed a total surgical cost of about $50,000, with an average length of hospitalization of 8 days.[35] The highest individual cost was for implants (24% of total costs), and the second highest was for inpatient room and intensive care (22%). Independent predictors of higher cost were more severe major and minor structural curves, higher total number of levels fused, and longer hospital stay. No reported studies have examined the indirect costs associated with the management of patients with neuromuscular scoliosis, such as the costs of manual and powered wheelchairs, orthoses, multiple visits to medical experts, and caregiver burden and loss of opportunity.

30.6 Alternative Approaches to Management

It is interesting that the approach to managing neuromuscular spinal deformity has gone largely unchanged for decades, especially in the setting of a medically complex and frail patient population and a history of exceedingly high rates of surgical complications, major intraoperative blood loss, and perioperative morbidity and mortality. Apart from modifications to the instrumentation techniques, as for idiopathic scoliosis, posterior spinal fusion remains the treatment of choice. In patients who have severe neuromuscular disease with a GMFCS level of 4 or higher, the construct is recommended to span from the pelvis to the upper thoracic spine. Research efforts have historically been focused on providing evidence of curve correction and restoration of pelvic obliquity, but recent reports emphasizing effects on patient quality of life have not confirmed the importance of cosmesis and sitting balance.

Advances have been made in the management of young children with early onset idiopathic scoliosis. We have learned that early definitive spinal fusion has been fraught with complications requiring revision surgery in up to 40% of cases, and that restrictive pulmonary disease may result.[36] These findings may be extrapolated to the population of patients with neuromuscular scoliosis, and thus the application of growing constructs has gained favor, with a wide variability in construct choice and levels of instrumentation.[37] The vertical expandable prosthetic titanium rib (VEPTR) has been used to control neuromuscular deformity, and early reports have demonstrated its radiographic success as a spine-to-spine and rib-to-pelvis growing rod construct.[38,39] Similarly, a single submuscular growing rod construct has been shown to control deformity effectively while allowing the spine to continue growing in a cohort including patients with neuromuscular scoliosis.[40] Further research into skeletal maturity will be required to substantiate these reports, but they represent thoughtful strategies in managing neuromuscular deformity while attempting to minimize perioperative co-morbidity and complications.

30.7 Limited Staged Fusion

It has been our observation that neuromuscular curves treated with extended periods of bracing or casting pending skeletal maturity often become rigid and at times partially fused, interfering with correction at the time of definitive spinal fusion. Correction of these deformities requires segmental instrumentation from the upper thoracic spine to the pelvis and multilevel osteotomies, both of which entail prolonged surgical time and increased blood loss. Furthermore, blood loss becomes increasingly difficult to control during the later stages of the operation, probably because of increasingly disordered coagulation. Excessive blood loss appears to be related to a number of complications, including prolonged hospital and ICU stays. To mitigate these adverse factors in a complex and frail patient population, and given that the objective of operative intervention is primarily spinal stabilization rather than spectacular deformity correction, a novel approach of limited spinal fusion has been introduced in our institution.

The premise of this approach is to stabilize the spine in a staged and "least invasive as possible" fashion. The anesthesiologist and surgeon preoperatively agree on an upper limit for blood loss; usually, this is calculated as 40% of the estimated blood volume. The first stage is to anesthetize the patient successfully, and the second is to stabilize him or her in a prone position. In this stage, the lumbar spine and pelvis are exposed sufficiently to be instrumented with pelvic and pedicle screws and for bone to be grafted. Blood loss is then evaluated, and if the patient is hemodynamically stable with acceptable blood loss, the operation proceeds to the next stage. Here, the upper thoracic spine is exposed sufficiently for a minimum of six pedicle screws to be inserted and for bone to be grafted. The next stage is to insert precontoured rods, which are tunneled submuscularly from proximal to distal fixation points and secured. Limited in situ contouring may be performed. If, at the end of any stage, blood loss is deemed to be too great, the procedure is terminated at that point and a second procedure is planned once the patient returns to baseline physiology; in most cases, this is 7 to 10 days later. Preoperative and intraoperative communication with both the anesthesiology and blood salvage teams is critical to this approach to ensure that accurate measurements of blood loss are made.

This unconventional approach has some drawbacks. There is an obvious risk for pseudarthrosis and implant failure, which require revision surgery. However, this risk is tempered by our belief that in children with a GMFCS level of 4 or 5, the axial spine is not loaded as much as in fully active children. Thus, there exists the distinct possibility that the fused proximal and distal segments with the intervening rod and the stiff or even spontaneously fused scoliotic spine may resist failure. The patient and patient's family must be warned of this potential complication and the risk for required revision surgery, which may involve exposure of the region of the spine where the rods have broken and where a pseudarthrosis has been identified. Such rod fracture occurred on one occasion, and in earlier cases, in which we used proximally tapered rods, they were more likely to fail. Another drawback is the potential for the need of an additional anesthetic if the primary procedure is abandoned because of increased blood loss. This situation occurred in one patient in our series, and hemostasis was meticulous during the remainder of the procedures. Nevertheless, it is our feeling that administering a second anesthetic for the completion of second-stage surgery in a physiologically resuscitated patient is a better option than proceeding under potentially pathologic hemostatic conditions and risking hazardous blood loss.

30.8 Case Presentations

30.8.1 Case 1

A girl with severe global developmental delay, hypotonia, and central apnea who walked independently, thus GMFCS level 2, presented at the age of 11 years and 9 months. She had a collapsing thoracolumbar curve with a Cobb angle of 113 degrees, pelvic obliquity of 22 degrees (▶ Fig. 30.1), and sagittal hypokyphosis (▶ Fig. 30.2) preoperatively. Supine bending radiographs revealed a rigid thoracic curve with a Cobb angle of 97 degrees (▶ Fig. 30.3) and a flexible lumbar curve (▶ Fig. 30.4). The patient was managed with the limited fusion approach; her lumbar spine was instrumented from L3 to L5 (▶ Fig. 30.5 and ▶ Fig. 30.6) and her thoracic spine from T2 to T5 (▶ Fig. 30.7 and ▶ Fig. 30.8), followed by submuscular placement of a tunneled rod and bone grafting. Follow-up radiographs at 1 and 3 years demonstrate

satisfactory correction of the coronal deformity with a Cobb angle of 60 degrees, pelvic obliquity of 17 degrees, and restoration of her sagittal profile (▶ Fig. 30.9, ▶ Fig. 30.10, ▶ Fig. 30.11, ▶ Fig. 30.12). She continues to walk independently and has had no postoperative complications.

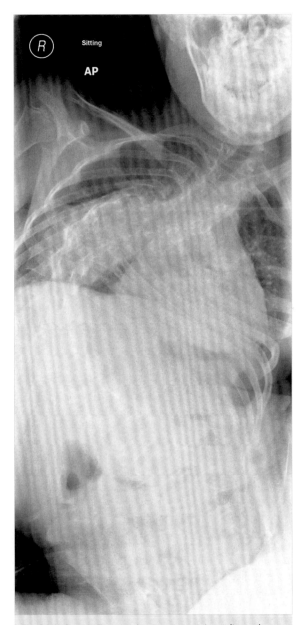

Fig. 30.1 Case 1: Preoperative anteroposterior radiograph demonstrating collapsing thoracolumbar scoliosis with a Cobb angle of 113 degrees and pelvic obliquity of 22 degrees.

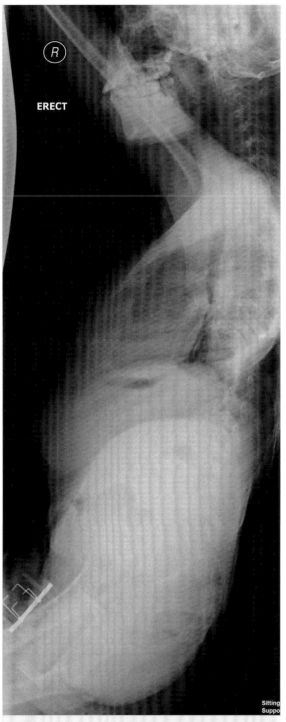

Fig. 30.2 Case 1: Preoperative lateral radiograph demonstrating global sagittal hypokyphosis.

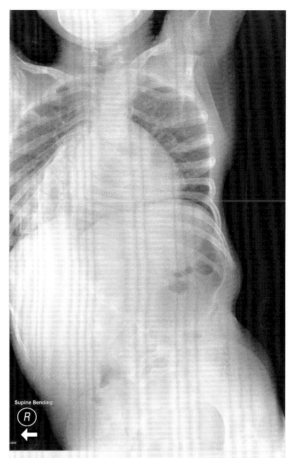

Fig. 30.3 Case 1: Preoperative supine bending radiograph demonstrating a rigid thoracic curve with a Cobb angle of 97 degrees.

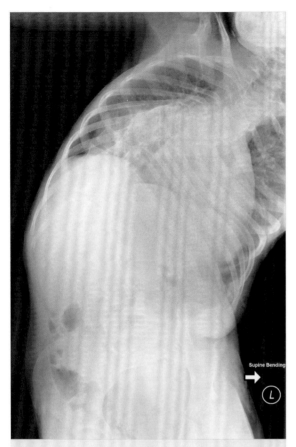

Fig. 30.4 Case 1: Preoperative supine bending radiograph demonstrating a flexible lumbar curve.

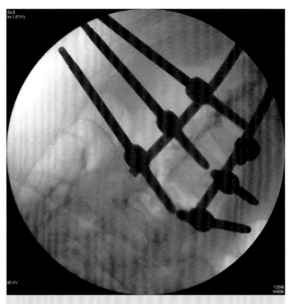

Fig. 30.5 Case 1: Intraoperative anteroposterior fluoroscopic image demonstrating selective lumbar instrumentation from L3 to L5.

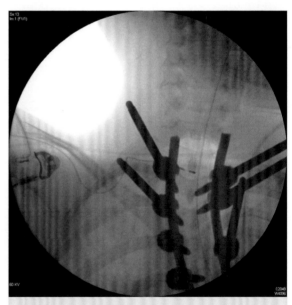

Fig. 30.7 Case 1: Intraoperative anteroposterior fluoroscopic image demonstrating selective thoracic instrumentation from T2 to T5.

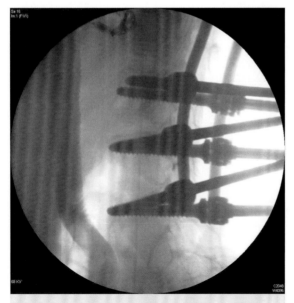

Fig. 30.6 Case 1: Intraoperative lateral fluoroscopic image demonstrating selective lumbar instrumentation from L3 to L5.

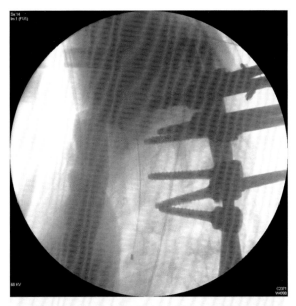

Fig. 30.8 Case 1: Intraoperative lateral fluoroscopic image demonstrating selective thoracic instrumentation from T2 to T5.

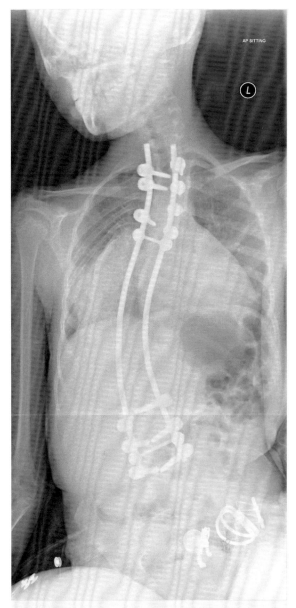

Fig. 30.9 Case 1: Anteroposterior radiograph at 1 year post-operatively demonstrating thoracolumbar stabilization with a Cobb angle of 60 degrees and pelvic obliquity of 17 degrees.

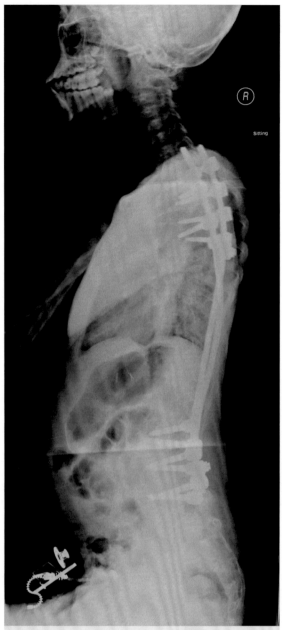

Fig. 30.10 Case 1: Lateral radiograph at 1 year postoperatively demonstrating satisfactory restoration of sagittal kyphosis.

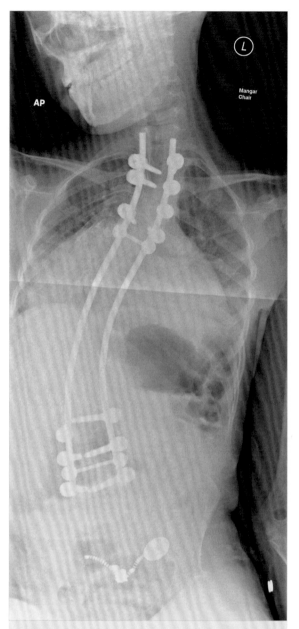

Fig. 30.11 Case 1: Anteroposterior radiograph at 3 years postoperatively demonstrating thoracolumbar stabilization with a maintained Cobb angle of 60 degrees and pelvic obliquity of 17 degrees.

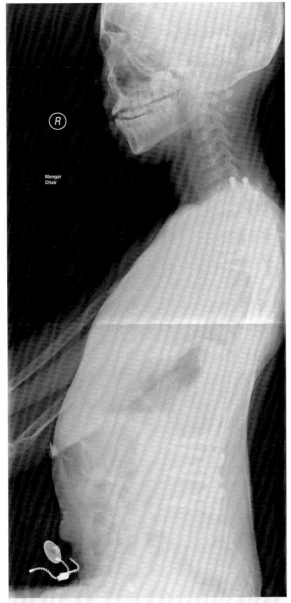

Fig. 30.12 Case 1: Lateral radiograph at 3 years postoperatively demonstrating a maintained neutral sagittal profile.

30.8.2 Case 2

A girl with total-body spastic quadriplegic cerebral palsy, GMFCS level 5, presented at the age of 11 years and 3 months with thoracolumbar scoliosis. She had global developmental delay, microcephaly, seizure disorder, visual impairment, cognitive dysfunction, and extremity

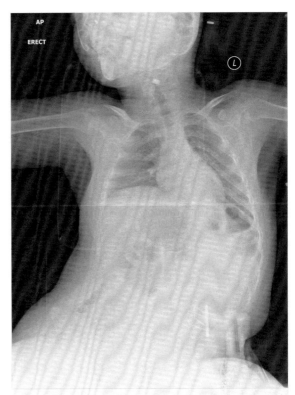

Fig. 30.13 Case 2: Preoperative anteroposterior radiograph demonstrating thoracolumbar scoliosis with a Cobb angle of 63 degrees and pelvic obliquity of 13 degrees.

involvement, and she was fed via a percutaneous endoscopic gastrostomy tube. Her preoperative coronal Cobb angle measured 63 degrees, her pelvic obliquity was 13 degrees (▶ Fig. 30.13), and her sagittal profile was normal (▶ Fig. 30.14). She was managed with the limited fusion approach. Her lumbopelvic instrumentation spanned from L2 to S1 with iliac bolts (▶ Fig. 30.15, ▶ Fig. 30.16, ▶ Fig. 30.17). Her upper thoracic spine could not be instrumented with pedicle screws, so sublaminar wires were placed segmentally from T2 to T4. Follow-up radiographs at 1 and 2 years demonstrate satisfactory correction of the coronal deformity with a Cobb angle of 37 degrees, pelvic obliquity of 3 degrees, and a normal sagittal profile (▶ Fig. 30.18, ▶ Fig. 30.19, ▶ Fig. 30.20, ▶ Fig. 30.21). Her postoperative course was complicated by a lumbar deep wound infection requiring débridement, washout, soft tissue reconstruction, and prolonged antibiotic prophylaxis. She continues to do well 4 years postoperatively, and her family is satisfied with the deformity correction.

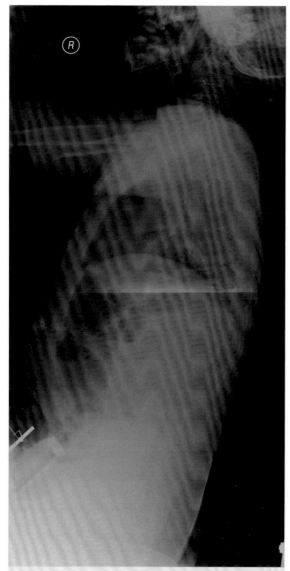

Fig. 30.14 Case 2: Preoperative lateral radiograph demonstrating a normal sagittal profile.

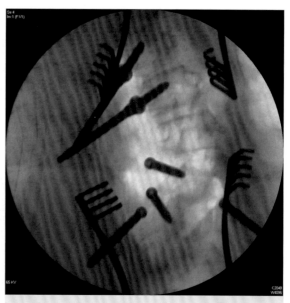

Fig. 30.15 Case 2: Intraoperative anteroposterior fluoroscopic image demonstrating unilateral selective lumbar instrumentation from L2 to S1 and the ilium.

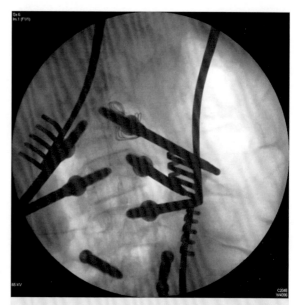

Fig. 30.16 Case 2: Intraoperative anteroposterior fluoroscopic image demonstrating completed bilateral selective lumbar instrumentation from L2 to S1.

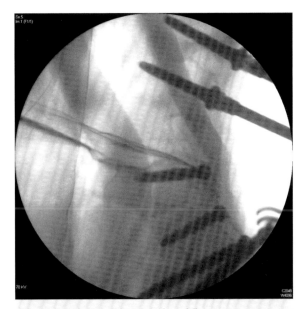

Fig. 30.17 Case 2: Intraoperative lateral fluoroscopic image demonstrating selective lumbar instrumentation from L2 to S1 and the ilium.

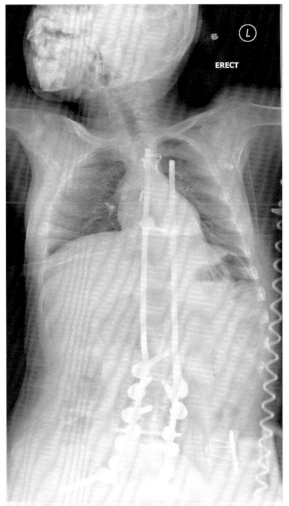

Fig. 30.18 Case 2: Anteroposterior radiograph at 1 year post-operatively demonstrating upper thoracic (sublaminar wire fixation) to pelvic stabilization with a Cobb angle of 37 degrees and pelvic obliquity of 3 degrees.

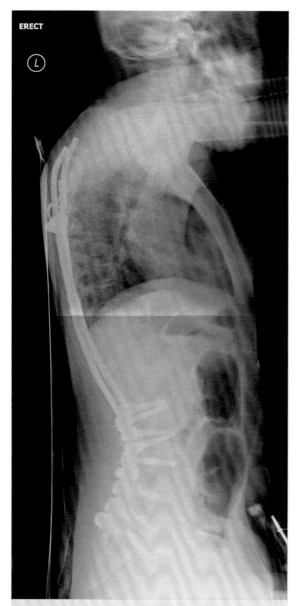

Fig. 30.19 Case 2: Lateral radiograph at 1 year postoperatively demonstrating a maintained neutral sagittal profile.

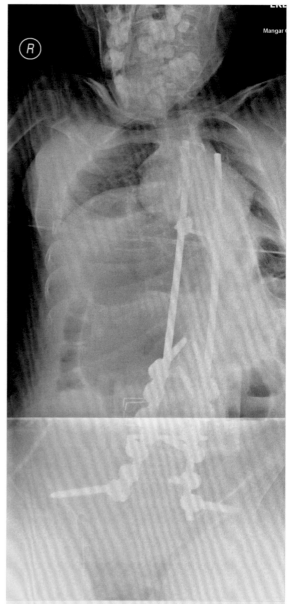

Fig. 30.20 Case 2: Anteroposterior radiograph at 2 years postoperatively demonstrating upper thoracic to pelvic stabilization with a maintained Cobb angle of 37 degrees and pelvic obliquity of 3 degrees.

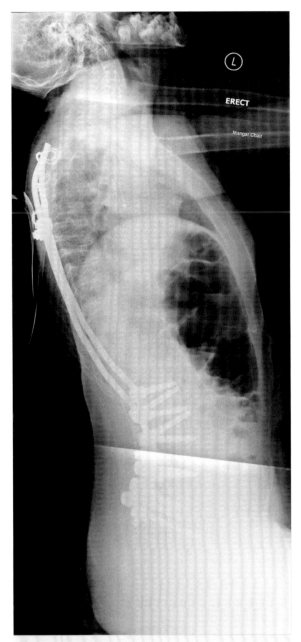

Fig. 30.21 Case 2: Lateral radiograph at 2 years postoperatively demonstrating a maintained neutral sagittal profile.

30.9 Conclusion

Pediatric patients with neuromuscular scoliosis are medically complex and require multidisciplinary care. The management of spinal deformity is challenging, as the definitive procedure is fraught with a high rate of perioperative morbidity and mortality. Little has changed during recent years with respect to the technology for spinal deformity correction in this patient population. Furthermore, a standardized and robust quality-of-life

outcome measurement has yet to be developed to enhance our understanding of the effect of surgery on these patients. Our recently applied surgical technique aims to minimize perioperative morbidity and simultaneously achieve spinal stabilization. A series of patients who have undergone the limited fusion approach is nearing 2-year clinical and radiographic follow-up, and we look forward to publishing a compilation of the results and quality-of-life data. The future in neuromuscular scoliosis corrective surgery likely holds the promise of less invasive measures to achieve stabilization; perhaps the limited fusion approach will help make these measures a reality.

References

[1] Review of the paediatric and young adult spinal deformity service. Edinburgh, United Kingdom: National Services Division, NHS Scotland; February 2011

[2] Barsdorf AI, Sproule DM, Kaufmann P. Scoliosis surgery in children with neuromuscular disease: findings from the US National Inpatient Sample, 1997 to 2003. Arch Neurol 2010; 67: 231–235

[3] Hart DA, McDonald CM. Spinal deformity in progressive neuromuscular disease. Natural history and management. Phys Med Rehabil Clin N Am 1998; 9: 213–232, viii

[4] Lindseth RE. Spine deformity in myelomeningocele. Instr Course Lect 1991; 40: 273–279

[5] Majd ME, Muldowny DS, Holt RT. Natural history of scoliosis in the institutionalized adult cerebral palsy population. Spine 1997; 22: 1461–1466

[6] Saito N, Ebara S, Ohotsuka K, Kumeta H, Takaoka K. Natural history of scoliosis in spastic cerebral palsy. Lancet 1998; 351: 1687–1692

[7] Miller A, Temple T, Miller F. Impact of orthoses on the rate of scoliosis progression in children with cerebral palsy. J Pediatr Orthop 1996; 16: 332–335

[8] Olafsson Y, Saraste H, Al-Dabbagh Z. Brace treatment in neuromuscular spine deformity. J Pediatr Orthop 1999; 19: 376–379

[9] Lonstein JE, Akbarnia A. Operative treatment of spinal deformities in patients with cerebral palsy or mental retardation. An analysis of one hundred and seven cases. J Bone Joint Surg Am 1983; 65: 43–55

[10] Comstock CP, Leach J, Wenger DR. Scoliosis in total-body-involvement cerebral palsy. Analysis of surgical treatment and patient and caregiver satisfaction. Spine 1998; 23: 1412–1424, discussion 1424–1425

[11] Tsirikos AI, Lipton G, Chang WN, Dabney KW, Miller F. Surgical correction of scoliosis in pediatric patients with cerebral palsy using the unit rod instrumentation. Spine 2008; 33: 1133–1140

[12] Lonstein JE, Koop SE, Novachek TF, Perra JH. Results and complications after spinal fusion for neuromuscular scoliosis in cerebral palsy and static encephalopathy using luque galveston instrumentation: experience in 93 patients. Spine 2012; 37: 583–591

[13] Reames DL, Smith JS, Fu KM et al. Scoliosis Research Society Morbidity and Mortality Committee. Complications in the surgical treatment of 19,360 cases of pediatric scoliosis: a review of the Scoliosis Research Society Morbidity and Mortality database. Spine 2011; 36: 1484–1491

[14] Piazzolla A, Solarino G, De Giorgi S, Mori CM, Moretti L, De Giorgi G. Cotrel-Dubousset instrumentation in neuromuscular scoliosis. Eur Spine J 2011; 20 Suppl 1: S75–S84

[15] Modi HN, Suh SW, Hong JY, Park YH, Yang JH. Surgical correction of paralytic neuromuscular scoliosis with poor pulmonary functions. J Spinal Disord Tech 2011; 24: 325–333

[16] Granata C, Merlini L, Cervellati S et al. Long-term results of spine surgery in Duchenne muscular dystrophy. Neuromuscul Disord 1996; 6: 61–68

[17] Szpalski M, Gunzburg R, Aebi M, Weiskopf R. Research and evidence about blood sparing in spine surgery. Eur Spine J 2004; 13 Suppl 1: S1–S2

[18] Shapiro F, Sethna N. Blood loss in pediatric spine surgery. Eur Spine J 2004; 13 Suppl 1: S6–S17

[19] McLeod LM, French B, Flynn JM, Dormans JP, Keren R. Antifibrinolytic use and blood transfusions in pediatric scoliosis surgeries performed at US children's hospitals [published online ahead of print October 30, 2013]. J Spinal Disord Tech

[20] Dhawale AA, Shah SA, Sponseller PD et al. Are antifibrinolytics helpful in decreasing blood loss and transfusions during spinal fusion surgery in children with cerebral palsy scoliosis? Spine 2012; 37: E549–E555

[21] Pruitt DW, Tsai T. Common medical comorbidities associated with cerebral palsy. Phys Med Rehabil Clin N Am 2009; 20: 453–467

[22] Tsirikos AI, Chang WN, Dabney KW, Miller F, Glutting J. Life expectancy in pediatric patients with cerebral palsy and neuromuscular scoliosis who underwent spinal fusion. Dev Med Child Neurol 2003; 45: 677–682

[23] Erickson MA, Baulesh DM. Pathways that distinguish simple from complex scoliosis repair and their outcomes. Curr Opin Pediatr 2011; 23: 339–345

[24] Miller NH, Benefield E, Hasting L, Carry P, Pan Z, Erickson MA. Evaluation of high-risk patients undergoing spinal surgery: a matched case series. J Pediatr Orthop 2010; 30: 496–502

[25] Almenrader N, Patel D. Spinal fusion surgery in children with non-idiopathic scoliosis: is there a need for routine postoperative ventilation? Br J Anaesth 2006; 97: 851–857

[26] Abu-Kishk I, Kozer E, Hod-Feins R et al. Pediatric scoliosis surgery—is postoperative intensive care unit admission really necessary? Paediatr Anaesth 2013; 23: 271–277

[27] James S, Ziviani J, Boyd R. A systematic review of activities of daily living measures for children and adolescents with cerebral palsy. Dev Med Child Neurol 201 4: 233–244

[28] Bagó J, Climent JM, Pérez-Grueso FJS, Pellisé F. Outcome instruments to assess scoliosis surgery. Eur Spine J 2013; 22 Suppl 2: S195–S202

[29] Ersberg A, Gerdhem P. Pre- and postoperative quality of life in patients treated for scoliosis. Acta Orthop 2013; 84: 537–543

[30] Watanabe K, Lenke LG, Daubs MD et al. Is spine deformity surgery in patients with spastic cerebral palsy truly beneficial?: a patient/parent evaluation. Spine 2009; 34: 2222–2232

[31] Obid P, Bevot A, Goll A, Leichtle C, Wülker N, Niemeyer T. Quality of life after surgery for neuromuscular scoliosis. Orthop Rev (Pavia) 2013; 5: e1

[32] Cassidy C, Craig CL, Perry A, Karlin LI, Goldberg MJ. A reassessment of spinal stabilization in severe cerebral palsy. J Pediatr Orthop 1994; 14: 731–739

[33] Tsirikos AI, Chang WN, Dabney KW, Miller F. Comparison of parents' and caregivers' satisfaction after spinal fusion in children with cerebral palsy. J Pediatr Orthop 2004; 24: 54–58

[34] Jones KB, Sponseller PD, Shindle MK, McCarthy ML. Longitudinal parental perceptions of spinal fusion for neuromuscular spine deformity in patients with totally involved cerebral palsy. J Pediatr Orthop 2003; 23: 143–149

[35] Diefenbach C, Ialenti MN, Lonner BS, Kamerlink JR, Verma K, Errico TJ. Hospital cost analysis of neuromuscular scoliosis surgery. Bull Hosp Jt Dis (2013) 2013; 71: 272–277

[36] Karol LA. Early definitive spinal fusion in young children: what we have learned. Clin Orthop Relat Res 2011; 469: 1323–1329

[37] Vitale MG, Gomez JA, Matsumoto H, Roye DP Jr. Chest Wall and Spine Deformity Study Group. Variability of expert opinion in treatment of early-onset scoliosis. Clin Orthop Relat Res 2011; 469: 1317–1322

[38] White KK, Song KMD, Frost N, Daines BK. VEPTR™ growing rods for early-onset neuromuscular scoliosis: feasible and effective. Clin Orthop Relat Res 2011; 469: 1335–1341

[39] Abol Oyoun N, Stuecker R. Bilateral rib-to-pelvis Eiffel Tower VEPTR construct for children with neuromuscular scoliosis: a preliminary report. Spine J 201 4; 14: 1183–1191

[40] Farooq N, Garrido E, Altaf F et al. Minimizing complications with single submuscular growing rods: a review of technique and results on 88 patients with minimum two-year follow-up. Spine 2010; 35: 2252–2258

Part 9

The Future

31 Clinical Trials: Holy Grail or Poisoned Chalice?

Colin Nnadi and Jeremy C.T. Fairbank

Clinical trials for surgical devices are often the bane of an orthopedic surgeon's life. This is not for want of enthusiasm about research; rather, it can largely be attributed to the burdensome and often bureaucratic process involved in obtaining (and maintaining!) authorization for a trial. In a regulatory environment that is rightly placing an increasing emphasis on patient safety, and with an increasingly litigious patient population, the need for a thorough vetting process of the medical devices used in clinical care is more pressing than ever.

Unfortunately, the regulatory requirements for placing a medical device on the market are rather unsatisfactory. Although drugs may be approved by a single body (the European Medicines Agency) after proof of safety and efficacy in controlled trials, there is no such centralized body in relation to medical devices. Instead, the Notified Body[1] in each European country must approve the CE (European Conformity) mark before the device may be marketed throughout Europe. Despite the aim of European legislation to harmonize regulation in this area, the lack of a central body to approve medical devices introduces a level of uncertainty to the process, and it inevitably increases the time and cost required to introduce a new medical device to the European market. Furthermore, unlike the position with regard to drugs, there is no need for proof of clinical efficacy of a medical device before its general use is allowed in Europe. Indeed, the regulatory body in the United Kingdom, the Medicines and Healthcare Products Regulatory Agency (MHRA), has highlighted the poor evidence base for most medical devices.[1,2]

Under The Medical Devices Regulations 2002,[3] there are four main risk-based categories for medical devices: I, IIa, IIb, and III. The level of risk to the patient increases from class I to class III. Device classification depends on the intended use of the device and the indications for use. The lowest-risk devices, such as stethoscopes, are in class I. Dental fillings are a class IIa device. Medical implants are always classified as IIb or III. Orthopedic devices are class III because they "support or sustain human life, are of substantial importance in preventing impairment of human health, or [prevent] a potential, unreasonable risk of illness or injury."[4]

In the United States, class III medical devices are regulated by the U.S. Food and Drug Administration (FDA) and are available for general use after going through one of two possible routes to authorization: either premarket authorization or submission of a 510(k) Premarket Notification Form to demonstrate that the device is at least as safe and effective as a legally marketed device that is not subject to premarket approval. The former route involves proof that the device is both safe and effective for its intended use (obtained through clinical trials). The latter involves demonstration that the medical device is substantially equivalent to an existing product on the market, known as the Predicate Device. Ninety percent of medical devices on the North American market have been approved through the 510(k) route.

The fundamental difference between the European[5] and American systems is the reliance on postmarketing surveillance by the European system, as opposed to premarket testing by the U.S. system. However, the FDA also cites postmarketing surveillance as a condition of approval,[6] whereas in Europe, manufacturers are guided by a medical device vigilance system.[2] In the United Kingdom, this vigilance is regulated by the MHRA.

Each system has its advantages and disadvantages. The U.S. system requires a device not only to be safe but also to demonstrate that it alters the outcome of the condition it is intended to treat. While this arguably limits adverse events, one could also argue that this premarket stringency stifles innovation. The European system, on the other hand, encourages innovation because the medical device is more readily accessible for patient benefit provided it is monitored post marketing. It is the nature of this vigilance that has caused concern. Firstly, postmarketing surveillance in Europe is obligatory, but there is no punishment if the surveillance is not performed, and secondly, such vigilance is usually carried out informally through feedback from users. I am of the belief that postmarketing surveillance should be performed in a strictly regulated environment, such as that provided by a clinical trial. This would allow surgeons to evaluate the risks and benefits of a device and would also enhance both surgeon and patient decision making in regard to treatment.

The Oxford Spine Unit recently set up a postmarketing surveillance study to evaluate a new device used in the treatment of early onset scoliosis, and I wish to share our trials and tribulations with the reader. This chapter may inspire the reader to immerse himself or herself in the intricate complexities and nuances of clinical research to complement an illustrious career as a spinal surgeon. On the other hand, the thought of unheard-of acronyms, mountains of forms to be filled out and letters to be written, and numerous meetings with bureaucrats may consign the idea of undertaking a surgical clinical trial to the darkest corners of the memory forever. I will leave the reader to judge.

31.1 The MAGEC Clinical Trial

The Spine Unit of the Oxford University Hospitals (OUH) recently introduced a new medical device for the treatment of early onset scoliosis: the MAGEC (magnetic expansion control) Remote Control Spinal Deformity

System (Ellipse Technologies, Irvine, California). This product makes it possible to lengthen a growing rod non-invasively with a remotely controlled device. The decision to use this device was based on the fact that the need for repeated surgeries is eliminated, with a corresponding reduction in patient morbidity, in addition to psychosocial benefits to the patient and family. The potential cost savings were also a significant factor.

31.2 Basics of Setting Up a Clinical Trial

31.2.1 Approval from the Children's Directorate

The first stage involved obtaining approval and support from the Women's and Children's Directorate of the OUH. Following preliminary discussions with the Clinical Director of the Women's and Children's Directorate, it was apparent that an application for approval to the OUH Technology Advisory Group would be first required. This group, which is part of the Clinical Governance Support Unit, was established to inform the OUH about new clinical technologic developments that might be beneficial to patients. Each application to the Technology Advisory Group is assessed according to three criteria: clinical effectiveness (benefit vs. risk), technical suitability (safety standards), and competency (training and competency evaluation). It consists of several submissions: background paper, competency and training, evidence on cost-effectiveness, ethical and consent processes, and presentation.

Background Paper

The background paper provides information about the device and discusses whether it is used in current practice, and if so the indications for its use. The paper then goes on to describe how the device will be used in the trial and considers whether there will be any effects on provision of service, including potential implications for other services. The level of risk to the patient both with and without the device, and alternative treatments, are also discussed.

Competency and Training

Research data with the relevant references are provided. Questions regarding proven benefits, the size of the benefit, improvement in quality of life, whether certain patients benefit more than others, and any evidence of risk are all assessed and addressed.

Evidence on Cost-effectiveness

Evidence of cost-effectiveness is made available, and comparisons with similar treatments are made.

Ethical and Consent Processes

Patient choice and view are central to the introduction of any new device, and therefore consideration is given to the ethical and consent processes.

Presentation

A presentation to a panel is undertaken and questions are asked. The Technology Advisory Group panel consists of up to 10 members. A final decision is made within 2 weeks of the session.

Once formal approval was given by the Technology Advisory Group, a submission was then made to the Women's and Children's Directorate Planning and Budgetary Office for further discussion with the health commissioners. An Options Appraisal Template was used to advance the case for the trial.

31.2.2 Quality Assurance Model

Once we had approval from the hospital management team and had agreed on funding streams with the health commissioners, the next stage of the process involved setting up a quality assurance model in line with Technology Advisory Group guidance. Initial consensus was that an ethics committee application would not be necessary because the device was being used for its intended purpose and had a track record in other centers in the United Kingdom. However, in order to optimize the evaluation of the safety and performance of the device, we felt that the trial had to be done in a regulated environment, as would be the case with a formal study. Because of the paucity of cases of early onset scoliosis in general, it was felt that a multicenter study would be the best option.

Our first port of call in deciding on a quality assurance model was the National Institute for Health Research (NIHR) via the Clinical Research Network. The NIHR was set up in 2006 by the U.K. government to create a high-quality health system within the National Health Service (NHS), and the Clinical Research Network is part of this organization. The NIHR model revolves around the principle of the Portfolio, which is a collection of high-quality clinical studies that benefit from the infrastructure provided by the Clinical Research Network. The first step in using the NIHR model involves applying to the Coordinated System for Gaining NHS Permission (CSP). In past multicenter studies, investigators had to make a separate application to each participating hospital. The CSP is intended to avoid bureaucracy by allowing study details to be entered only once. The CSP then coordinates further review across all participating hospitals. Despite these noble intentions, there is still a considerable amount of time spent filling out forms.

A lead Comprehensive Local Research Network (CLRN) is then assigned to the study, which provides a single point of contact for up-to-date developments in the study. There are 25 CLRNs making up the Comprehensive Clinical Research Network (CCRN). Together, they facilitate and coordinate clinical research across England. Advice on Research Management and Governance is also provided by the CCRN.

There is a cost burden to the health service for running clinical studies consisting of three categories: research, service support, and treatment costs. Studies in the Portfolio receive coordinated NHS support not only in the form of research nurse / allied health professional time but also of liaison with other recruiting centers to ensure adequate and appropriate research support. There is also help available for problem solving.

An initial meeting takes place to discuss this support and to agree on goals and escalation policies. Contact points are decided and future meetings are planned. It was at this meeting that I was introduced to the acronym-laden world of clinical research. The path to glory was strewn with CIs, PIs, GCPs, ISFs, SAEs, SARs, and SADEs. TMFs and SOPs were also thrown in for good measure.

31.2.3 Good Clinical Practice

The first step of the journey toward inclusion in the Portfolio required training in Good Clinical Practice (GCP)[7] so that I could familiarize myself with the nuances of clinical research and gain acquaintance with the many acronyms one is expected to reel off with ease. It is a legal requirement in the United Kingdom to conduct all clinical trials according to the principles of GCP as defined by The Medicines for Human Use (Clinical Trials) Regulations 2004.[8]

GCP is an international ethical and scientific quality standard for designing, conducting, recording, and reporting trials that involve the participation of human subjects. It is based on 14 principles of GCP set forth by the International Conference on Harmonisation of Technical Requirements for Registration of Pharmaceuticals for Human Use (ICH). Compliance with GCP ensures first and foremost that study participants (patients) are protected, and secondly that the data produced are credible. The 14 principles are listed below:

1. The rights, safety, and well-being of the trial subjects shall prevail over the interests of science and society.
2. Each individual involved in conducting a trial shall be qualified by education, training, and experience to perform his tasks.
3. Clinical trials shall be scientifically sound and guided by ethical principles in all their aspects.
4. The necessary procedures to secure the quality of every aspect of the trial shall be complied with.
5. The available nonclinical and clinical information on an investigational medicinal product shall be adequate to support the proposed clinical trial.
6. Clinical trials shall be conducted in accordance with the principles of the Declaration of Helsinki.
7. The protocol shall provide for the definition of inclusion and exclusion of subjects participating in a clinical trial, monitoring, and publication policy.
8. The investigator and sponsor shall consider all relevant guidance with respect to commencing and conducting a clinical trial.
9. All clinical information shall be recorded, handled, and stored in such a way that it can be accurately reported, interpreted, and verified while the confidentiality of the records of the trial subjects remains protected.
10. Before the trial is initiated, foreseeable risks and inconveniences have been weighed against the anticipated benefit for the individual trial subject and other present and future patients. A trial should be initiated and continued only if the anticipated benefits justify the risks.
11. The medical care given to, and medical decisions made on behalf of, subjects shall always be the responsibility of an appropriately qualified doctor or, when appropriate, of a qualified dentist.
12. A trial shall be initiated only if an ethics committee and the licensing authority come to the conclusion that the anticipated therapeutic and public health benefits justify the risks and may be continued only if compliance with this requirement is permanently monitored.
13. The rights of each subject to physical and mental integrity, to privacy, and to the protection of the data concerning him in accordance with the Data Protection Act 1998 are safeguarded.
14. Provision has been made for insurance or indemnity to cover the liability of the investigator and sponsor which may arise in relation to the clinical trial.

For further guidance in this area, readers are referred to *10 Golden Rules for Pharmacists* by David Hutchinson (Canary Publications, 1999).

31.2.4 Trial Protocol

Compliance with GCP begins with a GCP-compliant protocol. This is a document that describes the objective, design, methodology, statistical considerations, and organization of a trial.

The first part of the protocol contains the study outline, which summarizes the study in terms of design, inclusion and exclusion criteria, and end points. A detailed protocol is then written to ensure that the reader can easily understand what the study is about. It comprises the following sections:

Detailed Protocol

- General Information
- Background Information
- Trial Purpose and Objectives
- Trial Design
- Selection and Withdrawal of Subjects
- Treatment of Subjects
- Assessment of Efficacy
- Assessment of Safety
- Statistics
- Direct Access to Source Data / Documents
- Quality Control and Assurance
- Ethics
- Data Handling and Record Keeping
- Finance and Insurance
- Publication Policy
- Supplements

A Gantz chart (▶ Table 31.1) provides a summary of the expected timeline for each phase of the study.

31.2.5 Other Documents

Once the protocol has been finalized, associated documents can be drafted.

Patient Information Sheet

The patient information sheet (PIS) details the object of the study in plain English and a format that is easy to understand. It should discuss the risks and benefits of the treatment, as well as alternative treatment options. It should also provide assurance to the patient that opting out of or into the study will not affect the standard of care. Occasionally, there may be groups of patients—for example, children—whose level of understanding may differ from one age group to another. In such circumstances, a separate PIS is provided for each group. Pictures, drawings, or even videos are advised for children younger than 5 years of age.

Consent Form

A customized trial consent form is to be used instead of a standard clinical consent form (▶ Table 31.2). It should contain a short title of the study, the name of the Principal Investigator (PI), the ethics reference number, the date, and the document version number. A signature is obtained from the participant, or on behalf of the participant in the case of a minor, and from the person taking consent. One copy is then given to the participant, one is stored in the Research Site File, and one is kept in the patient's medical notes.

General Practitioner Letter

It is important that the general practitioner (GP) be made aware that his or her patient is undergoing procedures that are not standard clinical practice.

Case Report Form

The case report form (CRF) is used to collect study data. It is good practice to have CRF completion guidelines detailing, for example, the order in which initials are used (e.g., for John Smith, JS or SJ) and the manner of writing dates (e.g., DDMMYY).

31.2.6 National Research Ethics Service Opinion

No study involving human subjects should be commenced without obtaining approval from the National Research Ethics Service (NRES).[5] The Declaration of Helsinki, which was first adopted in 1964, provides ethical guidance to physicians and other participants in medical research involving human subjects. Its principles are based on patient safety, risk management, informed consent, and compliance with research protocol.

The aim of gaining a favorable opinion from the Ethics Committee is to ensure that the trial complies with the stated principles of the Declaration of Helsinki. The U.K. NHS Research Ethics Committees (RECs) are under the auspices of the NRES, which in turn is managed by the National Patient Safety Agency (NPSA). Independent Review Boards carry out a similar function in the United States.

The process is commenced by applying online through the Integrated Research Application System (IRAS) website. The IRAS is the sole system for gaining approval for health and social / community care research in the United Kingdom. It uses a filter system to avoid data collection / study type mismatch. It also ensures that regulatory and governance requirements are met. For a surgical study, relevant information is captured by the IRAS for review by the following bodies:
1. Administration of Radioactive Substance Advisory Committee (ARSAC);
2. Medicines and Healthcare Products Regulatory Agency (MHRA);
3. Ministry of Justice (MoJ);
4. NHS Health & Safety Commission (HSC) R&D offices;
5. NRES / NHS / HSC Research Ethics Committees; and
6. National Information Governance Board (NIGB).

There are four parts to the application.
Part A
Part A comprises core study information in the form of Chief Investigator (CI) and Sponsor details. Reference numbers for the study must also be given. A summary

Table 31.1 Gantz chart

Research activities	N	D	J	F	M	A	M	J	J	A	S	O	N	D	J	F	M	A	M	J	J	A	S	O	N	D	J
Steering committee meeting																											
Recruitment of sites																											
Recruitment of participants																											
Outcome measures																											
Imaging																											
Surgery																											
Physiotherapy																											
Follow-up in outpatient department																											
Data monitoring																											
Baseline data collection																											
Data collection periods																											
Data entry and cleaning																											
Data analysis																											
Writing and dissemination																											
Feedback																											

Table 31.2 Consent form

Hospital Name	
Telephone: 00000000	
Fax: 00000000	
Date: _____	
Center Number: _____	
Study Number: _____	
Patient Identification Number for this trial: _____	
Consent Form	
Title of Project: _____	
Name of Researcher: _____	
1. I confirm that I have read and understand the information sheet dated _____ (version x) for the above study. I have had the opportunity to consider the information and ask questions, and I have had these answered satisfactorily.	
2. I understand that our participation is voluntary and that we are free to withdraw at any time without giving any reason, without my medical care or legal rights being affected.	
3. I understand that relevant sections of my child's medical notes and data collected during the study may be looked at by individuals from X when it is relevant to our taking part in this research. I give permission for these individuals to have access to my records.	
4. I agree to our GP being informed of our participation in the study	
5. I agree to my child taking part in the above study	

_____	_____	_____
Name of Parent	Date	Signature on Behalf of Child
Child's Name _____		
_____	_____	_____
Name of Person	Date	Signature of Person Taking

When completed: one copy for participant, one for researcher site file, one (original) to be kept in medical notes.

and background of the research are provided, together with a description of its purpose and methodology. A single principle question to be answered should be identified and supplemented with secondary questions. The structure of the sample group and inclusivity criteria are stated. Details of any procedures performed on participants, and whether these are above and beyond the normal standard of care, must be provided. The number of procedures performed, and by whom, must also be given. The method of recruitment and patient consent for the study is supplied. The confidentiality of the participant data is paramount, and therefore arrangements must be in place for the secure storage of data both during and after the study. Conflicts of interest and financial incentives must be declared. The intention to notify other professionals, such as GPs, should also be confirmed. Details of plans for the scientific review, publication, and dissemination of the research must be provided. These requirements fulfill Article 19 of the World Medical Association Declaration of Helsinki, adopted in 2008, which states that

"every clinical trial must be registered on a publicly accessible database before recruitment of the first subject."

Collaborator details as well as insurance and indemnity arrangements should be specified. The local R&D contact should be identified. Information on the CE status of the device is documented.

Part B

Part B contains the details of the medical device to be used in the study. Manufacturer details along with the device identification name and number are mandatory. The length of time since the device came into use must be stated. The key questions are the following:

1. Is this a new device?
2. Is the device being used within its CE mark intended purpose?
3. Is the device being used outside the terms of its CE mark intended purpose?

The next section of Part B assesses the level of risk for exposure to radiation to study participants. There are four categories of risk, in order of increasing severity: I, IIa, IIb, and III. Category III indicates a moderate cancer risk (i.e., 1 in 1,000) from a substantial effective dose of radiation. The category assigned to the medical device must be reviewed by a medical physicist and countersigned by a radiologist.

Part B also contains a section on children that identifies the potential age range of the children who will be included in the study and the reasons for their taking part. Arrangements for obtaining informed consent from parents / legal guardians are identified. In certain age groups, when applicable, the process for providing information and taking consent is outlined.

Part C

Part C provides an overview of other research sites or host organizations involved in the study. The PIs at each site should be identified.

Part D

Finally, Part D contains declarations signed by the CI and the Sponsor's Representatives, who undertake that they will submit annual progress reports, safety reports, an end-of-study declaration, and an end-of-study report.

The completed application form is then submitted after the allocation of a reference number by the REC. The receipt of application forms is acknowledged within 5 days. At the same time, each PI from the other hospital sites taking part in the study submits a Site Specific Information (SSI) document (which contains information specific to the research site) to the local R&D office for a Site Specific Assessment (SSA). An opinion must be given by the R&D office within 30 days of submission.

31.2.7 Agreements

> **Box 1 Sponsor Responsibilities**
>
> - Quality assurance and quality control
> - Delegating duties
> - Trial design
> - Trial management, data handling, and record keeping
> - Compensation / indemnity
> - Finance arrangements
> - Regulatory submission / notification
> - Ethics confirmation
> - Manufacturing, packaging, labeling, and coding of investigational products
> - Record management and access

These are legally binding documents that make clear each party's obligations and responsibilities in relation to the research study. Their use depends on the type of study, and there are different types of agreement depending on the structure of the trial. Our Sponsors signed a Clinical Trial Agreement (CTA) with the institution (OUH). This agreement specified the legal requirements, conditions, and obligations pertaining to the study. Box 1 and Box 2 below indicate the expected responsibilities of the Sponsor and Investigator.

> **Box 2 Investigator Responsibilities**
>
> - Appropriately qualified
> - Assessment of resources
> - Continued medical care
> - Ethics communication
> - Protocol compliance
> - Drug accountability
> - Informed consent
> - Record keeping
> - Reports
> - Trial termination / suspension

Once a favorable ethical opinion has been advised, NHS permission can be given for the study to begin.

31.2.8 Trial Master File

All the documentation described thus far must be stored and kept in the Trial Master File (TMF). This is a collection of all the essential documents relating to the study, which enables evaluation of the conduct of the study and the quality of data produced. The TMF is looked after by the CI, who has overall responsibility for the research (including that carried out at other sites in multicenter studies). The Sponsor, which may be an individual, company, or institution, may wish to audit the study to ensure full compliance with regulations. The Sponsor initiates, finances, and manages the study. Regulatory authorities, such as the MHRA or the local R&D, may also wish to audit the study. In a multicenter study, each local site has an Investigator Site File (ISF) containing essential documents.

The TMF will contain the following documents:
1. Approvals and sponsorship;
2. Protocol and participant information;
3. Site details;
4. Contracts and agreements;
5. Recruitment and reporting;
6. Data management;
7. Investigational device and machino-vigilance;
8. Monitoring, audit, and trial committees; and
9. End-of-study report and closure.

31.2.9 Initiation Meeting

Before the trial can proceed, an initiation meeting must take place at which all members of the research team are present. Standard Operating Procedures (SOPs) should have been drafted at this stage. These serve to standardize study procedures. During the MAGEC trial, our experience was that the most relevant SOPs for a surgical device study are those to do with safety reporting, informed consent, and the completion of paperwork.

31.2.10 Safety Reporting

The safety of the research participants is of primary concern. In pediatric spine surgery, most implants have not been through a premarket approval process. They may have been tested in the laboratory or in animal models, but this does not guarantee fail-safe behavior. There are well-documented cases in which new implants have been introduced to the market and then subsequently and unceremoniously withdrawn because of complications. To ensure that any potential problems with a trial product are identified as early as possible, Adverse Event (AE) reporting is mandatory for any clinical trial. Learning from AEs promotes good practice and enhances the ethical and scientific quality of research. Most importantly, it safeguards the public.

Safety reporting requires an essential knowledge of the basic definitions and time scales for reporting. Traditionally, AEs are defined for use in drug trials. More conventional definitions concerning safety reporting are as outlined below.

Adverse Event (AE)

An AE is any untoward medical occurrence in a participant who has been administered a medicinal product that does not necessarily have a causal relationship with the intervention. These events are recorded on CRFs and are reported within 24 hours to the local R&D and the Sponsor.

Serious Adverse Event (SAE)

An SAE is any AE that results in death, threat to life, hospital admission or prolongation of hospital admission, congenital birth defect, or other important medical events.

Serious Adverse Reaction (SAR)

This is an SAE believed with reasonable probability to have a causal relationship with a study intervention. SARs should be reported to the MHRA, Ethics Committee, and local R&D in an Annual Safety Report (ASR).

Suspected Unexpected Serious Adverse Reaction (SUSAR)

This is a disproportionate and unexpected SAR to the investigational product or device that is not consistent with the Summary of Product Characteristics (SPC) (for an authorized product) or the Investigator's Brochure (IB) (for an unauthorized medicinal product).

SUSARs must be reported to the regulatory bodies immediately (the MHRA in the United Kingdom). If they are fatal or life-threatening, the authorities must be informed within 7 days and must be provided with follow-up information within a further 8 days. Other SUSARs should be reported within 15 days of awareness.

In the MAGEC study, some modified definitions of AEs were required to reflect the use of a device in the study: Adverse Device Effect (ADE), Serious Adverse Device Effect (SADE), and Unexpected Adverse Device Effect (UADE).

Adverse Device Effect (ADE)

An ADE is any untoward and unintended response to a medical device. This definition includes any event resulting from insufficiencies or inadequacies in the instructions for use or deployment of the device, or any event that is a result of a user error.

Serious Adverse Device Effect (SADE)

An SADE is an ADE that resulted in any of the consequences characteristic of an SAE or that might have led to death or a serious deterioration in the health of a subject or any other person if suitable action had not been taken. The definition of SADE includes incidents and near-incidents.

Unexpected Adverse Device Effect (UADE)

A UADE is any SADE on the health or safety or any life-threatening problem or death caused by, or associated with, a device if that effect was not previously identified in nature, severity, or degree of incidence in the Investigational Plan or Application (including a supplementary plan or application), or any other unanticipated serious problem associated with a device that relates to the rights, safety, or welfare of the subject.

The CI is responsible for recording AEs and reporting SAEs through the appropriate pathways. In multicenter studies, safety reporting can be delegated to the PIs of the individual sites. The PIs should have undergone GCP training and be well versed in safety reporting. The Sponsor is responsible for evaluating the safety of the device and for communicating any specific concerns. There must be a clear and well-defined pathway for updates and reporting. Monitoring visits by the Sponsor should occur on a regular basis.

One of the difficulties we experienced was in assessing the expectedness of an SAE or SAR in a medical device, as opposed to a medicinal drug, which is usually accompanied by an IB or an SPC. An IB is a collection of clinical and nonclinical data gathered in the developmental stage of a drug. Under circumstances in which a licensed drug is being trialed for another indication, an IB is also made available. Licensed drugs have an SPC, which provides information on all known side effects and reactions. These documents make it easier to assess the expectedness of an SAE or SAR for that drug. The difficulty with most orthopedic devices is the overlap between the developmental phase and market entry. A significant number of implants go through several design modifications, even while in clinical use. These changes may involve the surface geometry or finishing, and different materials may be used, which can give rise to dissimilar mechanical properties. This situation can lead to confusion about whether to use an IB or an SPC.

All SAEs should be reported to the Sponsor and local R&D within 24 hours of awareness of the event. A description of the event, its expectedness, and time of resolution should be clearly stated. Expectedness indicates the probability of an SAE occurring, taking into account a preexisting condition or the known risks associated with a particular intervention. For instance, rod breakage in a growing rod system requiring hospital admission is an expected SAE. Likewise, patients with diabetes can have complications arising from unstable blood sugar levels, which require admission to hospital. This distinction between types of expectedness should be made during the protocol development stage.

31.2.11 Informed Consent

This is deemed to occur when a competent individual willingly confirms his or her readiness to take part in a study, having fully understood all aspects of the study and what that means in reality. Consent is an ongoing process and is not to be considered only at the time when a signature is placed on the dotted line. Depending on how participants are identified, an ethics-approved invitation letter may be given to determine whether potential participants are interested and would like further information. For the MAGEC trial, we identified participants at outpatient consultations; clinical examination findings and radiographs were used as screening tools. Often in orthopedic surgery, there are close similarities between the clinical and research care pathways, and consequently a clear research consent process is needed. A PIS, written in lay language and detailing all the information needed for the participant to give informed consent to the study, should be provided to the participant. Time should be allowed for this information to be considered. There should then be a consent interview at which the content of the PIS is discussed. It is paramount that this information be fully understood by the participant. It is also very important that the participant understand that he or she can withdraw consent at any time without negative ramifications regarding care. Only once this process is completed can written consent be obtained. A copy of the signed form is given to the participant, one goes into the medical records, and one into the TMF. In the case of vulnerable participants, such as children, a responsible adult should give consent on their behalf, but children should also give their "assent" after age-appropriate information is provided (▶ Table 31.3).

The person taking consent must have a thorough understanding of the study, intervention risks, and side effects of the condition; should be qualified by experience; and should have received appropriate and documented training.

Consent indicates willingness to take part, but not enrollment, in the trial. Enrollment occurs, after valid consent has been given, by entering the participant's details into an enrollment log. These should also be written in the participant's medical notes. A sticker placed on the front of the medical notes detailing the name of the study and the enrollment date is good practice. Participants should also be given cards indicating that they are in the study and containing contact details for the trial team. The GP should also be notified of the participant's enrollment in the study.

31.3 Considerations after Setup

31.3.1 Monitoring, Data Collection, and Audit

So far, we have described the processes involved in setting up a clinical trial for a medical device. These took approximately 9 months. Once the study is up and running, consideration then needs to be given to monitoring, data collection, and audit trails. Time management and organization are essential tools required to run any study. Always allow enough time to see participants, and always be prepared with the paperwork. The delegation of different responsibilities should be recorded in the delegation log, and therefore research team members should be on hand to collect data. The credibility and accuracy of the data are ensured by monitoring visits by the Sponsor. The safety of participants is also enhanced by these visits. The Sponsor, in our case the U.K. distributor company, conducts these visits at regular intervals. Both sides have a responsibility to ensure that the study is run according to stated protocol, guidelines, and regulations. Any breaches in protocol are subject to audit review. Commercial studies in orthopedic surgery are usually carried out as part of postmarketing surveillance, whereas in drug trials, such studies are undertaken as part of the premarketing authorization process.

The degree of monitoring to be carried out in the study depends on the number of sites involved and their proximity to one another. Monitoring is straightforward if there is only one site, but when multiple sites are involved, monitoring can pose difficulties. Two main forms of monitoring are used: central, in which data are transferred to the central site, and peripheral, in which a reciprocal arrangement exists by which a member of the staff from one site monitors another site, and vice versa. Central monitoring raises the issue of data protection

Table 31.3 Assent form for children

Hospital Name
Telephone: 00000000
Fax: 00000000
Date: _____
Assent Form for Children
Version x
(to be completed by the child and the child's parent or guardian)
Project Title:
Child (or if unable, parent on their behalf) / young person to circle all they agree with:
Has somebody else explained this project to you? Yes / No
Do you understand what this project is about? Yes / No
Have you asked all the questions you want? Yes / No
Have you had your questions answered in a way you understand? Yes / No
Do you understand it's OK to stop taking part at any time? Yes / No
Are you happy to take part? Yes / No
If any of your answers are no or if you don't want to take part, don't sign your name!
If you do want to take part, you can write your name below.
Your Name _____
Date _____
The doctor who explained this project to you needs to sign too:
Print Name _____
Sign _____
Date _____
Thank you for your help.

during the transfer of patient-identifiable data. Participant consent is therefore required. A strategy detailing which aspects of the study to target during the visit should be agreed upon. It is sensible to monitor a study involving a surgical device for safety reporting, consent, and completion of study paperwork.

All data and any changes must be recorded meticulously so as to leave a legible paper trail. As stated previously, consent is an ongoing process, and this should be reconfirmed on a continual basis throughout the study. Any AEs and concomitant medications must be diligently recorded.

31.3.2 Amendments

There are occasions when amendments to the approved protocol or any associated supporting documents are necessary. These may be minor amendments, in which case approval from the Ethics Committee is not necessary.

Examples of minor amendments are changes in funding arrangements, correction of typing errors, extensions to the duration of the study, and minor changes to the protocol.

Substantial amendments are those that will affect the following aspects of the study: participant safety, scientific value of the derived data, SOPs, safety of any device or medicinal product under investigation, and change of the CI or a PI. All substantial amendments should be reported to the Ethics Committee that approved the study. A Notice of Substantial Amendments Form should be completed indicating the changes made and the reasons for the changes. Document version numbers and dates should be updated to reflect the amendments. A copy of the amended document and the new version should be submitted in addition to the Notice of Amendment. All members of the research team should be made aware of the changes. The R&D department should also be notified.

31.3.3 Clinical Study Plan

A summary of the processes involved in running a study can be detailed in a Clinical Study Plan. This can be used to outline specific information relating to the study and for training purposes at other sites. It also serves as a reference tool for members of the research team.

31.4 Conclusion

In the last decade, many advances have been made in the regulation of hip implants in orthopedic surgery. Hip registries have ensured that outcomes and complication rates are monitored. Implant characteristics that lead to higher failure rates have been identified and considered in the design process. However, despite these controls and improvements, there have been instances in which the regulatory process has failed.[9,10,11] Unfortunately, pediatric orthopedic spinal surgery is still an evolving field, although it has progressed in leaps and bounds over the last 10 years. It is imperative that we learn from the hip arthroplasty experience. The pediatric spinal patient cohort is much younger, and poorly performing devices are therefore likely to have dire consequences for patients and, indirectly, the health care system in the long term. The patients have a longer life span during which the results of failure can be expressed. At worst, such failure may be in the form of multiple revision surgeries or morbidity from neurologic complications. Failure has significant socioeconomic consequences for both patients and society.

The process of setting up a clinical trial to evaluate a new device, as described above, is laborious and strewn with bureaucratic red tape if it is carried out properly. There is also an inadvertent bias toward clinical drug trials with courses designed to teach GCP, which leaves the surgeon feeling isolated and misunderstood. However, as requests from surgeons to be involved in clinical device trials increase and intensify, it is increasingly likely that the process will become more considerate of the specialist needs of the surgeons running the trials.

The process cannot work without willing commercial partners, and I would like to say a special thank you to Carolyn Burke of Surgi C, Birmingham, United Kingdom, for her role in facilitating the setup of the MAGEC study. Our experience has led me to believe that spinal device companies should include clinical trials as part of their budget planning when they introduce new implants to the health care sector. Spinal device registries should be set up to report outcomes and failure rates. At present, there are numerous devices on the market with no long-term survivorship data. The current state of affairs needs to change to reflect a greater and ever-increasing emphasis on patient safety.

Would I run another clinical trial?

To be, or not to be, that is the question—
Whether 'tis Nobler in the mind to suffer
The Slings and Arrows of outrageous Fortune,
Or to take Arms against a sea of troubles,
And by opposing end them?
–William Shakespeare, Hamlet

References

[1] The Notified Body: Bulletin No. 6, MHRA, January 2006
[2] House of Commons Science and Technology Committee. Fifth report of session 2012–13. Regulation of medical implants in the EU and UK. http://www.publications.parliament.uk/pa/cm201213/cmselect/cmsctech/163/163.pdf. Accessed July 22, 2014
[3] The Medical Devices Regulations 2002. Accessed July 23, 2014.
[4] Council Directive 93/42/EEC of 14 June 1993 concerning medical devices. Official Journal L 169, 12/07/1993 P. 0001 – 0043. . Accessed July 22, 2014
[5] European Observatory on Health Systems and Policies. Accessed November 19, 2014
[6] US Food and Drug Administration. Postmarket surveillance studies. . Updated November 3, 2014. Accessed November 19, 2014
[7] GCP. University of Oxford. Available from:
[8] The Medicines for Human Use (Clinical Trials) Regulations 2004. Accessed July 22, 2014
[9] Cohen D. Out of joint: the story of the ASR. BMJ 2011; 342: d2905
[10] Langton DJ, Jameson SS, Joyce TJ et al. Accelerating failure rate of the ASR total hip replacement. J Bone Joint Surg Br 2011; 93: 1011–1016
[11] Thomas SR, Shukla D, Latham PD. Corrosion of cemented titanium femoral stems. J Bone Joint Surg Br 2004; 86: 974–978

32 Is There a Gold-Standard Surgical Option?

Ahmed Abdelaal and Colin Nnadi

Defined as scoliotic spinal deformity of any etiology presenting before the age of 5 years, early onset scoliosis is one of the most challenging problems to treat in the world of pediatric orthopedic surgery. Dickson was the first to use the term *early onset* to reflect the establishment of scoliosis by 5 years of age.[1] Early onset scoliosis has a long list of possible etiologies. These include congenital, idiopathic, and neuromuscular conditions, as well as various syndromes. Nevertheless, the use of the term *early onset scoliosis* to describe these disorders collectively, regardless of the etiology, highlights an important concept: the age of the patient at onset is a crucial factor when treatment is considered because a deformed spine has major effects on the developing thorax and cardiopulmonary system.[2]

Left untreated, early onset scoliosis has grave cardiopulmonary and skeletal consequences that were observed and documented as early as the middle of the last century. James et al, in 1959, reported that progressive early onset scoliosis "develops rapidly and relentlessly, causing the severest form of orthopaedic cripple with dreadful deformity, marked dwarfing and shortening of life."[3] In 2003, Campbell et al used the term *thoracic insufficiency syndrome* to describe the compromised pulmonary development associated with severe early onset scoliosis. They defined thoracic insufficiency syndrome as the inability of the thorax to support normal lung growth and respiration. Disabling or life-threatening respiratory failure as a result of thoracic insufficiency syndrome is relatively common at, or before, late middle age.[4,5,6]

The ultimate goal in the treatment of early onset scoliosis is to control the progression of deformity while allowing the development and growth of the spine, lungs, and thorax, thereby improving pulmonary function and providing a better quality of life.[2,7] Conservative options, such as casting, bracing, or a combination of both, are commonly employed as the first line of treatment. However, severe, relapsing, or progressing deformities may require early surgical intervention to protect the inherent growth potential for spinal height and lung development. For decades, a prevailing belief that a spine that was "short and straight" as a result of early fusion was preferable to one that was "longer but crooked" had been supported.[8,9,10] Therefore, the concept of early definitive fusion as a treatment was embraced. However, spinal fusion was not without its complications. The crankshaft phenomenon, described by Dubousset et al, and thoracic insufficiency syndrome, recognized by Campbell et al in young children who had undergone early spinal fusion

for early onset scoliosis, have both prompted attempts to discover new modalities of treatment.

Skaggs classified fusionless surgical procedures into distraction-based, guided-growth, and tension-based systems.[7] Each of these strategies follows different principles, has different biomechanical characteristics, and has variable ability to correct deformity and maintain the correction while protecting the potential for growth. However, each strategy continues to evolve. Since the beginning of the last decade, we have witnessed a rapid expansion of the philosophy of treatment for early onset scoliosis. This has resulted in a better understanding and continued modifications of the widely accepted distraction-based systems (growth rods, vertical expandable prosthetic titanium rib [VEPTR]) as standard treatments. Additionally, there has been a revival of interest in the abandoned guided-growth systems following the emergence of newer techniques (modern Luque trolley, Shilla technique). Finally, the innovative tension-based systems (staples and tethers) also show exciting potential.

Despite the wide range of surgical treatment options for progressive early onset scoliosis, no solution has emerged as the single gold-standard option. The intention of this review is not to make treatment recommendations, but to document the options available to date and to examine the supporting evidence for each.

32.1 Methods

The keywords *scoliosis* and *early onset* were used in an electronic search of both PubMed and MEDLINE conducted on April 1, 2012. Inclusion criteria were that articles had been written in the English language and published after the year 2000 because since 2000, new surgical options have arisen while older methods have fallen out of favor.

The search for *scoliosis* yielded 5,764 titles, which were not all necessarily relevant to the objective of this particular review. When the term *early onset* was added as a keyword, 116 articles were found. The titles and abstracts of all 116 articles were examined to determine which were relevant to the quest for "surgical treatment methods." Articles published in nursing journals, case reports, genetic reports, biomechanical studies, and reviews were then excluded. Articles on specific rare syndromes, such as neurofibromatosis and spinal muscular atrophy (SMA), as well as articles about scoliosis with a specific etiology (e.g., congenital or neuromuscular scoliosis), were also excluded from the review. A copy of the full article was obtained for each of the remaining titles. The references for all included articles were examined and checked for any relevant papers, and these papers were included.

A total of 19 articles were included in the final review. These were classified according to the modality of treatment they considered: (1) distraction-based, (2) guided-growth, or (3) tension-based systems. Thus, 13 papers were found to report distraction-based systems, two papers on guided-growth systems, and four papers on tension-based systems. The included articles in this review comprise case series as well as some experimental studies of new modalities. No randomized controlled studies were found.

32.2 Review

Although an algorithm for managing early onset scoliosis has been proposed by Gillingham et al,[4] no rigid indications for the different surgical interventions currently exist. Numerous options are available and at the disposal of the treating surgeon. Vitale et al investigated variability in decision making with regard to the treatment of early onset scoliosis among a group of 13 experienced pediatric spinal surgeons.[11] They reported a wide variation in choice of construct type, number of constructs, and level of instrumentation. This review describes the systems based on three surgical principles (distraction, guided growth, and tension), with particular attention given to reporting recent advances and their updated outcomes.

32.3 Distraction-Based Systems

32.3.1 Growing Rods

The concept of using growing rods in the management of early onset scoliosis has been around since the 1960s. Harrington was the first to report on the technique in 1962.[12] He connected a single rod to the spine with a single hook proximally and a single hook distally and performed periodic lengthening. Since then, several modifications have been introduced to improve outcomes, and up until 2004, several authors reported on their results, including Moe et al,[13] Klemme et al,[14] Blakemore et al,[15] and Mineiro and Weinstein.[16] Their articles described the same principle of active distraction with a single rod. They all reported variable but high complication rates. It was not until 2005 that Akbarnia et al published their first report on the dual growing rod technique.[17] Since the introduction of this concept (dual rods instead of a single rod), focus has shifted away from single rods, and multiple reports and experiments have been published. Because the aim of this review is to examine current practice, we considered the earlier reports on single growing rods to be beyond its scope and excluded them. Seven articles on dual growing rods were found in our search, and these are the subject of this part of the review (▶ Table 32.1).

Table 32.1 Summary of included studies on growing rods

Author (reference)	Year	No.	Intervention	Follow-up (range)	Deformity correction, %	Complications, No. (%)
Akbarnia et al[17]	2005	23	DGRs	4.7 yrs (2–9)	54%	11 (48%)
Akbarnia et al[18]	2008	13 (lengthening <6 months [7] and >6 months [6])	DGRs	3–11 yrs	64%	6 (46%)
Sankar et al[19]	2011	38	DGRs	3.3. yrs (2–7)	52%	
Bess et al[20]	2010	69	DGRs	53.8 months (24–126)	48.7%	38 (55%)
Schroerlucke et al[21]	2012	90 (26 K–, 35 N, 29 K+)	DGRs (64) SGRs (26)	>2 yrs		12 in K– (46%) 12 in N (34%) 18 in K+ (62%)
Sponseller et al[22]	2009	36 (severe deformity extending to pelvis)	DGRs (30) SGRs (6) All fixed to pelvis distally	40 months (± 20)	44%	
Yang et al[23]	2011	327	DGRs (206) SGRs (121)			Only rod fractures (11% in DGRs, 26% in SGRs)

Abbreviations: DGRs, dual growing rods; K–, hypokyphosis; N, normal sagittal balance; K+, hyperkyphosis; SGRs, single growing rods.

In 2005, Akbarnia et al published their first retrospective review of their case series, reporting on the technique and its early results.[17] They used dual growing rods to treat 23 children with early onset scoliosis of various etiologies between 1993 and 2001, with a minimum of 2 years of follow-up (average, 4.7 years). They described the technique of connecting two upper and two lower rods to the upper and lower regions of the spine, respectively, with two or more vertebral levels used at each end as foundations. The upper and lower rods were then connected with a tandem connector at the thoracolumbar junction. All instrumentation was done through a limited subperiosteal exposure. Distraction was applied, and the tandem connector was tightened. This procedure was followed by serial lengthening procedures at an average of 7.4-month intervals. Akbarnia et al reported 56% improvement in the Cobb angle (from an average of 82 degrees preoperatively to 36 degrees at the latest follow-up). There were 13 complications in 11 patients (48%) during the treatment period.

In 2008, Akbarnia et al reported on their series of 13 children with noncongenital early onset scoliosis who had completed dual growing rod treatment before final fusion.[18] They found even better results after the final fusion (64% improvement in the Cobb angle and 45% increase in the T1-S1 length). In this report, they examined the effect of frequency of lengthening and found that patients who underwent lengthening at intervals of less than 6 months had a higher annual growth rate (1.84 vs. 1.02 cm) and even a significantly greater correction of scoliosis (from 89 to 20 degrees, or 78%) than those who underwent lengthening less frequently (48%). More recently, Sankar et al[19] reported the overall results of their study, which were comparable with those in previous reports by Akbarnia et al (Cobb angle correction from 74 to 35 degrees and T1-S1 growth of 1.74 cm per year). They also noticed a "law of diminishing returns" in T1-S1 growth with repeated lengthening procedures (1.04 cm after the first lengthening but only 4 mm after the seventh) as a result of autofusion. As in previous studies, correction of the Cobb angle was achieved predominantly following the initial instrumentation. These findings are significant in a number of ways. They warn us not to expect too much distraction intraoperatively in a child who has undergone multiple lengthening procedures, and so to avoid excessive distraction and subsequent instrumentation failure. Also, they suggest delaying the initial surgery and stopping treatment after fewer lengthening procedures to prevent early autofusion and reduce the risk for complications from unnecessary surgeries.

Variable but high complication rates following dual growing rod surgery have been reported, including wound problems (superficial and deep infections); implant problems (fracture, loss of fixation, and implant prominence); alignment complications (kyphosis and curve progression); and general complications.[20] Because the Growing Spine Study Group (GSSG) is a multicenter international organization that houses a registry of patients with early onset scoliosis, it is not surprising that they have published the largest and most inclusive evaluations of complications. Bess et al in 2010 reported on 140 patients treated with growing rods (single and dual) over 18 years.[20] Of these, 69 were treated with dual growing rods, and they are a subject of interest in this review. Of the 69 children, 38 (55%) had 83 complications (average of 1.2 complications per patient) requiring 32 unplanned procedures. Two factors were found to increase the risk for a complication: the number of surgical procedures (24% increased risk with each additional procedure beyond the index surgery) and younger age at the time of index surgery (13% reduction in risk for each year of increase in age). Two points are worth noting here. First, in some of the children, the growing rods were implanted subcutaneously, and these children had the highest rate of complications. The subcutaneous placement of rods is not recommended anymore, and the complication rate might have been less if all rods had been implanted submuscularly. Secondly, as highlighted by Karol,[24] only 14 children had undergone final fusion at the time of the report. Therefore, the reported risk rate is likely to increase as the remaining children undergo further lengthening procedures.

The GSSG continued to investigate the outcome of growing rod surgery. Schroerlucke et al studied the effect of preoperative thoracic kyphosis on the complication rate.[21] They reported a 3.1 times greater risk for a complication in children with kyphosis of more than 40 degrees than in children with normal kyphosis. They also found an increased risk for implant-related complications (especially rod fractures) in the group with hyperkyphosis. Even though this increase was not statistically significant, it surely is of clinical importance. Yang et al[23] reported a 15% rate of rod fractures (31 fractures in 206 children treated with dual growing rods). In their study of 327 children treated with growing rods (single and dual), they identified ambulation, syndromic diagnosis, single rods, stainless steel rods, small-diameter rods, and small tandem connectors as risk factors for rod fractures. Interestingly, preoperative hyperkyphosis was not found to be a risk factor in the analysis of Yang et al (contradictory to the findings of Schroerlucke et al).

Growing rods have proved to be a very effective, versatile, and reproducible treatment for early onset scoliosis. However, a number of questions remained unanswered. Can we avoid the high risk for complications associated with repeated lengthening surgeries? Can growing rods be used in severe early onset scoliosis extending to the pelvis? Can we somehow avoid proximal thoracic fusion and preserve motion? And apart from their known effect on the growing spine, do growing rods influence the thoracic geometry as well? Investigators undertook a quest to find answers to these questions.

In 2010, Sabourin et al developed a special imaging system to create a three-dimensional reconstruction of the spine and rib cage.[25] They evaluated seven children who had undergone growing rod treatment and found that growing rods corrected not only spinal deformity but also chest wall deformity (rib orientation), thoracic axial rotation, and thoracic asymmetry. Sponseller et al reviewed the results of growing rods anchored distally to the pelvis in 36 children.[22] The indications for such a procedure were either severe early onset scoliosis extending to the pelvis or a lack of alternative anchor points in the lumbar spine. Once again, growing rods (especially dual rods) lived up to their expectations. The children showed substantial improvement in coronal and sagittal balance as well as pelvic obliquity and spinal growth. The rods were well tolerated without any increase in the rate of complications.

Repeated lengthening operations remain a big obstacle to reducing the rate of complications in growing rod surgery. However, very exciting reports have emerged recently indicating the beginning of a new era in the development of growing rods. A noninvasive, remotely distractible, magnetically controlled growing rod system has been developed.[26] Akbarnia et al first evaluated its safety and efficacy in an animal model, and the results were very encouraging.[27] Currently, the magnetically controlled growing rod system is being applied in multiple centers around the world, and preliminary results are promising.[26] This technique allows noninvasive lengthening of the rods with precise incremental distraction. Two systems currently exist: the MAGEC rod and the Phenix rod. The MAGEC Remote Control Spinal Deformity System (Ellipse Technologies, Irvine, California) is supplied sterile and can be implanted as a single rod or as dual rods. If dual rods are implanted, each can be individually adjusted with an external remote controller. Rod lengthening is done as an outpatient procedure, usually on a monthly basis. The Phenix rod, on the other hand, is used as a single rod. It is delivered clean but nonsterile. The rod is custom-made to specifications determined by the

child's spinal deformity. Parents are given a magnetic device that they hold over the child's back and rotate to extend the rod. They turn the magnet once a day to lengthen the rod by 0.2 mm.

32.3.2 Vertical Expandable Prosthetic Titanium Rod

The vertical expandable prosthetic titanium rib (VEPTR) was first introduced by Campbell and Smith in 1989.[28] Since then, it has proved to be a very effective treatment for children with thoracic insufficiency syndrome related to congenital anomalies of the spine and thoracic cavity.[28] It increases the chest volume and allows lung growth while indirectly correcting scoliosis.[29] The effect of the VEPTR on respiratory function has been, and indeed is still being, investigated by both surgeons and chest physicians, an issue that is beyond the scope of this review. However, as a summary, in 2009 Motoyama et al presented the results of their extensive work on this topic.[30] They reported a significant increase in lung volume in most patients treated with VEPTR, especially in children younger than 6 years of age.

The VEPTR follows the same principle of distraction as growing rods, but it has the advantage that spinal instrumentation, and so the possibility of autofusion, a problem usually encountered with spinal instrumentation, is avoided. Proximally, the ribs are used as anchor points, while ribs, spine, or pelvis is employed distally. The ability to control complex spinal deformities has encouraged surgeons to expand the indications for use of the VEPTR to include early onset scoliosis of noncongenital causes.[31] In our search, six articles were found pertaining to use of the VEPTR as a primary tool for the correction of spinal deformity in early onset scoliosis (▶ Table 32.2).

All reports demonstrated the ability of the VEPTR to preserve the space available for lung and to maintain thoracic kyphosis at acceptable values while stimulating spinal growth. Ramirez et al reported a 59% improvement

Table 32.2 Summary of included studies on the VEPTR

Author (reference)	Year	No.	Intervention	Follow-up (range)	Deformity correction, %	Complications, No. (%)
Ramirez et al[32]	2009	17	VEPTR	25 months (12–38)	59%	6 (35%)
Hasler et al[31]	2010	23	VEPTR	3.6 yrs (2–5.8)	25%	9 (40%)
Smith[33]	2011	37 (A 18, NA 19)	Bilateral rib-to-pelvis VEPTR	(A) 84 months (8–153) (NA) 64 months (8–153)	(A) 26% (NA) 30%	(A) 14 (77%) (NA) 10 (55%)
Latalski et al[34]	2011	12	VEPTR	30 months (10–48)	–	8 (66%)
White et al[35]	2011	14	Spine-to-spine VEPTR	35 months (2–4)	22%	6 (42%)
Reinker et al[36]	2011	14	VEPTR	5.7 yrs (1.7–12.8)	–	

Abbreviations: A, ambulatory; NA, nonambulatory; VEPTR, vertical expandable prosthetic titanium rib.

in the Cobb angle in a group of 17 patients.[32] However, other authors (Hasler et al,[31] White et al,[35] and Smith et al[33]) reported more modest percentages of correction ranging between 22% and 30% in their reviews of 23, 14, and 37 patients, respectively. It is worth noting at this point that all children in these latter reviews had noncongenital early onset scoliosis, compared with only 4 children in the report of Ramirez et al.

VEPTR-related complications included rib fractures, failure of anchor points to the ribs, brachial plexus injuries, chest wall problems (scarring and stiffness), and sagittal balance problems. Complication rates ranged between 35% and 77%.[31,32,33,34,35] However, it is also noted that the VEPTR constructs used varied, which may explain the wide range in the complication rates. As Schroerlucke et al did in their report on growing rods, Reinker et al studied the effect of preoperative kyphosis on the outcome of VEPTR surgery.[36] In their group of 14 patients with severe kyphoscoliosis treated with VEPTR, total kyphosis worsened, from 68 to 90 degrees, during the course of treatment, with detrimental effect on thoracic growth. They also noted association with anchor point failures.

32.4 Guided-Growth Systems

In an attempt to control spinal deformity and protect spinal growth while reducing the number of operations and avoiding external immobilization, Luque developed the concept of segmental spinal instrumentation without fusion.[37] Sublaminar wires were passed into the spine in a segmental fashion through extraperiosteal spinal exposure.[38] The wires were then connected to *l*- or *u*-shaped rods. The principle was that as the spine grew, the rods would "guide" growth while maintaining deformity correction.[38] Luque and McAfee et al reported excellent initial results.[37,39] However, others (Rinsky et al, Eberle et al, Mardjetko et al[40,41,42]) subsequently reported very poor results, with a high incidence of loss of correction and implant failure, modest spinal growth, and a 100% rate of spontaneous fusion (which rendered fusion surgery technically very difficult). The Luque trolley was subsequently abandoned.[42]

Recently, attempts have been made to revive the principle of guided growth. Although they are not routine practice, these attempts have been included in this review because they provide insight into some future directions in the management of early onset scoliosis. Two articles (and one abstract) were found to be relevant.

Appreciating the shortfalls of the Luque trolley, Ouellet modified the original idea by using a different approach and newer implants.[38] A minimally invasive approach with extraperiosteal dissection avoided the need to strip the periosteum off the lamina, and the use of low-profile implants aimed to minimize the risk for autofusion. Ouellet reported the results of his "modern Luque trolley" in a group of 5 children with early onset scoliosis. There was a 65% improvement in the Cobb angle (from an average of 60 degrees initially to 21 degrees at final follow-up at an average of 4 years). The average total spinal growth was 3 cm, representing 73% of the expected values. Revision surgery was required in three patients, in two because they outgrew their constructs and in one because of recurrence of the deformity and spontaneous fusion. All three patients experienced improvement following revision surgery. No wound problems or clinically important implant failures were encountered.

A deeper look into the figures in this report reveals some interesting observations. It is clear that the figures of a single patient have skewed the entire results of the study. This patient achieved 45% deformity correction and grew only 26% of the expected value, findings that inevitably raise the suspicion that the construct was not ideal for this patient. If the results for this patient are dismissed, the figures show 70% deformity correction and an astonishing 94% of expected growth. However, the small sample size, the inclusion of patients with scoliosis of different etiologies, and the lack of long-term follow-up make it impossible to deduce any statistical significance or make any clinical recommendations. The inability to control rotational deformity, the risk for autofusion, the risk for junctional kyphosis, and the generation of debris particles across the gliding interfaces all need to be thoroughly and individually investigated. The results do justify further exploration of this technique.

Another technique of growth guidance is the Shilla system. This technique corrects the apex of the deformity with a limited fusion and fixes the fused segment to dual rods, while allowing the ends of the spine to grow.[43] Growth guidance at both ends of the spine occurs through implanted pedicle screws, which slide along the rods at both ends of the construct. McCarthy et al published the results of their pilot study of the Shilla system in an animal model (goats).[43] This study demonstrated the ability of the system to protect growth. However, as expected, wear particles were observed around the gliding surfaces. At the 2nd International Congress on Early Onset Scoliosis and Growing Spine, McCarthy et al presented their preliminary results of implanting Shilla rods in 10 children.[44] They reported a 50% improvement in the Cobb angle (from 70 to 34 degrees) and improvements in space available for lung and truncal height of 13% and 12%, respectively. An additional five unplanned operations for complications were needed in five children.

32.5 Tension-Based Systems

The Hueter–Volkmann law states that a growth plate subjected to increased pressure will grow more slowly than a similar growth plate subjected to less pressure.[45] This axiom is the main principle behind the use of tension-based systems in growth modulation. The use of staples to halt the aberrant growth of the convex side, yet allow the lagging growth of the concave side to continue, can theoretically correct a deformity.[46]

This principle was first applied in the treatment of scoliosis more than 50 years ago, but results were disappointing.[47] In the 1990s, interest in the principle of growth modulation was renewed. Stainless steel staples were used, but again with poor results, and subsequently the technique was abandoned.[47] Over the last decade, the development of shape memory alloy materials has provided a novel platform for improving vertebral staples. The results of preclinical (animal models) and clinical trials of nitinol (shape memory alloy) staples and of other innovative techniques (tethers) are included in this review.

Two papers on animal studies and two on clinical trials were found in our search. It is worth mentioning that the use of tension-based systems in early onset scoliosis has not been attempted or recommended. However, the continued interest in their use may be grounds for consideration as a future option. This review aims only to highlight the important milestones in their development.

Animal models were integral in the development of tension-based systems. In a goat model,[46] Braun et al demonstrated the efficacy of nitinol staples in halting deformity progression. They later described even greater control of deformity in another goat model treated with flexible tethers attached to bone anchors.[48] In 2003, Betz et al used vertebral body stapling to treat 21 adolescents with scoliosis.[49] They concluded that vertebral body stapling is feasible, safe, and effective in controlling deformity. In 2010, Betz et al published 3-year follow-up results in a group of 28 patients.[50] They demonstrated the ability of vertebral body stapling to control lumbar curves and thoracic curves of less than 35 degrees, with 87% and 79% success rates, respectively. However, they did not recommend the use of vertebral body stapling in thoracic curves larger than 35 degrees. These results are preliminary, and follow-up to skeletal maturity will be needed.

32.6 Conclusion

Early onset scoliosis typically presents before the age of 5 years. Progressive curves treated with conventional spinal fusion usually result in the same deleterious effects as completely untreated deformities.[51] The resulting skeletal and cardiopulmonary compromise renders definitive fusion at this age for this condition a nonviable option.

The purpose of this review has been to examine the surgical options currently available to treating surgeons. Since being developed by Akbarnia and Marks, the dual growing rod system has proved its usefulness in treating a very complex and difficult condition. It has also produced consistent results and is safe. In collating the literature for this article, we found the average overall deformity correction rate to range from 52 to 64% and

complication rates to range from 48 to 55%. Statistical analysis of the complications identified young age at initial surgery and a high number of surgical procedures as the two main risk factors.[20] However, there is conflicting evidence on the effect of hyperkyphosis.[21,23] Because of the potentially grave effects of deformity on a vulnerable group of patients, all authors considered these complication rates to be acceptable. Growing rods have also proved effective in more difficult situations, such as severe early onset scoliosis extending to the pelvis.[22]

Although the VEPTR was originally designed to treat children with thoracic insufficiency syndrome resulting from congenital spinal and thoracic deformities, attempts have been made to use it in patients with early onset scoliosis of noncongenital origin. The avoidance of autofusion, which is associated with other techniques of spinal instrumentation, is the main advantage. However, in comparison with dual growing rods, the VEPTR provides modest deformity control (22–30%) and has a higher complication rate (35–77%).

Guided-growth systems were developed initially in an attempt to avoid repeated surgeries and thus reduce the risk for complications. However, early results with them were disappointing, and their use was subsequently abandoned. The modification of Luque trolley by Ouellet and the development of the new alternative Shilla system by McCarthy are recent attempts to revive the principle of growth guidance. Although both have demonstrated promising initial results, they should be interpreted with caution. The small sample size, short follow-up, and uncertainties about the effects of these systems on local tissues all produce more questions than answers at this stage.

Tension-based systems (staples and tethers) have shown great success in the treatment of skeletal limb deformities. However, the results of their use in scoliosis should be interpreted with caution. Preclinical and clinical studies demonstrated their ability to control, but not correct, scoliotic deformity. This ability was demonstrated only in adolescents and was limited to patients with mild and moderate deformities.

32.7 Statement of Opinion

In this review, the evidence behind the different surgical options has been explored. Tension-based systems have proved to be an effective alternative to bracing in adolescents with certain deformities (thoracic deformity of < 35 degrees and lumbar deformity). However, to date, they do not have a role in the younger group of patients with early onset scoliosis. The modern Luque trolley and the Shilla system offer an attractive prospect for correcting deformity and guiding spinal growth with a minimal number of procedures. However, results are preliminary, and more extensive studies with a larger sample size and longer follow-up are needed to evaluate their efficacy as well as safety.

Distraction systems were found to have the most solid body of evidence to support their efficacy. They delivered consistent results and are the most widely used modality. The VEPTR produced the best results when used in congenital or thoracogenic scoliosis, and indeed it is the gold-standard line of treatment for thoracic insufficiency syndrome.[31] However, when investigated as an option for early onset scoliosis of spinal origin, dual growing rods were even better. Dual growing rods have proved their ability to achieve treatment goals. They correct deformity and maintain the correction while allowing spinal growth to continue. Complication rates are high, but acceptable. On analysis of the complications in different reports, it is universally agreed that the high number of procedures strongly predicts that complications will be encountered. However, with promising advances in the development of magnetically controlled growing rod systems, this hurdle may be cleared in the near future.

The consensus from this review is that dual growing rods have the best body of evidence to support their use in the surgical treatment of progressive early onset scoliosis of noncongenital origin, whereas the VEPTR appears to have the best results for the treatment of thoracic insufficiency syndrome. However, because of the lack of randomized controlled studies on the surgical treatment of early onset scoliosis, it is difficult to define with any degree of certainty the gold standard of treatment.

References

[1] Dickson RA. Conservative treatment for idiopathic scoliosis. J Bone Joint Surg Br 1985; 67: 176–181

[2] Akbarnia BA. Management themes in early onset scoliosis. J Bone Joint Surg Am 2007; 89 Suppl 1: 42–54

[3] James JI, Lloyd-Roberts GC, Pilcher MF. Infantile structural scoliosis. J Bone Joint Surg Br 1959; 41-B: 719–735

[4] Gillingham BL, Fan RA, Akbarnia BA. Early onset idiopathic scoliosis. J Am Acad Orthop Surg 2006; 14: 101–112

[5] Branthwaite MA. Cardiorespiratory consequences of unfused idiopathic scoliosis. Br J Dis Chest 1986; 80: 360–369

[6] Pehrsson K, Larsson S, Oden A, Nachemson A. Long-term follow-up of patients with untreated scoliosis. A study of mortality, causes of death, and symptoms. Spine 1992; 17: 1091–1096

[7] Skaggs DL, Akbarnia BA, Flynn JM JB, Myung KS, Sponseller PD, Vitale MG Chest Wall and Spine Deformity Study Group. Growing Spine Study Group. Pediatric Orthopaedic Society of North America. Scoliosis Research Society Growing Spine Study Committee. A classification of growth friendly spine implants. J Pediatr Orthop 2014; 34: 260–274

[8] Karol LA. Early definitive spinal fusion in young children: what we have learned. Clin Orthop Relat Res 2011; 469: 1323–1329

[9] Day GA, Upadhyay SS, Ho EK, Leong JC, Ip M. Pulmonary functions in congenital scoliosis. Spine 1994; 19: 1027–1031

[10] Winter RB, Moe JH. The results of spinal arthrodesis for congenital spinal deformity in patients younger than five years old. J Bone Joint Surg Am 1982; 64: 419–432

[11] Vitale MG, Gomez JA, Matsumoto H, Roye DP Jr. Chest Wall and Spine Deformity Study Group. Variability of expert opinion in treatment of early-onset scoliosis. Clin Orthop Relat Res 2011; 469: 1317–1322

[12] Harrington PR. Treatment of scoliosis. Correction and internal fixation by spine instrumentation. J Bone Joint Surg Am 1962; 44-A: 591–610

[13] Moe JH, Kharrat K, Winter RB, Cummine JL. Harrington instrumentation without fusion plus external orthotic support for the treatment of difficult curvature problems in young children. Clin Orthop Relat Res 1984; 185: 35–45

[14] Klemme WR, Denis F, Winter RB, Lonstein JW, Koop SE. Spinal instrumentation without fusion for progressive scoliosis in young children. J Pediatr Orthop 1997; 17: 734–742

[15] Blakemore LC, Scoles PV, Poe-Kochert C, Thompson GH. Submuscular Isola rod with or without limited apical fusion in the management of severe spinal deformities in young children: preliminary report. Spine 2001; 26: 2044–2048

[16] Mineiro J, Weinstein SL. Subcutaneous rodding for progressive spinal curvatures: early results. J Pediatr Orthop 2002; 22: 290–295

[17] Akbarnia BA, Marks DS, Boachie-Adjei O, Thompson AG, Asher MA. Dual growing rod technique for the treatment of progressive early-onset scoliosis: a multicenter study. Spine 2005; 30 Suppl: S46–S57

[18] Akbarnia BA, Breakwell LM, Marks DS et al. Growing Spine Study Group. Dual growing rod technique followed for three to eleven years until final fusion: the effect of frequency of lengthening. Spine 2008; 33: 984–990

[19] Sankar WN, Skaggs DL, Yazici M et al. Lengthening of dual growing rods and the law of diminishing returns. Spine 2011; 36: 806–809

[20] Bess S, Akbarnia BA, Thompson GH et al. Complications of growing-rod treatment for early-onset scoliosis: analysis of one hundred and forty patients. J Bone Joint Surg Am 2010; 92: 2533–2543

[21] Schroerlucke SR, Akbarnia BA, Pawelek JB et al. Growing Spine Study Group. How does thoracic kyphosis affect patient outcomes in growing rod surgery? Spine 2012; 37: 1303–1309

[22] Sponseller PD, Yang JS, Thompson GH et al. Pelvic fixation of growing rods: comparison of constructs. Spine 2009; 34: 1706–1710

[23] Yang JS, Sponseller PD, Thompson GH et al. Growing Spine Study Group. Growing rod fractures: risk factors and opportunities for prevention. Spine 2011; 36: 1639–1644

[24] Karol LA. Commentary on an article by S. Bess, MD, et al.: "Complications of growing-rod treatment for early-onset scoliosis. Analysis of one hundred and forty patients". J Bone Joint Surg Am 2010; 92: e27

[25] Sabourin M, Jolivet E, Miladi L, Wicart P, Rampal V, Skalli W. Three-dimensional stereoradiographic modeling of rib cage before and after spinal growing rod procedures in early-onset scoliosis. Clin Biomech (Bristol, Avon) 2010; 25: 284–291

[26] Cheung KM, Cheung JP, Samartzis D et al. Magnetically controlled growing rods for severe spinal curvature in young children: a prospective case series. Lancet 2012; 379: 1967–1974

[27] Akbarnia BA, Mundis GM Jr Salari P, Yaszay B, Pawelek JB. Innovation in growing rod technique: a study of safety and efficacy of a magnetically controlled growing rod in a porcine model. Spine 2012; 37: 1109–1114

[28] Campbell RM Jr Smith MD, Hell-Vocke AK. Expansion thoracoplasty: the surgical technique of opening-wedge thoracostomy. Surgical technique. J Bone Joint Surg Am 2004; 86-A Suppl 1: 51–64

[29] Campbell RM Jr Smith MD. Thoracic insufficiency syndrome and exotic scoliosis. J Bone Joint Surg Am 2007; 89 Suppl 1: 108–122

[30] Motoyama EK, Yang CI, Deeney VF. Thoracic malformation with early-onset scoliosis: effect of serial VEPTR expansion thoracoplasty on lung growth and function in children. Paediatr Respir Rev 2009; 10: 12–17

[31] Hasler CC, Mehrkens A, Hefti F. Efficacy and safety of VEPTR instrumentation for progressive spine deformities in young children without rib fusions. Eur Spine J 2010; 19: 400–408

[32] Ramirez N, Flynn JM, Serrano JA, Carlo S, Cornier AS. The Vertical Expandable Prosthetic Titanium Rib in the treatment of spinal deformity due to progressive early onset scoliosis. J Pediatr Orthop B 2009; 18: 197–203

[33] Smith JT. Bilateral rib-to-pelvis technique for managing early-onset scoliosis. Clin Orthop Relat Res 2011; 469: 1349–1355

[34] Latalski M, Fatyga M, Gregosiewicz A. Problems and complications in VEPTR-based treatment. Ortop Traumatol Rehabil 2011; 13: 449–455

[35] White KK, Song KM, Frost N, Daines BK. VEPTR™ growing rods for early-onset neuromuscular scoliosis: feasible and effective. Clin Orthop Relat Res 2011; 469: 1335–1341

[36] Reinker K, Simmons JW, Patil V, Stinson Z. Can VEPTR(®) control progression of early-onset kyphoscoliosis? A cohort study of VEPTR(®) patients with severe kyphoscoliosis. Clin Orthop Relat Res 2011; 469: 1342–1348

[37] Luque ER. Segmental spinal instrumentation for correction of scoliosis. Clin Orthop Relat Res 1982: 192–198

[38] Ouellet J. Surgical technique: modern Luqué trolley, a self-growing rod technique. Clin Orthop Relat Res 2011; 469: 1356–1367

[39] McAfee PC, Lubicky JP, Werner FW. The use of segmental spinal instrumentation to preserve longitudinal spinal growth. An experimental study. J Bone Joint Surg Am 1983; 65: 935–942

[40] Rinsky LA, Gamble JG, Bleck EE. Segmental instrumentation without fusion in children with progressive scoliosis. J Pediatr Orthop 1985; 5: 687–690

[41] Eberle CF. Failure of fixation after segmental spinal instrumentation without arthrodesis in the management of paralyticscoliosis. J Bone Joint Surg Am 1988; 70: 696–703

[42] Mardjetko SM, Hammerberg KW, Lubicky JP, Fister JS. The Luque trolley revisited. Review of nine cases requiring revision. Spine 1992; 17: 582–589

[43] McCarthy RE, Sucato D, Turner JL, Zhang H, Henson MAW, McCarthy K. Shilla growing rods in a caprine animal model: a pilot study. Clin Orthop Relat Res 2010; 468: 705–710

[44] McCarthy R, Luhmann S, Lenke L. Greater than two year follow-up Shilla growth enhancing system for the treatment of scoliosis in children. Presented at: 2nd International Congress on Early Onset Scoliosis and Growing Spine; November 7–8, 2008; Montreal, Canada

[45] Cunningham ME, Frelinghuysen PHB, Roh JS, Boachie-Adjei O, Green DW. Fusionless scoliosis surgery. Curr Opin Pediatr 2005; 17: 48–53

[46] Braun JT, Ogilvie JW, Akyuz E, Brodke DS, Bachus KN. Fusionless scoliosis correction using a shape memory alloy staple in the anterior thoracic spine of the immature goat. Spine 2004; 29: 1980–1989

[47] Hoh DJ, Elder JB, Wang MY. Principles of growth modulation in the treatment of scoliotic deformities. Neurosurgery 2008; 63 Suppl: 211–221

[48] Braun JT, Akyuz E, Ogilvie JW, Bachus KN. The efficacy and integrity of shape memory alloy staples and bone anchors with ligament tethers in the fusionless treatment of experimental scoliosis. J Bone Joint Surg Am 2005; 87: 2038–2051

[49] Betz RR, Kim J, D'Andrea LP, Mulcahey MJ, Balsara RK, Clements DH. An innovative technique of vertebral body stapling for the treatment of patients with adolescent idiopathic scoliosis: a feasibility, safety, and utility study. Spine 2003; 28: S255–S265

[50] Betz RR, Ranade A, Samdani AF et al. Vertebral body stapling: a fusionless treatment option for a growing child with moderate idiopathic scoliosis. Spine 2010; 35: 169–176

[51] Johnston CE. Early onset scoliosis: editorial comment. Clin Orthop Relat Res 2011; 469: 1315–1316

33 Magnetic Growing Rods

N.S. Harshavardhana, M.H. Hilali Noordeen

33.1 Case 1: Magnetic Growing Rods to Improve Pulmonary Function in Early Onset Scoliosis Secondary to a Neuromuscular Disorder

Spinal muscular atrophy (SMA) is an autosomal recessive disorder caused by homozygous deletion of the survival motor neuron 1 gene (*SMN1*) located on chromosome 5.[1] The incidence is reported to be from 1 in 6,000 to 1 in 10,000 in European populations.[2] The selective destruction of anterior motor neurons manifests as proximal muscle weakness with progressive pulmonary deterioration. The clinical spectrum varies from early death during infancy to nearly normal life expectancy, depending on the severity of the disease. The most common orthopedic manifestation is scoliosis, which is seen in 65 to 95% of affected individuals.[3] In addition, hip subluxation and dislocation develop in a large proportion of patients. Depending on the age at onset and time of diagnosis, SMA is classified mainly into three types[4]:

- Type 1 (Werdnig–Hoffmann disease), the most severe form, has an onset within the first 6 months of life. Patients usually die by the first decade.
- Type 2 (intermediate type) is usually characterized by an onset after 2 years. It accounts for most of the spinal deformities seen in early onset scoliosis clinics. The majority of patients are wheelchair–bound by the end of first decade, and survival beyond the second decade is uncommon
- Type 3 (Kugelberg–Welander syndrome) has a late onset, and patients survive up to and beyond the fourth decade. They usually retain ambulatory potential beyond adolescence and into adulthood.

33.1.1 Case Summary

A 5-year-old Caucasian girl was referred by her pediatrician to the senior author [MHHN] for evaluation because of concerns about the development of scoliosis. She had been born at full term to non-consanguineous parents. Her Apgar scores were 8 and 10 at 1 and 5 minutes after birth. Her developmental milestones had been normal up to her first birthday. Subsequently, recurrent chest infections and emergency admissions to a pediatric intensive care unit for a couple of years warranted investigations for cystic fibrosis and other genetic / inherited conditions. Extensive work-up by pediatricians and geneticists revealed a diagnosis of type 2 SMA. By her fourth and fifth birthdays, she was lagging in motor milestones, with frequent falls, and had a Gowers sign (suggestive of proximal trunk and lower extremity muscle weakness).

At her first clinic visit, she was in the 70% percentile for weight and age and the 75% percentile for height. On clinical examination, she had unequal shoulders and sat leaning to the left side. She was capable of walking a few steps with support. Plain radiographs revealed a left sided thoracolumbar scoliosis of 65 degrees, which was largely flexible. She was prescribed a TLSO (thoracolumbosacral orthosis), to be worn full-time (at least 22 hours per day), and it was arranged for her to be seen at 4-month intervals. By her sixth birthday, despite her compliance with full-time brace wear, the scoliosis had worsened to 85 degrees (▶ Fig. 33.1). Pulmonary function tests revealed the FEV$_1$ (forced expiratory volume in 1 second) to be 20% of the predicted value, and the FVC (forced vital capacity) was 23% of the predicted value. Surgery was offered, and the parents were counseled about the importance of arresting progression of the deformity. Discussion among anesthesiologists, pediatricians, and intensive care physicians at multidisciplinary team meetings yielded a consensus that her pulmonary function was too

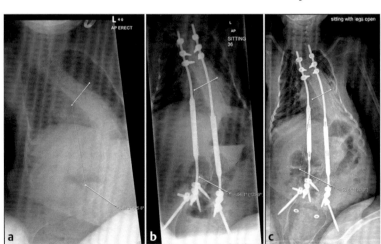

Fig. 33.1 Spinal muscular atrophy type 2. An 85-degree curve just before surgery has a correction of 30 degrees (to 55 degrees) postoperatively. Anteroposterior radiographs immediately preoperatively (**a**), immediately postoperatively (**b**), and 2 years postoperatively (**c**).

poor for her to withstand conventional growing rod surgeries and regular 6-monthly distractions under general anesthesia. She was discussed at the multi-disciplinary meeting and a collective decision was made for her to have the novel implant inserted. Thereafter, she was enrolled into the magnetic growing rods program to have dual growing rods inserted submuscularly from T2 to the pelvis.

33.1.2 Surgical Technique

The patient was placed in the prone position on a Montreal mattress with adequate padding of all pressure points. It was ensured that there was no compression on the eyes. General anesthesia was administered via endotracheal intubation. Special care was taken to avoid hyperextension of the upper extremities to avoid the risk of causing brachial plexopathy / traction neuropraxia. After preparation with 2% chlorhexidine and draping under strict asepsis, two incisions were made in the midline over the proximal thoracic spine to expose the T2-T5 vertebrae and over the distal lumbar spine to expose the L3-S1 vertebral segments by subperiosteal dissection. A freehand technique was used to insert 4.5 × 25-mm pedicle screws at the T3 and T4 vertebrae bilaterally. Two down-going transverse process hooks were inserted into T2. The transverse process hooks exert laterally directed forces, protecting the spinal cord from the screws by preventing medial migration if they happen to loosen with time. Two 5 × 30-mm pedicle screws were then inserted into the L4 and L5 pedicles. Two 7.5-mm-diameter iliac wing screws were then inserted into the pelvis under C-arm image intensifier guidance. A flexible rod template was used to measure the length of rod needed, and the magnetic growing rod was cut to the desired length. The actuator area containing the magnet measures 9 cm in length and 9 mm in diameter. Appropriate sagittal contouring was done proximal and distal to the actuator area to ensure that the actuator area remained straight and to facilitate ease of insertion. The magnetic coil was tested with the handheld device before it was inserted.

A 20-gauge chest tube was used to railroad the rod submuscularly in a caudocranial direction on the concave side. The rod was then attached to the pedicle screws and iliac bolts (with the use of lateral connectors). Cranially, the rod was attached to the hybrid construct (hooks and pedicle screws). The procedure was repeated on the convex side, and all anchors were tightened with gentle distraction on the concave side to level the pelvis and correct the scoliosis. Finally, a cross-link was attached at the proximal end to link the two rods as a single unit.

The posterior elements were then decorticated and mixed with bone marrow aspirate obtained at the time of pedicle screw insertions. Silicated calcium phosphate (Actifuse granules; Baxter BioSurgery, Deerfield, Illinois) was mixed with native / host bone and laid over both the proximal and distal fixation anchors. Hemostasis was secured, and the wound was closed in layers with absorbable sutures and no drains were used.

33.1.3 Postoperative Care and Rehabilitation

The child was allowed to sit up erect with effect from postoperative day 1 and to mobilize from day 3. No brace was needed at the time of discharge. She was seen at regular 3-monthly intervals in the office by the senior author, who also performed serial 3-monthly distractions. The initial 3 months of close observation was needed to ensure adequate arthrodesis at the anchor sites, to facilitate regular serial distractions. The patient underwent lengthening on an outpatient basis wherein a handheld magnetic wand was used to identify the precise area of the magnetic coil. Low-dose radiography was used after each distraction to confirm that the spine had indeed lengthened.

Profound improvement in her health was noted 1 year postoperatively, by which time she had undergone four lengthening procedures and gained 12 mm in height. There was a significant improvement in her quality of life, with markedly fewer visits to the accident and emergency department. Her occasional episodes of pneumonia were very few and far between. At the end of 2 years postoperatively, she had an FEV_1 of 50% predicted and an FVC of 55% predicted (statistically significant difference; $p < 0.0002$). Elongation of the right-sided convex rod was 23.2 mm, and elongation of the left-sided concave rod was 32.4 mm (▶ Fig. 33.2). The parents were extremely satisfied with the clinical results.

33.1.4 Discussion

The natural history of type 2 SMA is progressive proximal muscle weakness with deterioration in pulmonary function over time.[5] Mortality is inevitable by the end of the second decade. The evolving *parasol deformity* of the chest (i.e., vertical positioning of ribs with development of a bell-shaped thorax due to weak intercostal muscles and a strong diaphragm) causes volume depletion deformity of thorax, resulting in thoracic insufficiency syndrome.[6] Conventional growing rods require regular 6-monthly distractions under general anesthesia, which is not without complications (i.e., risk for aspiration and psychological stress for the child, parents, and extended family).[7] The vertebral expandable prosthetic titanium rib (VEPTR) is an alternative option wherein the VEPTR gantry supports the collapsing chest cage (parasol deformity). However, it is also fraught with multiple complications (at least 25%) and an increased risk for wound dehiscence.[8]

Although a dramatic improvement in pulmonary function was seen in this child, we do not believe that magnetic growing rods alter the natural history of SMA. They

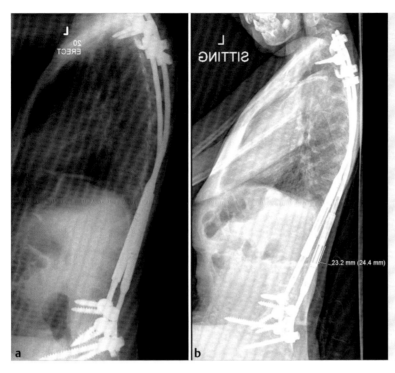

Fig. 33.2 Spinal muscular atrophy type 2. Lateral radiographs immediately postoperatively (**a**) and 2 years postoperatively (**b**) show 23.2 mm of achieved lengthening.

do, however, significantly delay the rate of pulmonary deterioration, which creates a spurious impression of improvement during pulmonary function testing. This is the first report of a case of type 2 SMA in the world with a 2-year follow-up that has reported an improvement in pulmonary function.

33.2 Case 2: Magnetic Growing Rods for Early Onset Idiopathic Scoliosis

Early onset scoliosis is characterized by the manifestation of spinal deformity in children younger than 5 years of age.[9] The etiology can be congenital, neuromuscular, syndromic, or idiopathic. The characteristics of idiopathic early onset scoliosis differ from those of adolescent idiopathic scoliosis in that the former may be associated with long-term pulmonary morbidity.[10] The inability of the chest cage and thorax to support normal breathing results in pathophysiology that manifests as thoracic insufficiency syndrome.[11] Lung compliance, vital capacity, and alveolar maturation are closely linked to growth and development of the thoracic cage and spine.

Diverse options are available to treat idiopathic early onset scoliosis. The key principle is to guide spinal growth with mechanical adjuncts to facilitate normal pulmonary maturation. Early definitive spinal fusion is unacceptable and strongly discouraged because it leads to a disproportionate ratio of the upper segment to the lower segment and restrictive lung disease with a significant reduction

in pulmonary vital capacity.[12] The traditional treatment has been casting and bracing. However, significant proportions of children are unresponsive to this form of therapy, and the rapid progression of scoliosis compels surgical intervention. Numerous growth-sparing modalities exist to treat early onset scoliosis:

1. Growing rods;
2. Vertebral expandable prosthetic titanium rib (VEPTR);
3. Vertebral stapling / convex tether;
4. Shilla technique.

Self-growing expandable rods are a novel solution for addressing rapidly progressive curves that are refractory to brace therapy. They eliminate the need for multiple procedures requiring anesthesia and the psychological trauma associated with frequent hospital admissions.[13] Recent reports have highlighted the cognitive impairment and learning disabilities associated with multiple exposures of the immature brain to general anesthesia.[14] We report here the case of a patient who had idiopathic early onset scoliosis treated by the senior author with a single submuscular magnetic growing rod and followed for 2 years.

33.2.1 Case Summary

A 7.5-year-old girl of Asian ethnicity was referred by her family physician to the senior author for evaluation because of concerns about the development of scoliosis. She had been born at full term to non-consanguineous parents. Her Apgar scores were 9 and 10 at 1 and 5 minutes after birth. Her motor and verbal developmental milestones had been normal. She started to crawl at age 6 months and to stand with support by 9 to 11 months. She was able to walk by 13 to 15 months and to build a tower of six cubes by her third birthday. Her scholastic progress at primary school was appropriate for her age. An aunt observed her "crooked" spine while she was in a swimming suit during a family holiday at the beach. Subsequently, her mother pointed this out to her pediatrician, who noticed shoulder asymmetry and scoliosis and promptly referred the child to be seen by a specialist.

At the first clinic visit, her weight was in the 70% percentile for age and her height was in the 95% percentile. She was lean and had a body mass index (BMI) of 16.2. On clinical examination, she had unequal shoulders, with the right shoulder higher than the left. The clavicular angle measured 11 degrees. A posteroanterior radiograph at the first clinic visit revealed a right thoracic scoliosis that measured 42 degrees. Magnetic resonance imaging of the neuraxis did not reveal any intraspinal anomaly. She was prescribed a brace (thoracolumbosacral orthosis) to be worn full-time (at least 22 hours per day), and it was arranged for her to be seen at 6-month intervals. By her ninth birthday, despite her compliance with full-time brace wear, the scoliosis had worsened to 62 degrees. The convex bending radiograph revealed a fairly rigid curve that corrected to 50 degrees (▶ Fig. 33.3). The flexibility index was 20%. There had been a progression of 20 degrees in 2 years. Surgery was offered, and the parents were counseled about the importance of arresting progression of the deformity. They were given the choice of either conventional growing rods or the newer magnetic growing rods, which would eliminate the need for multiple surgeries and serial hospital admissions at 6-month intervals for lengthening procedures that could interfere with the child's attendance at school and academic commitments. The parents were also given an opportunity to speak with patient advocates (i.e., other parents whose children had had conventional growing rods or magnetic

growing rods inserted). The parents voluntarily chose to have magnetic growing rods inserted. According to the caregivers' wishes, at 9.5 years of age, the patient was enrolled in the magnetic growing rods program to have a single growing rod inserted submuscularly from T2 to L1. The senior author prefers that the vertebra within the curve that is just touched by the central sacral vertical line (CSVL) be the caudal instrumented vertebra.

33.2.2 Surgical Technique

The patient was placed in a prone position on a Montreal mattress with adequate padding of all pressure points. It was ensured that there was no compression on the eyes. General anesthesia was administered via endotracheal intubation. Special care was taken to avoid hyperextension of the upper extremities to avoid the risk of causing brachial plexopathy / traction neuropraxia.[15] After preparation with 2% chlorhexidine and draping under strict asepsis, two incisions were made in the midline over the proximal thoracic spine to expose the T2-T5 vertebrae and over the distal lumbar spine to expose the T11-L1 vertebral segments by subperiosteal dissection. A freehand technique was used to insert 5×25-mm pedicle screws at the T3 and T4 vertebrae bilaterally. Two downgoing transverse process hooks were inserted into T2. The transverse process hooks exert laterally directed forces, protecting the spinal cord from the screws by preventing medial migration should they happen to loosen with time. Two 5.5×30-mm pedicle screws were then inserted into the T12 and L1 pedicles. A flexible rod template was used to measure the length of rod needed, and the magnetic growing rod was cut to the desired length. The actuator area containing the magnet measures 9 cm in length and 9 mm in diameter. Appropriate sagittal contouring was done to ensure that the actuator area remained straight. The magnetic coil was tested with the handheld device before it was inserted to be certain that it was working properly.

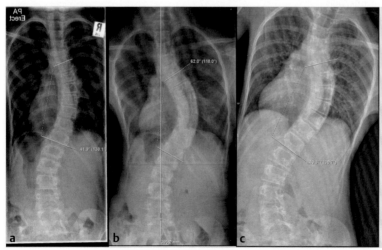

Fig. 33.3 Early onset scoliosis (idiopathic). Posteroanterior radiographs at the first visit and immediately preoperatively show a curve of 62 degrees (correcting to 50 degrees on convex bending). Radiographs at the first clinic visit (**a**) and immediately preoperatively (**b**) show 20 degrees of progression in 2 years. Preoperative convex bending (**c**).

A 20-gauge chest tube was used to railroad the rod submuscularly in a caudocranial direction on the concave side. The rod was then attached to the distal pedicle screw anchors. Cranially, the rod was attached to the hybrid construct (hooks and pedicle screws). The posterior elements were then decorticated and mixed with bone marrow aspirate obtained at the time of pedicle screw insertions. Silicated calcium phosphate (20 mg of Actifuse granules) was mixed with native / host bone and laid over both the proximal and distal fixation anchors. Hemostasis was secured, and the wound was closed in layers with absorbable sutures.

33.2.3 Postoperative Care and Rehabilitation

The child was allowed to sit up erect with effect from postoperative day 2 and to mobilize from day 3. No brace was needed at the time of discharge. Contact sports and horseback riding were prohibited for at least 6 months. She was seen at regular 3-month intervals in the office by the senior author, who also performed serial 3-month distractions. The initial 3 months of close observation was needed to ensure adequate arthrodesis at the anchor sites before regular serial distractions were begun. The patient underwent lengthening on an outpatient basis wherein a handheld magnetic wand was used to identify the precise area of the magnetic coil. Low-dose radiography was used after each distraction to confirm that the spine had lengthened.

Improvement in the patient's coronal balance was noted, and the shoulder asymmetry had completely disappeared at 6 months postoperatively. At 1 year postoperatively, by which time she had undergone four lengthening procedures, she had gained 11 mm in height. The elongation of the magnetic rod at final follow-up of 25 months was 28 mm (▶ Fig. 33.4). The Cobb angle at last follow-up measured 36 degrees. The overall Cobb angle correction from time since surgery was 26 degrees. She was Risser grade 4 radiologically and postmenarchal at last follow-up. Her parents were extremely satisfied with the clinical results, and the scope for performing a definitive spinal fusion within the coming year or two was discussed.

33.2.4 Discussion

Growing rods are a popular treatment option and have revolutionized the surgical management of early onset scoliosis that is refractory to all conservative modalities of management.[16] The rods act as internal scaffolds, guiding the growth of the spine with time and minimizing coronal deformity. However, they are not without complications, and in a series of 910 growing rod surgeries, Bess et al reported a complication rate of 20%.[17] The most commonly observed complications were implant failure,

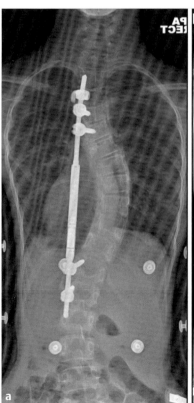
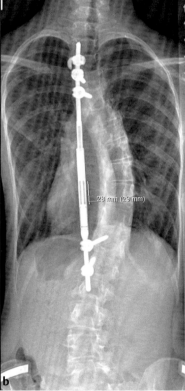

Fig. 33.4 Early onset scoliosis (idiopathic). Posteroanterior radiographs immediately postoperatively (**a**) and 2 years postoperatively (**b**) show 28 mm of lengthening.

rod breakage, and anchor dislodgment. The use of dual rods minimized, if not completely eliminated, these risks. In addition, according to the "law of diminishing returns," the results of surgery eventually plateau, either because of spinal arthrodesis after multiple exposures or because of spinal noncompliance.[18] Noordeen et al reported that in vivo distractive forces doubled by the fifth distraction and that the inferior migration of pedicle screws (i.e., distal anchors) with elongation of the pedicles was a common phenomenon.[19]

The VEPTR was developed by Campbell et al to address thoracic insufficiency syndrome and is commonly employed to treat early onset scoliosis with a congenital or syndromic etiology.[11,20] The VEPTR is particularly helpful when expansion thoracoplasty is performed to manage fused ribs and spine in very young children and to address different types of volume depletion deformities of the lung. Its use in purely idiopathic scoliosis is controversial, and further evidence is desired before it can be routinely recommended for this particular clinical condition. An attractive feature of the VEPTR is that the surgeon has the option to leave the spine completely untouched cranially by using rib anchors as proximal fixation constructs.

The Shilla technique was developed by McCarthy et al, who performed a short-segment apical fusion and used nonlocking polyaxial screws proximally and distally to guide a long rod to correct spinal curvature.[21] These rods were intentionally left long to accommodate spinal growth. Their results at best were comparable with those of conventional growing rods.

Magnetic growing rods are novel, noninvasive lengthening devices with a built-in magnetic coil that can be operated with a handheld device in the office, eliminating the need for multiple, repeated procedures under anesthesia.[14] Recent publications by the senior author from his own personal series and multicentric studies do confirm fewer complications and a more cost-effective alternative in the long run.[22,23] This is one of the earliest cases of magnetic growing rod insertion for idiopathic early onset scoliosis with a 2-year follow-up.

References

[1] Munsat TL. The spinal muscular atrophies. In: Appel SH, ed. Current Neurology. St. Louis, MO: Mosby; 1994:55–71

[2] Feldkötter M, Schwarzer V, Wirth R, Wienker TF, Wirth B. Quantitative analyses of SMN1 and SMN2 based on real-time lightCycler PCR: fast and highly reliable carrier testing and prediction of severity of spinal muscular atrophy. Am J Hum Genet 2002; 70: 358–368

[3] Granata C, Merlini L, Magni E, Marini ML, Stagni SB. Spinal muscular atrophy: natural history and orthopaedic treatment of scoliosis. Spine 1989; 14: 760–762

[4] Wang CH, Finkel RS, Bertini ES et al. Participants of the International Conference on SMA Standard of Care. Consensus statement for standard of care in spinal muscular atrophy. J Child Neurol 2007; 22: 1027–1049

[5] Zerres K, Rudnik-Schöneborn S, Forrest E, Lusakowska A, Borkowska J, Hausmanowa-Petrusewicz I. A collaborative study on the natural history of childhood and juvenile onset proximal spinal muscular atrophy (type II and III SMA): 569 patients. J Neurol Sci 1997; 146: 67–72

[6] Schroth MK. Special considerations in the respiratory management of spinal muscular atrophy. Pediatrics 2009; 123 Suppl 4: S245–S249

[7] McElroy MJ, Shaner AC, Crawford TO et al. Growing rods for scoliosis in spinal muscular atrophy: structural effects, complications, and hospital stays. Spine 2011; 36: 1305–1311

[8] Ing C, DiMaggio C, Whitehouse A et al. Long-term differences in language and cognitive function after childhood exposure to anesthesia. Pediatrics 2012; 130: e476–e485

[9] Dickson RA. Early-onset idiopathic scoliosis. In: Weinstein S, ed. The Pediatric Spine: Principles and Practice. New York, NY: Raven Press; 1994:421–429

[10] Fletcher ND, Bruce RW. Early onset scoliosis: current concepts and controversies. Curr Rev Musculoskelet Med 2012; 5: 102–110

[11] Redding GJ. Thoracic insufficiency syndrome. In: Akbarnia BA, Yazici M, Thompson GH. The Growing Spine. New York, NY: Springer; 2010:79–86

[12] Karol LA, Johnston C, Mladenov K, Schochet P, Walters P, Browne RH. Pulmonary function following early thoracic fusion in non-neuromuscular scoliosis. J Bone Joint Surg Am 2008; 90: 1272–1281

[13] Akbarnia BA, Mundis GM Jr Salari P, Yaszay B, Pawelek JB. Innovation in growing rod technique: a study of safety and efficacy of a magnetically controlled growing rod in a porcine model. Spine 2012; 37: 1109–1114

[14] Flick RP, Katusic SK, Colligan RC et al. Cognitive and behavioral outcomes after early exposure to anesthesia and surgery. Pediatrics 2011; 128: e1053–e1061

[15] Schwartz DM, Drummond DS, Hahn M, Ecker ML, Dormans JP. Prevention of positional brachial plexopathy during surgical correction of scoliosis. J Spinal Disord 2000; 13: 178–182

[16] Akbarnia BA. Instrumentation with limited arthrodesis for the treatment of progressive early-onset scoliosis. Spine: State Art Rev 2000; 14: 181–189

[17] Bess S, Akbarnia BA, Thompson GH et al. Complications of growing-rod treatment for early-onset scoliosis: analysis of one hundred and forty patients. J Bone Joint Surg Am 2010; 92: 2533–2543

[18] Sankar WN, Skaggs DL, Yazici M et al. Lengthening of dual growing rods and the law of diminishing returns. Spine 2011; 36: 806–809

[19] Noordeen HM, Shah SA, Elsebaie HB, Garrido E, Farooq N, Al-Mukhtar M. In vivo distraction force and length measurements of growing rods: which factors influence the ability to lengthen? Spine 2011; 36: 2299–2303

[20] Campbell RM Jr Smith MD, Mayes TC et al. The characteristics of thoracic insufficiency syndrome associated with fused ribs and congenital scoliosis. J Bone Joint Surg Am 2003; 85-A: 399–408

[21] McCarthy RE, Luhmann S, Lenke L, McCullough FL. The Shilla growth guidance technique for early-onset spinal deformities at 2-year follow-up: a preliminary report. J Pediatr Orthop 2014; 34: 1–7

[22] Akbarnia BA, Cheung K, Noordeen H et al. Next generation of growth-sparing techniques: preliminary clinical results of a magnetically controlled growing rod in 14 patients with early-onset scoliosis. Spine 2013; 38: 665–670

[23] Dannawi Z, Altaf F, Harshavardhana NS, El Sebaie H, Noordeen H. Early results of a remotely-operated magnetic growth rod in early-onset scoliosis. Bone Joint J 2013; 95-B: 75–80

34 Current Gaps in Knowledge: What Should Research Provide for the Future?

Richard E. McCarthy

The present status of research in early onset scoliosis is much like the story of the blind man describing the elephant, with each of the researchers describing a different component, different aspect, or a different part of the whole process. Certainly the ability to step back and see the whole picture of the elephant would allow us better clarity in designing treatment modalities for our future patients.

As practitioners, what is it we need so that we can best describe and treat our patients who have early onset scoliosis?

34.1 Area One

We need a clear and concise method to classify and describe our patients in a manner that allows practitioners to communicate accurately. This classification system should apply to the untreated patient, but a classification is also necessary for our treatment methods. Concerning the etiology, the symptoms we can readily see are the deformities of the skeletal system, but of a more subtle nature, what is the position of the body habitus with regard to balance and gait, the ambulatory status, and the sagittal alignment, and of greatest importance, what is the impact of the deformity upon the lungs?

Many of the children with these disorders whom we treat do not follow the usual rules for normal progression through the phases of skeletal maturity; how does this aberration fit into our classification systems? The physiologic development of the respiratory tree is an important factor in the treatment of patients with early onset scoliosis because we are aware that the major part of parenchymal cell duplication occurs before the age of 8 years, so the importance of instituting a treatment method before this age becomes critical. Is there also a difference in the maturational age of the lung parenchyma in children who have a delay in their skeletal maturation? How do we place these factors into a classification system that includes DeMeglio's caution to use the fourth dimension of respiratory capacity—namely, the expansion of the ribs that encircle the lungs and provide a cavity in which the lungs develop and prosper?[1,2] The three-dimensional impact of a scoliotic deformity upon respiration is indeed complex. The spine, ribs, and lungs have been characterized by Robert Campbell as analogous to the structural components of a room where for many years spinal surgeons have focused on the corner of the room—namely, the spine—while neglecting the growth capacity of the walls (ribs) attached to the corner and the enormous importance of what happens inside the room itself (respiratory function).[3]

With this in mind, if a classification system is based upon the severity of lung dysfunction, how is lung function to be measured? Pulmonary function studies in children before the age of 6 years, as we perform them now, are suspect at best.[4] Do computed tomographic (CT) scans of the lungs truly correlate with lung function? Does improved space lead to improved breathing? Dr. Campbell has further encouraged us to look closely at dynamic magnetic resonance images to truly understand the function of the respiratory tree and its association with spinal deformity. How is this to be calibrated? What metric should we use? This is indeed an area for further exploration because there is little understanding of how to measure respiratory function in children, especially those too young or cognitively unable to cooperate with pulmonary function studies.

Dr. Vitale and his group have made a first attempt to arrive at a consensus on the important components of a classification system. Through a process known as equipoise, in which experts, through a series of encounters over time, are able to arrive at a point of agreement upon the key essentials that best permit the description of a specific deformity, they have settled upon five components (age, etiology, size of curve, kyphosis, and progression) that fulfill this requirement with the greatest succinctness.[5] Whether the classification system will be adopted universally has yet to be proved. It does not include measures of curve flexibility or metrics reflecting a child's nutrition. Neither does it describe three-dimensional deformity of the chest and torso. It does not consider, in any manner, the respiratory function of an individual. All of these components are intimately involved in and affect a child's treatment.

34.2 Area Two

A second area where research needs to help practitioners who treat patients with early onset scoliosis is the development of better imaging techniques. Presently, most practitioners rely heavily upon two-dimensional radiographs obtained with the patient in a coronal and a sagittal position, while understanding the three-dimensional components of the curve is left to the imagination. Only with a CT scan can we appreciate in the axial plane rotational deformities about the spine in which the chest is invaded by the rotated vertebral bodies and the lung fields are compressed by rib deformities that effectively crush the lungs. CT scans in young children have the capability of exposing the growing skeleton to a great deal of irradiation, with the worrisome problem of irradiation-induced carcinomas later. Low-dose irradiation systems, such as the sterEOS Imaging System (EOS Imaging, Paris, France), hold promise because they allow patients to be examined in the standing position, and the amount of exposure to irradiation is less than with current plane systems.[6,7] Will the acceptance of this technique be expanded? Is the cost of the system justified, or is it something that we just have to accept as we develop classification systems based upon three-dimensional imaging?

The Scoliosis Research Society has slowly been making progress in devising a system for looking at three-dimensional imaging diagrammatically. Through its efforts, the Da Vinci projection has been developed, which allows one to see a spinal deformity in its entirety as visualized from above and describe the amount of rotational deviation as colored triangles associated with each curve. The projection also allows us to visualize the effect of our treatments by comparing diagrams obtained before and after treatment.[6,8]

34.3 Area Three

A third area in which research needs to help us is in developing a better way to describe in a global sense the effects our treatment methods have upon the children whom we send into adulthood—not only in regard to whether they are able to manage physically and functionally, but whether they are able to participate in activities of daily living, recreational activities, and social situations. How intelligent are they? Do our treatment modalities produce adults lacking cognitive abilities? This is a legitimate issue to analyze because some of the literature from our anesthesia colleagues indicates a decrease in cognitive ability among those patients who are repeatedly and regularly subjected to anesthesia at a young age.[9] Additionally, what emotional effects are we inflicting upon our young children and their families when they repeatedly undergo surgery? Are they emotionally well balanced? Some of the seemingly least important things we do can be of great import in a child's mind. Dr. Mel Smith, one of the innovators in the development of the vertical expandable titanium prosthetic rib (VEPTR) system, made the observation that the most objectionable part of the lengthening procedure in the opinion of his VEPTR patients was the removal of the tape on bandages after the surgery. In response to this concern, he developed a simple method of wrapping a child's torso with a gauze bandage rather than using tape, which was much appreciated by his patients. Sometimes, these efforts toward making our treatments more palatable for children do have a lasting positive effect. Most importantly,

what metric do we use to measure these capacities for maturity in our children? How well do they fit into society? A clear sign of some of the effects of treatment is the regressive behavior that many parents note around the time of surgery with regard to toileting, acting out, and emotional lability. The long-term effects of lengthening surgery every 6 months are unknown. With regard to the physical effects of surgery, they seem obvious, but in fact are they? The scars are obvious, characterized by poor blood supply and an increased risk for breakdown and infection, but the emotional effects and the effects of anesthesia can also be long-reaching in the deficits they cause. Possibly the more widespread use of magnetic self-lengthening rods without hospitalizations will prove efficacious.

34.4 Area Four

The metallosis associated with all growing rod systems is a topic rarely discussed when we consider children who have early onset scoliosis. Additionally, in fact, little research on this topic is done in children. Studies looking at the effects of metallosis in adults deal primarily with total joint procedures. Some of the animal research seems to indicate that titanium is a metal that pervasively spreads through all the organ systems in animals and, in all likelihood, in humans as well. This is contrasted with the effects of stainless steel, which are seen in the local tissues surrounding moving parts in growing rods; however, stainless steel molecules remain local, are absorbed through the lymphatic tissue, and are thought not to travel beyond to major organ systems.[10] We simply do not know the long-term effects of metal molecules in the organs of individuals with an expected life span of 80 years.

34.5 Area 5

What we need most from scientific research is a model, either an animal model or a computer simulation, for studying the long-term effects of all of our treatment modalities in a short period of time. We haven't found the perfect animal model as yet; we have certainly tried to make porcine and bovine animals into models of scoliosis, but whether the information learned from four-legged animals can be transported to and reproduced in humans is still to be proved. Much is yet to be learned, and future generations of spine surgeons will depend upon the foundations that we have laid for them to build upon.

References

[1] Charles YP, Diméglio A, Marcoul M, Bourgin JF, Marcoul A, Bozonnat MC. Influence of idiopathic scoliosis on three-dimensional thoracic growth. Spine 2008; 33: 1209–1218

[2] DiMeglio A, Canavese F, Charles YP. Growth and adolescent idiopathic scoliosis: when and how much? J Pediatr Orthop 2011; 31 Suppl: S28–S36

[3] Campbell RM Jr Smith MD, Mayes TC et al. The characteristics of thoracic insufficiency syndrome associated with fused ribs and congenital scoliosis. J Bone Joint Surg Am 2003; 85-A: 399–408

[4] Campbell RM Jr Smith MD. Thoracic insufficiency syndrome and exotic scoliosis. J Bone Joint Surg Am 2007; 89 Suppl 1: 108–122

[5] Williams B, Akbarnia B, Blakemore L, et al. Organizing chaos: development of a consensus-based early onset scoliosis classification schema. Presented at: 5th International Congress on Early Onset. Scoliosis and Growing Spine (ICEOS); November 18–19, 2011; Orlando, FL

[6] Labelle H, Aubin CE, Jackson R, Lenke L, Newton P, Parent S. Seeing the spine in 3D: how will it change what we do? J Pediatr Orthop 2011; 31 Suppl: S37–S45

[7] McKenna C, Wade R, Faria R et al. EOS 2D/3D X-ray imaging system: a systematic review and economic evaluation. Health Technol Assess 2012; 16: 1–188

[8] Sangole AP, Aubin CE, Labelle H et al. Three-dimensional classification of thoracic scoliotic curves. Spine 2009; 34: 91–99

[9] Flynn JM, Matsumoto H, Torres F, Ramirez N, Vitale MG. Psychological dysfunction in children who require repetitive surgery for early onset scoliosis. J Pediatr Orthop 2012; 32: 594–599

[10] McCarthy RE, Sucato D, Turner JL, Zhang H, Henson MA, McCarthy K. Shilla growing rods in a caprine animal model: a pilot study. Clin Orthop Relat Res 2010; 468: 705–710

Index